GOWNED AND GLOVED SURGERY

D1088133

Gowned and Gloved Surgery: Introduction to Common Procedures

Robert E. Roses, MD
Resident
Department of Surgery
University of Pennsylvania School of Medicine
Hospital of the University of Pennsylvania
Philadelphia, Pennsylvania

E. Carter Paulson, MD
Resident
Department of Surgery
University of Pennsylvania School of Medicine
Hospital of the University of Pennsylvania
Philadelphia, Pennsylvania

Suhail K. Kanchwala, MD
Resident, Division of Plastic and Reconstructive Surgery
Department of Surgery
University of Pennsylvania School of Medicine
Hospital of the University of Pennsylvania
Philadelphia, Pennsylvania

Jon B. Morris, MD
Professor and Vice Chair for Education
Program Director for General Surgery
Department of Surgery
University of Pennsylvania School of Medicine;
Attending Surgeon
Department of Surgery
Hospital of the University of Pennsylvania
Philadelphia, Pennsylvania

SERIES EDITORS

Neil P. Sheth, MD
Instructor
Department of Othopaedic Surgery
Hospital of the University of Pennsylvania
Philadelphia, Pennsylvania

Jess H. Lonner, MD
Director of Knee Replacement Surgery
Booth Bartolozzi Balderston Orthopaedics
Pennsylvania Hospital;
Medical Director
Philadelphia Center for Minimally Invasive Knee
   Surgery
Philadelphia, Pennsylvania

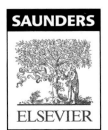

SAUNDERS

ELSEVIER

SAUNDERS

ELSEVIER

1600 John F. Kennedy Boulevard
Suite 1800
Philadelphia, PA 19103-2899

GOWNED AND GLOVED SURGERY:
INTRODUCTION TO COMMON PROCEDURES   ISBN: 978-1-4160-5356-9
Copyright © 2009 by Saunders, an imprint of Elsevier Inc.

All rights reserved. No part of this publication may be reproduced or transmitted in any form or by any means, electronic or mechanical, including photocopying, recording, or any information storage and retrieval system, without permission in writing from the publisher. Permissions may be sought directly from Elsevier's Rights Department: phone: (+1) 215 239 3804 (U.S.) or (+44) 1865 843830 (UK); fax: (+44) 1865 85333; e-mail: healthpermissions@elsevier.com. You may also complete your request online via the Elsevier website at http://www.elsevier.com.

Notice

Knowledge and best practice in this field are constantly changing. As new research and experience broaden our knowledge, changes in practice, treatment and drug therapy may become necessary or appropriate. Readers are advised to check the most current information provided (i) on procedures featured or (ii) by the manufacturer of each product to be administered, to verify the recommended dose or formula, the method and duration of administration, and contraindications. It is the responsibility of the practitioner, relying on their own experience and knowledge of the patient, to make diagnoses, to determine dosages and the best treatment for each individual patient, and to take all appropriate safety precautions. To the fullest extent of the law, neither the Publisher nor the Editors assume any liability for any injury and/or damage to persons or property arising out or related to any use of the material contained in this book.

The Publisher

Library of Congress Cataloging-in-Publication Data

Gowned and gloved surgery : introduction to common procedures /
[edited by] Robert E. Roses . . . [et al.].—1st ed.
    p. ; cm.—(Gowned and gloved)
  Includes bibliographical references.
  ISBN 978-1-4160-5356-9
1. Surgery–Textbooks.   I. Roses, Robert E.   II. Series.
  [DNLM: 1. Surgical Procedures, Operative. WO 500 G723 2009]
RD31.G73 2009
617–dc22

                                                    2008023592

Acquisitions Editor: James Merritt
Developmental Editor: Andrea Vosburgh
Project Manager: Bryan Hayward
Design Direction: Gene Harris
Marketing Manager: Alyson Sherby

Working together to grow
libraries in developing countries

www.elsevier.com | www.bookaid.org | www.sabre.org

ELSEVIER   BOOK AID International   Sabre Foundation

Printed in China

Last digit is the print number: 9 8 7 6 5 4 3 2 1

CONTRIBUTORS

IBRAHIM ABDULLAH, MD
Resident
Department of Surgery
University of Pennsylvania School of Medicine
Hospital of the University of Pennsylvania
Philadelphia, Pennsylvania

DONNA J. BARBOT, MD
Clinical Associate Professor
Department of Surgery
University of Pennsylvania School of Medicine;
Chief
Department of Surgery
Chestnut Hill Hospital, University of Pennsylvania
   Health System Affiliate
Philadelphia, Pennsylvania

BENJAMIN BRASLOW, MD
Assistant Professor
Division of Trauma/Surgical Critical Care
Department of Surgery
University of Pennsylvania School of Medicine;
Attending Surgeon
Department of Surgery
Hospital of the University of Pennsylvania
Philadelphia, Pennsylvania

CLAYTON J. BRINSTER, MD
Resident
Department of Surgery
University of Pennsylvania School of Medicine
Hospital of the University of Pennsylvania
Philadelphia, Pennsylvania

LOUIS P. BUCKY, MD, FACS
Associate Professor of Surgery
Division of Plastic and Reconstructive Surgery
Department of Surgery
University of Pennsylvania School of Medicine;
Chief, Division of Plastic and Reconstructive Surgery
Department of Surgery
Pennsylvania Hospital;
Attending Surgeon
Division of Plastic and Reconstructive Surgery
Department of Surgery
Hospital of the University of Pennsylvania
Philadelphia, Pennsylvania

JO BUYSKE, MD
Associate Executive Director
American Board of Surgery;
Adjunct Professor of Surgery
Department of Surgery
University of Pennsylvania School of Medicine
Philadelphia, Pennsylvania

JEFFREY P. CARPENTER, MD
Professor of Surgery
Department of Surgery
University of Pennsylvania School of Medicine;
Attending Surgeon
Department of Surgery
Hospital of the University of Pennsylvania
Philadelphia, Pennsylvania

BRIAN J. CZERNIECKI, MD, PHD
Associate Professor of Surgery
Department of Surgery
University of Pennsylvania School of Medicine;
Attending Surgeon
Department of Surgery
Hospital of the University of Pennsylvania
Philadelphia, Pennsylvania

JEFFREY A. DREBIN, MD, PHD
William M. Measey Professor
Chief, Division of Gastrointestinal Surgery
Vice Chairman
Department of Surgery
University of Pennsylvania School of Medicine;
Attending Surgeon
Chief of Gastrointestinal Surgery
Department of Surgery
Hospital of the University of Pennsylvania
Philadelphia, Pennsylvania

KRISTOFFEL R. DUMON, MD
Assistant Professor of Surgery
Department of Surgery
University of Pennsylvania School of Medicine;
Attending Surgeon
Department of Surgery
Hospital of the University of Pennsylvania
Philadelphia, Pennsylvania

RONALD M. FAIRMAN, MD

Professor of Surgery
Chief, Division of Vascular Surgery and Endovascular
    Surgery
Department of Surgery
University of Pennsylvania School of Medicine;
Attending Surgeon
Department of Surgery
Hospital of the University of Pennsylvania
Philadelphia, Pennsylvania

PAUL J. FOLEY, MD

Resident
Department of Surgery
University of Pennsylvania School of Medicine
Hospital of the University of Pennsylvania
Philadelphia, Pennsylvania

JOSHUA FOSNOT, MD

Resident
Department of Surgery
University of Pennsylvania School of Medicine
Hospital of the University of Pennsylvania
Philadelphia, Pennsylvania

DOUGLAS L. FRAKER, MD

Jonathan Rhoads Associate Professor of Surgery
Vice Chair, Clinical Affairs
Department of Surgery
University of Pennsylvania School of Medicine;
Attending Surgeon
Department of Surgery
Hospital of the University of Pennsylvania
Philadelphia, Pennsylvania

MICHAEL E. FRISCIA, MD

Resident
Department of Surgery
University of Pennsylvania School of Medicine
Hospital of the University of Pennsylvania
Philadelphia, Pennsylvania

DALE HAN, MD

Resident
Department of Surgery
University of Pennsylvania School of Medicine
Hospital of the University of Pennsylvania
Philadelphia, Pennsylvania

BENJAMIN HERDRICH, MD

Resident
Department of Surgery
University of Pennsylvania School of Medicine
Hospital of the University of Pennsylvania
Philadelphia, Pennsylvania

BENJAMIN M. JACKSON, MD, MS

Fellow, Division of Vascular Surgery
Department of Surgery
University of Pennsylvania School of Medicine
Hospital of the University of Pennsylvania
Philadelphia, Pennsylvania

SUHAIL K. KANCHWALA, MD

Resident, Division of Plastic and Reconstructive Surgery
Department of Surgery
University of Pennsylvania School of Medicine
Hospital of the University of Pennsylvania
Philadelphia, Pennsylvania

GIORGOS C. KARAKOUSIS, MD

Resident
Department of Surgery
University of Pennsylvania School of Medicine
Hospital of the University of Pennsylvania
Philadelphia, Pennsylvania

RACHEL R. KELZ, MD, MSCE

Assistant Professor of Clinical Surgery
Department of Surgery
University of Pennsylvania School of Medicine;
Attending Surgeon
Department of Surgery
Hospital of the University of Pennsylvania
Philadelphia, Pennsylvania

MATT L. KIRKLAND III, MD

Clinical Assistant Professor
Department of Surgery
University of Pennsylvania School of Medicine;
Attending Surgeon
Department of Surgery
Pennsylvania Hospital
Philadelphia, Pennsylvania

ROBERT T. LEWIS, MD

Resident
Department of Surgery
University of Pennsylvania School of Medicine
Hospital of the University of Pennsylvania
Philadelphia, Pennsylvania

NAJJIA N. MAHMOUD, MD, FACS, FASCRS

Assistant Professor of Surgery
Department of Surgery
University of Pennsylvania School of Medicine;
Attending Surgeon
Department of Surgery
University of Pennsylvania Health System
Philadelphia, Pennsylvania

DAVID J. MARON, MD
Assistant Professor of Surgery
Division of Colon and Rectal Surgery
Department of Surgery
University of Pennsylvania School of Medicine;
Attending Surgeon
Division of Colon and Rectal Surgery
Department of Surgery
Penn Presbyterian Medical Center
Philadelphia, Pennsylvania

DEMETRI J. MERIANOS, MD
Resident
Department of Surgery
University of Pennsylvania School of Medicine
Hospital of the University of Pennsylvania
Philadelphia, Pennsylvania

JON B. MORRIS, MD
Professor and Vice Chair for Education
Program Director for General Surgery
Department of Surgery
University of Pennsylvania School of Medicine;
Attending Surgeon
Department of Surgery
Hospital of the University of Pennsylvania
Philadelphia, Pennsylvania

ANDREW S. NEWMAN, MD
Resident
Department of Surgery
University of Pennsylvania School of Medicine
Hospital of the University of Pennsylvania
Philadelphia, Pennsylvania

HOOMAN NOORCHASHM, MD, PHD
Resident
Department of Surgery
University of Pennsylvania School of Medicine
Hospital of the University of Pennsylvania
Philadelphia, Pennsylvania

KIM M. OLTHOFF, MD
Associate Professor of Surgery
Director, Liver Transplant Program
Division of Transplantation
Department of Surgery
University of Pennsylvania School of Medicine;
Attending Surgeon
Department of Surgery
Hospital of the University of Pennsylvania
Philadelphia, Pennsylvania

RONALD F. PARSONS, MD
Resident
Department of Surgery
University of Pennsylvania School of Medicine
Hospital of the University of Pennsylvania
Philadelphia, Pennsylvania

E. CARTER PAULSON, MD
Resident
Department of Surgery
University of Pennsylvania School of Medicine
Hospital of the University of Pennsylvania
Philadelphia, Pennsylvania

PAIGE M. PORRETT, MD
Resident
Department of Surgery
University of Pennsylvania School of Medicine
Hospital of the University of Pennsylvania
Philadelphia, Pennsylvania

STEVEN E. RAPER, MD
Professor of Surgery
Department of Surgery
University of Pennsylvania School of Medicine;
Attending Surgeon
Department of Surgery
Hospital of the University of Pennsylvania
Philadelphia, Pennsylvania

PATRICK M. REILLY, MD, FACS
Associate Professor of Surgery
Vice-Chief, Division of Trauma and Surgical Critical
  Care
Department of Surgery
University of Pennsylvania School of Medicine;
Attending Surgeon
Department of Surgery
Hospital of the University of Pennsylvania
Philadelphia, Pennsylvania

JOSEPH ANTHONY P. RODRIGUEZ, MD
Resident
Department of Surgery
University of Pennsylvania School of Medicine
Hospital of the University of Pennsylvania
Philadelphia, Pennsylvania

ERNEST F. ROSATO, MD
Professor of Surgery
Department of Surgery
University of Pennsylvania School of Medicine;
Attending Surgeon
Department of Surgery
Hospital of the University of Pennsylvania
Philadelphia, Pennsylvania

ROBERT E. ROSES, MD
Resident
Department of Surgery
University of Pennsylvania School of Medicine
Hospital of the University of Pennsylvania
Philadelphia, Pennsylvania

ALAN SCHURICHT, MD, FACS
Clinical Associate Professor
Department of Surgery
University of Pennsylvania School of Medicine;
Attending Surgeon
Department of Surgery
Pennsylvania Hospital
Philadelphia, Pennsylvania

JOSEPH M. SERLETTI, MD, FACS
Henry Royster–William Maul Measey Professor of
    Surgery and Chief
Division of Plastic Surgery
Department of Surgery
University of Pennsylvania School of Medicine;
Attending Surgeon
Division of Plastic Surgery
Department of Surgery
Philadelphia, Pennsylvania

FRANCIS R. SPITZ, MD
Associate Professor of Surgery
Department of Surgery
University of Pennsylvania School of Medicine;
Attending Surgeon
Department of Surgery
Hospital of the University of Pennsylvania
Philadelphia, Pennsylvania

GRACE J. WANG, MD
Fellow, Division of Vascular Surgery
Department of Surgery
University of Pennsylvania School of Medicine
Hospital of the University of Pennsylvania
Philadelphia, Pennsylvania

NOEL N. WILLIAMS, MD, FRCSI
Associate Professor
Associate Program Director
Department of Surgery
University of Pennsylvania School of Medicine;
Attending Surgeon
Director of Bariatric Surgery
Department of Surgery
Hospital of the University of Pennsylvania
Philadelphia, Pennsylvania

THOMAS A. WIXTED, MD
Resident
Department of Surgery
University of Pennsylvania School of Medicine
Hospital of the University of Pennsylvania
Philadelphia, Pennsylvania

EDWARD Y. WOO, MD
Assistant Professor and Program Director
Division of Vascular Surgery
Department of Surgery
University of Pennsylvania School of Medicine;
Attending Surgeon
Department of Surgery
Hospital of the University of Pennsylvania
Philadelphia, Pennsylvania

PREFACE

This text is the second volume in the *Gowned and Gloved* series. Modeled loosely on its predecessor in the series, which focused on orthopaedic surgery, this book aims to enhance the medical student's experience in the operating room by describing, in brief, the technical features of a given procedure and relevant pathophysiology and anatomy. We have included 26 chapters on common general surgical procedures, grouping related procedures within a given chapter when appropriate. Importantly, the list of procedures discussed is by no means comprehensive. In selecting the content of the text, we chose procedures that are both frequently performed and allow for a relatively broad discussion of surgical disease.

To the degree possible, we followed a consistent chapter format, allowing for subtle adjustments to accommodate the subject matter. Every chapter begins with a case study. While these cases are not explicitly referenced throughout the body of each chapter, they do introduce pertinent issues that influence perioperative and intraoperative care. It may be useful for the reader to consider the yellow text boxes, which focus on critical management decisions, in the context of a given chapter's opening case. The remaining sections of each chapter are largely self explanatory. It should be noted, however, that information common to all procedures is omitted from the individual chapters. Such information is the focus of the first chapter of the book, which should be read before the others. Important terms appear in bold throughout the text.

We hope that students will find this book a useful resource during their surgical clerkships or sub-internships. We are grateful to Neil P. Sheth, MD; Jess H. Lonner, MD; and the staff of Elsevier, Inc. for inviting us to edit this volume; in particular, we wish to acknowledge Andrea Vosburgh for her assistance in reviewing the contributions. Finally, we wish to extend our gratitude to the authors of the individual chapters, who contributed their knowledge and experience to this volume.

ROBERT E. ROSES
E. CARTER PAULSON
SUHAIL K. KANCHWALA
JON B. MORRIS

CONTENTS

Preoperative and Intraoperative Care

Robert E. Roses, Suhail K. Kanchwala, and Patrick M. Reilly

Case Study

A 72-year-old male presents to a surgeon's office after being diagnosed with a symptomatic right inguinal hernia. He notes progressive enlargement of the hernia over the course of several months and complains of associated discomfort. He reports a history of hypertension and a myocardial infarction (MI) at the age of 65 years. He takes aspirin and two antihypertensive medications. He smoked heavily for 40 years until the age of 60 years. On physical examination, a large, reducible, mildly tender right inguinal hernia is noted. He appears well otherwise.

He is sent for preoperative testing, including a chest radiograph and an electrocardiogram (ECG), and he is referred to a cardiologist for a preoperative assessment of his cardiac risk. At the cardiologist's instruction, he undergoes a radionuclide stress test, which reveals no reversible myocardial perfusion defects. The cardiologist classifies the patient's cardiac risk as intermediate and recommends perioperative adrenergic blockade and a postoperative ECG. The patient undergoes an uneventful inguinal hernia repair under regional anesthesia with conscious sedation.

PREOPERATIVE CARE

Indications for surgery must be weighed against the risks associated with the planned procedure. Principles that guide this evaluation and preoperative planning are the subject of the first part of this chapter.

Preoperative Evaluation

All patients undergo a general evaluation before elective surgery, the primary aim of which is to identify and quantify comorbidities that may influence surgical outcomes. The scope of this evaluation is dictated by a number of factors, including patient age and medical history and the risks associated with the planned procedure. Frequently ordered preoperative tests include: an ECG; a chest radiograph; hemoglobin, creatinine, and glucose levels; a urinalysis; a pregnancy test; and coagulation studies. Not all of these are essential in all cases and some recommendations regarding their use are detailed in Table 1-1.

Additional Considerations

An aging population and advances in perioperative care with associated improvements in outcomes have lessened the number of absolute contraindications to surgical intervention. Patients with significant comorbidities, however, require a more extensive preoperative evaluation and, sometimes, preoperative interventions. Cardiovascular disease and pulmonary disease in particular often mandate special preoperative consideration.

   I. **Cardiovascular Disease**

      A. Approximately 30% of surgical patients have cardiac disease. A number of risk stratification tools (e.g., the Cardiac Risk Index and American College of

TABLE 1-1 Recommendations for Preoperative Screening Tests

Test	Age	Planned Procedure Type	Comorbid Disease or Condition
Electrocardiogram	Male > 40 years Female > 50 years	Cardiac Thoracic	Cardiovascular disease Hypertension Diabetes
Chest radiograph	>60 years	Cardiac Thoracic	Respiratory disease Cardiovascular disease Heavy smoker (relative)
Hemoglobin	—	Procedure with anticipated blood loss > 500 mL	Cardiovascular disease Renal disease Malignancy Diabetes Aspirin use Nonsteroidal anti-inflammatory drug use Anticoagulant use
Creatinine	>50 years	Procedure with associated risk of postoperative renal failure	Use of drugs with renal excretion Renal disease Cardiovascular disease Hypertension Diabetes Nonsteroidal anti-inflammatory drug use
Glucose	>45 years	—	Diabetes Steroid use
Urinalysis	—	Genitourinary Implantation of prosthesis (e.g., orthopedic implant or valve replacement)	Use of drugs with renal excretion Renal disease Cardiovascular disease Hypertension Diabetes
Pregnancy (qualitative human chorionic gonadotropin)	—	—	Women of childbearing age with uncertain pregnancy status
Coagulation studies	—	—	Bleeding risk/history Liver disease

Modified from Nierman E, Zakrewski K: Recognition and management of preoperative risk. Rheum Dis Clin North Am 25:587, 1999.

Cardiology/American Heart Association [ACC/AHA] Guidelines) are in use and take into account various clinical predictors, functional status, and planned procedure type to identify those patients who will benefit from a more extensive cardiac evaluation (Fig. 1-1). The preoperative history and physical examination should elicit signs and symptoms of coronary artery disease, valvular disease, congestive heart failure (CHF), and cardiac arrhythmias. Patients who have suffered from a recent MI (within 6 months) are at a substantially elevated risk for a perioperative MI. The timing of surgery for these patients must be given special consideration because this risk lessens with time.

B. Patients at elevated cardiac risk who have not undergone recent coronary revascularization (i.e., within the previous 5 years) are often referred for noninvasive testing (e.g., an echocardiogram and a stress test). Patients deemed high risk sometimes require coronary angiography to determine whether they can benefit from revascularization (i.e., coronary artery bypass or angioplasty) before elective surgery. Additionally, the cardiac evaluation can influence anesthetic choice and intraoperative monitoring strategies. Finally, β-blockers are often administered to decrease myocardial oxygen demand and reduce the risk of perioperative cardiac events in patients at elevated risk.

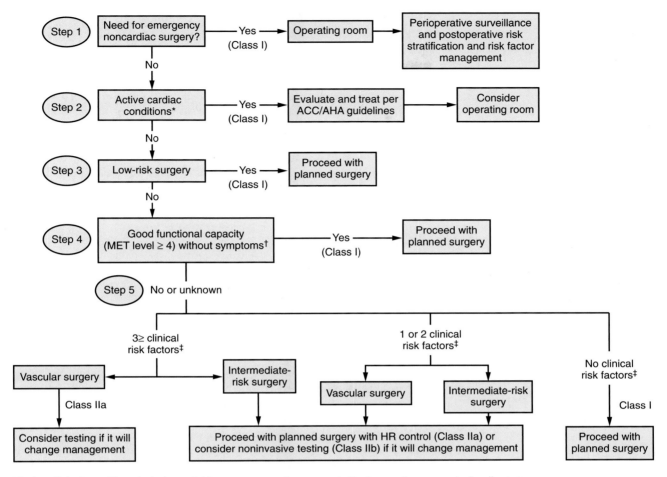

*Active clinical conditions include unstable coronary syndromes, arrhythmias, and severe valvular disease.

†Metabolic equivalents (METs) have been estimated for various activities (e.g., 1: can take care of oneself; 4: can climb a flight of stairs; 10: can engage in strenuous sports).

‡Clinical risk factors include ischemic heart disease, compensated or previous heart failure, diabetes mellitus, renal insufficiency, and cerebrovascular disease.

Figure 1-1

American College of Cardiology (ACC)/American Heart Association (AHA) 2007 Guidelines on Perioperative Cardiovascular Evaluation and Care for Noncardiac Surgery. The scope of the preoperative cardiac evaluation is determined by the clinical scenario and cardiac risk factors. HR, heart rate. (*Modified from Fleisher LA, Beckman JA, Brown KA, et al: ACC/AHA 2007 Guidelines on Perioperative Cardiovascular Evaluation and Care for Noncardiac Surgery: A Report of the American College of Cardiology/American Heart Association Task Force on Practice Guidelines [Writing Committee to Revise the 2002 Guidelines on Perioperative Cardiovascular Evaluation for Noncardiac Surgery]. Circulation 116: e418–e499, 2007.*)

II. **Pulmonary Disease**

A. Patients with significant pulmonary disease, specifically chronic obstructive pulmonary disease (COPD) and pulmonary hypertension, are at increased risk for postoperative complications, including respiratory failure (requiring mechanical ventilation > 48 hours), atelectasis, bronchospasm, and pneumonia. Pulmonary function tests (PFTs) are frequently obtained in patients with known pulmonary disease as well as in older patients (>60 years of age) with pulmonary symptoms or an extensive smoking history. Although poor pulmonary function may preclude pulmonary resection, guidelines are less definitive with regard to nonthoracic procedures. Pulmonary evaluation in nonthoracic surgical patients may, however, influence management (e.g., operative vs. nonoperative approach), choice of anesthesia (e.g., epidural vs. general), and surgical approach (palliative vs. curative).

B. Interventions that may decrease pulmonary complications include preoperative smoking cessation, the use of epidural anesthesia, bronchodilator therapy, and aggressive postoperative pulmonary toilet and rehabilitation.

III. **Review of Medications:** A thorough review of the patient's current medications is of critical import. Insulin, steroids, and anticoagulants are a few examples of widely prescribed agents that necessitate special consideration before surgery. In general, short-acting insulin preparations are substituted for long-acting ones or other antihyperglycemic agents. Long-term steroid therapy should be continued through the perioperative period, and administration of perioperative "stress-dose" steroids should be given consideration. When possible, aspirin and clopidogrel (Plavix) should be withheld for 7 to 10 days before surgery. Likewise, warfarin (Coumadin) should be withheld for several days before surgery to allow the international normalized ratio (INR) to fall to 1.5 or less.

Preparation for Surgery

I. **Fasting:** The American Society of Anesthesiologists (ASA) recommends a minimum interval of 2 hours without clear liquids and 6 hours without solid foods or unclear liquids before surgery. In practice, patients are generally instructed to abstain from eating after midnight the evening before surgery and to take important routine medications (e.g., antihypertensive agents) with a sip of water on the day of surgery.

II. **Antibiotic Prophylaxis:** Systemic administration of antibiotics before surgery significantly decreases the incidence of surgical site infections. The timing of antibiotic administration has proven to be critical; antibiotics should be administered before, but no more than 1 hour before, skin incision. The choice of antibiotics administered should reflect the nature of the procedure to be undertaken. Procedures may be classified as clean, clean-contaminated, contaminated, or dirty, and the risk of infection may be predicted based on this classification (Table 1-2). Antibiotic prophylaxis is generally unnecessary for clean cases except those involving placement of prosthetic material. Antibiotic prophylaxis should be given before class II, III, and IV procedures. Class III and IV procedures require coverage for aerobic and anaerobic infection. In the case of class IV procedures, antibiotics are often continued into the postoperative period as dictated by signs of ongoing infection (e.g., fever, tachycardia, and leukocytosis).

III. **Deep Vein Thrombosis Prophylaxis:** Acute deep vein thrombosis (DVT) and pulmonary embolism are major sources of perioperative morbidity and mortality. Virchow described the major factors that contribute to the pathogenesis of venous thrombosis (Virchow's triad [see text box]). Although the surgical patient is vulnerable to all of these, an increasingly aged, obese, and sedentary population, and the

Virchow's triad:
1. Venous stasis
2. Endothelial injury
3. Hypercoagulability

TABLE 1-2 Classification of Surgical Wounds		
Category	**Definition**	**Risk of Infection**
Clean (class I)	Respiratory, gastrointestinal, or genitourinary tract not entered	1%–3%
Clean-contaminated (class II)	Gastrointestinal or respiratory tract entered without significant spillage	5%–8%
Contaminated (class III)	Spillage from gastrointestinal tract or entrance into genitourinary or biliary tract in the presence of infected urine or bile Fresh traumatic wound	20%–25%
Dirty (class IV)	Acute bacterial infection encountered, delayed treatment of a traumatic wound Traumatic wound with retained devitalized tissue, foreign body, or fecal contamination	30%–40%

widespread use of central venous catheters have contributed further to the incidence of DVT. Little consensus exists regarding appropriate prophylaxis against DVT in surgical patients; however, perioperative use of sequential compression devices has been widely adopted for this purpose. These devices should be applied before the administration of anesthesia because induction may be associated with significant vasodilation and venous stasis. In patients deemed high risk, there may be a role for preoperative administration of subcutaneous heparin and even placement of a prophylactic inferior vena cava (IVC) filter.

IV. **Preparation of Blood Products:** Before procedures associated with a risk of significant surgical bleeding, a *type and screen* should be obtained to determine a patient's blood type (A, B, AB, or O) and to detect preformed antibodies to red blood cell–associated antigens. If the planned procedure is associated with a relatively high (>10%) likelihood of bleeding requiring transfusion, blood should be *crossmatched* for immediate use. If large-volume transfusion is anticipated, fresh frozen plasma (FFP) should be prepared in addition to packed red blood cells (pRBCs). Generally, 2 units of FFP should be prepared for every 5 units of pRBCs because large-volume transfusion of pRBCs alone is associated with coagulopathy resulting from dilution of clotting factors.

INTRAOPERATIVE CONSIDERATIONS

All surgical procedures require the coordinated effort of a team of surgeons, anesthesiologists, and support staff. The second part of this chapter focuses on *intraoperative* factors that influence surgical outcomes.

Anesthesia

Numerous anesthetic approaches exist; each has advantages and disadvantages. In choosing the most appropriate approach, the surgeon and anesthesiologist must consider several factors, including procedure type and length, anticipated blood loss, and patient comorbidities.

I. **General:** General anesthesia is defined as any form of anesthesia during which the patient no longer maintains consciousness. Induction of anesthesia is typically achieved with a combination of intravenous paralytics and sedatives, followed by maintenance with inhalational agents (e.g., halothane, desflurane, or isoflurane).

II. **Regional:** Regional anesthesia involves the delivery of an anesthetic agent to specific sensory nerves (e.g., epidural, interscalene, and pudendal blocks). Epidural anesthesia, in particular, is frequently administered during major abdominal and thoracic procedures, and may be used in conjunction with general anesthesia. Initiation of epidural anesthesia in the operating room may result in improved postoperative pain control and a more rapid recovery.

III. **Local:** Most commonly used as an adjunct for postoperative pain control, local anesthetics can be used as a primary method of anesthesia for minor procedures.

Airway

Airway management is a critical component of all anesthetic approaches. Deep sedation and the use of paralytics in conjunction with general anesthesia require ventilatory support. Endotracheal (ET) intubation is the most common method of securing the airway. ET tubes are inserted beyond the vocal cords and are equipped with a distal cuff. Inflation of the cuff protects against aspiration of gastrointestinal secretions and provides a seal to allow for ventilation. In contrast, laryngeal mask airways (LMAs) are equipped with a cuff that fits over the glottic opening (Fig. 1-2). LMAs are an alternative to ET tubes and are particularly useful for shorter procedures involving deep sedation. Because LMAs are more easily displaced and provide less protection against aspiration than do ET tubes, they should not be used for long procedures in which ventilatory support is necessary.

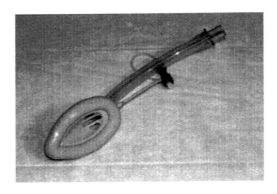

Figure 1-2
Laryngeal mask airway. *(From Cameron JL [ed]: Current Surgical Therapy, 8th ed, Philadelphia, Mosby, 2004.)*

Patient Preparation

After the induction of anesthesia, a variety of steps must be taken to prepare the patient for the operation. These may include the following:
  I. Urinary catheterization
 II. Placement of electrocautery grounding pads
III. Intravenous line placement
 IV. Invasive monitoring (e.g., Swan-Ganz and arterial catheterization)
  V. Placement of a nasogastric or orogastric tube
 VI. Patient positioning and application of the sterile preparation
VII. Application of drapes
VIII. Time-out for safety

Urinary Catheterization

| Is the anticipated operative time more than 3 hours? |

A urinary catheter should be placed before any procedure anticipated to take longer than 3 hours to allow for bladder decompression and urine output monitoring. The former is particularly important in laparoscopic cases, which require placement of a suprapubic port to prevent bladder injuries. Urinary catheterization is associated with several complications, the most prevalent of which is urinary tract infection (UTI). Strict adherence to sterile technique may limit infection rates, although duration of catheterization is the dominant predisposing factor for the development of UTIs. Rates of infection are estimated to be 4% to 7% per day of indwelling catheterization.

Gastric Decompression

| Will your patient require postoperative gastric decompression? |

Gastric decompression prevents gastric distention during intubation and enhances visualization during abdominal procedures. Either orogastric or nasogastric tubes may be used for these purposes. Orogastric tubes should be removed at the time of extubation. When a need for postextubation gastric decompression is anticipated, a nasogastric tube should be inserted.

Patient Positioning and Sterile Preparation

The patient is positioned to optimize visualization of the surgical field. Common positions include supine, prone jackknife (face down with the hips flexed), lateral decubitus, and Trendelenburg (head of the table tilted down). Pressure points should be padded to limit the incidence of pressure necrosis.

A variety of antiseptic solutions are commonly in use, including povidone-iodine (Betadine), alcohol, and chlorhexidene. The efficacy of betadine depends on the release of the active iodine from a carrier molecule. This requires several minutes after application; therefore, betadine should be allowed to dry before incision. The sterile preparation is typically applied in concentric circles, starting around the incision site and expanding outward. Three coats of preparation are applied before the application of sterile drapes.

Time-out for Safety

In an effort to minimize the small but devastating incidence of wrong-site, wrong-procedure, and wrong-person surgeries, hospitals have adopted the **time-out for safety.** Before incision, operating room personnel (including the surgeon, anesthesiologist, and nursing staff) confirm the patient's identity, the procedure type, and the operative site.

Dressing the Wound

At the conclusion of a procedure, a sterile dressing should be applied to the wound before removal of the sterile drapes. Theoretically, this dressing prevents bacterial colonization of the wound during the initial 24 to 48 hours of healing, allowing for epithelialization and limiting the risk of infection. Before application of the dressing, excess antiseptic solution should be washed off with sterile saline. In general, the dressing should be secured without the use of excessive tape, which may be irritating to the skin.

SUGGESTED READINGS

Fleisher LA, Beckman JA, Brown KA, et al: ACC/AHA 2007 Guidelines on Perioperative Cardiovascular Evaluation and Care for Noncardiac Surgery: A Report of the American College of Cardiology/American Heart Association Task Force on Practice Guidelines [Writing Committee to Revise the 2002 Guidelines on Perioperative Cardiovascular Evaluation for Noncardiac Surgery]. Circulation 116: e418–e499, 2007.

Marino PL: The ICU Book, 3rd ed. Philadelphia, Lippincott Williams & Wilkins, 2007.

Nierman E, Zakrewski K: Recognition and management of preoperative risk. Rheum Dis Clin North Am 25:587, 1999.

Weintraub SL, Wang Y, Hunt JP, O'Leary JP: Principles of preoperative and operative surgery. In Townsend CM (ed): Sabiston Textbook of Surgery: The Biologic Basis of Modern Surgical Practice, 17th ed. Philadelphia, Saunders, 2004, pp 221–241.

CHAPTER 2

Principles of Wound Closure

Suhail K. Kanchwala   and   Louis P. Bucky

Case Study

A 21-year-old male presents to the emergency room with right lower quadrant pain. He is taken to the operating room with the presumed diagnosis of appendicitis. Abdominal exploration through a right lower quadrant incision reveals perforated appendicitis. After appendectomy, the abdominal fascia is closed with interrupted absorbable sutures. The skin is left open and packed with moist gauze.

BACKGROUND

Normal wound healing progresses through three distinct but overlapping phases. The **inflammatory phase** of wound healing begins first and lasts between 3 and 7 days in the normal wound environment; the presence of significant devitalized tissue (e.g., in traumatic wounds) can prolong this phase. The inflammatory phase is characterized by the influx of neutrophils and macrophages. The **proliferative phase** of wound healing typically begins after 24 hours and may last for up to 3 weeks. The hallmark of the proliferative phase is the formation of **granulation tissue,** a dense network of fibroblasts, extracellular matrix, and newly formed blood vessels. The principal cell types involved in the proliferative phase are the keratinocyte and the fibroblast. The **remodeling phase** of wound healing begins after 2 weeks and may last as long as 1 year. In the remodeling phase, the wound begins to **contract** and the **collagen** present in the wound is reorganized. The principal cell type involved in wound contracture is the myofibroblast, whereas fibroblasts are responsible for depositing and reorganizing collagen (Fig. 2-1).

Wound management is an essential component of every surgical procedure. The majority of surgical wounds are closed primarily (i.e., tissues are reapproximated). Contaminated wounds, or those that cannot be closed without significant tension, are sometimes allowed to close by *secondary intention* (i.e., left open and allowed to fill with granulation tissue and contract over time). Alternatively, a wound may be left open initially and closed at a subsequent time, a procedure called *delayed primary closure.* The management of open wounds not amenable to immediate closure may include dressing changes or application of a *vacuum-assisted closure (VAC) dressing.* Large wounds that will not close on their own are sometimes covered with a *skin graft* or *flap.* These wound closure techniques are the focus of this chapter.

PREOPERATIVE EVALUATION

Generalized **malnutrition** as well as specific nutrient deficiencies (e.g., vitamin C, vitamin A, and zinc) significantly impair wound healing. If malnutrition is suspected preoperatively, albumin and prealbumin levels should be obtained and nutritional status should be optimized. This may involve delaying surgery to allow for nutritional support. Similarly, **diabetes,** prior local **radiation therapy,** and **immunosuppression** from other etiologies (e.g., steroid use) are associated with delayed wound healing and higher rates of infection. In diabetic patients, blood glucose levels should be tightly regulated in the perioperative

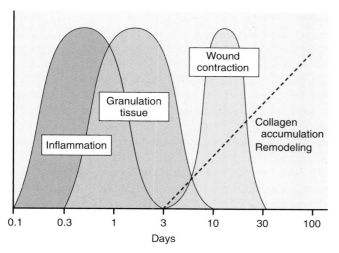

Figure 2-1
Phases of wound healing. *(Modified from Clark RAF: Wound repair. In Clark RAF [ed]: The Molecular and Cellular Biology of Wound Repair, 2nd ed. New York, Plenum Press, 1996, p 3.)*

period to lessen the risk of wound complications. Administration of vitamin A has been shown to improve wound healing in patients receiving steroids.

Is your patient immunosuppressed?

WOUND CLOSURE

Suture Materials

I.   **Suture Size:** Suture material is available in a variety of sizes. Sutures were originally manufactured in sizes ranging from #6 to #1, with #6 being the largest. As manufacturing techniques improved, #0 suture was introduced. Subsequently, smaller sizes were introduced and named according to the number of zeros they contained (i.e., 00 = 2-0, 000 = 3-0, etc.). The size of suture should reflect the application and the amount of tension on the wound. In general, the finest suture material that will maintain the approximation of tissues should be used.

II. **Absorbable versus Nonabsorbable:** A variety of permanent and absorbable suture materials are commonly available. In general, the suture material used should not absorb until the inherent tensile strength of the wound is sufficient to maintain tissue approximation. Tissues that take longer to heal (e.g., tendons or fascia) should be reapproximated with longer-lasting suture material. Skin, on the other hand, heals quickly and may be closed with rapidly absorbable suture material.

III. **Braided versus Monofilament:** Both absorbable and nonabsorbable suture materials are available in single-strand (monofilament) and braided varieties. The choice of which to use is often determined by surgeon preference. Braided suture tends to be easier to tie compared with monofilament suture; however, braided suture may cause a more substantial local tissue reaction, resulting in delayed healing.

IV. **Needle Type:** Suture material may be swedged onto needles of a variety of types and sizes to suit specific applications. The two most common needle types are tapered and cutting. **Cutting** needles have two sharp cutting edges. These needles are commonly used to place sutures into the skin because they make penetration easier. **Tapered** needles are round in cross-section and pass through tissue in a less traumatic fashion.

The following principles of wound closure should be adhered to when possible: 1. Skin closure without tension.   2. Closure of underlying dead space.   3. Close dermal approximation.

Suturing Techniques

I.   **Simple Interrupted:** The simple interrupted suture is among the most commonly used techniques; a limitation is that dermal apposition may be difficult to achieve.

CARE MUST BE TAKEN TO AVOID INVERTING THE SKIN EDGES WHEN USING SIMPLE INTERRUPTED SUTURES.

II. **Vertical Mattress:** The vertical mattress technique is commonly used to approximate tissues that are under tension. An advantage of the vertical mattress suture is that excellent dermal apposition is achieved without compromising the vascularity of the skin edges.

III. **Horizontal Mattress:** Like the vertical mattress suture, the horizontal mattress technique affords excellent dermal apposition; however, the horizontal mattress technique may result in a greater degree of wound ischemia compared with the vertical mattress technique.

IV. **Subcuticular:** This running stitch is buried in the superficial dermis and is used to closely reapproximate the epidermis.

V. **Over-and-Over** ("baseball stitch"): This technique may be used to close large incisions rapidly; the limitations are similar to those associated with simple interrupted sutures (i.e., poor dermal apposition). In addition, over-and-over sutures can compromise skin edge vascularity.

VI. **Skin Staples:** Surgical staples close large wounds efficiently and are commonly used after abdominal procedures. An advantage of stapled closure is that individual staples may be removed when a wound becomes infected without interrupting the remaining closure.

VII. **Skin Glue/Tape:** Skin glue (i.e., Dermabond) and skin tapes (Steri-Strips) can be used to approximate dermal lacerations that are not under significant tension or as an adjunct to other techniques (Fig. 2-2).

Alternative Closure Techniques

When the edges of a wound cannot be closed without significant tension, alternative methods of wound closure, such as local skin flaps or skin grafts, must be used. Importantly, flaps and skin grafts achieve wound closure at the cost of an additional wound.

I. **Local Skin Flaps:** A flap is defined as transposed tissue with an intact blood supply. Skin flaps use laxity in adjacent tissues to redistribute wound tension over a larger area. Skin flaps may be *rotated* or *advanced* to cover a wound (Fig. 2-3).

II. **Skin Grafts:** Skin grafting involves the harvest of skin from a *donor site* to cover a wound (i.e., the *recipient bed*). Because skin grafts rely on revascularation, an appropriate recipient bed is an important prerequisite for graft "take." Skin grafts will not survive in the presence of infection, ongoing trauma, or poor recipient site vascularity. The size of the wound that requires coverage and the availability of donor tissues determine whether a split-thickness or full-thickness graft is used.

A. **Split-thickness** skin grafting involves the harvest of epidermis and partial-thickness dermis from a donor site (commonly the thigh or buttocks). The donor site subsequently re-epithelializes from the dermal elements that remain. Split-thickness grafts may be meshed to allow greater expansion of the graft and coverage of a larger area; however, a disadvantage of split-thickness grafts is the significant amount of graft contracture seen postoperatively.

B. **Full-thickness** skin grafting involves harvest of the full epidermis and dermis. Full-thickness skin graft donor sites are typically closed primarily. Generally, full-thickness grafts are used to cover small wounds. Compared with split-thickness grafts, full-thickness grafts undergo little postoperative contraction.

| How large is the wound? |

POSTOPERATIVE CONSIDERATIONS: SURGICAL DRESSINGS

A variety of dressing types may be used in the management of surgical wounds.

I. Simple **dry dressings** serve to protect a wound from infection and absorb wound drainage. They are commonly applied to closed wounds. **Semipermeable, nonpermeable, hydrogel, and hydrocolloid** dressings maintain a moist environment and may facilitate healing of wounds that heal by epithelialization (e.g., skin graft donor sites).

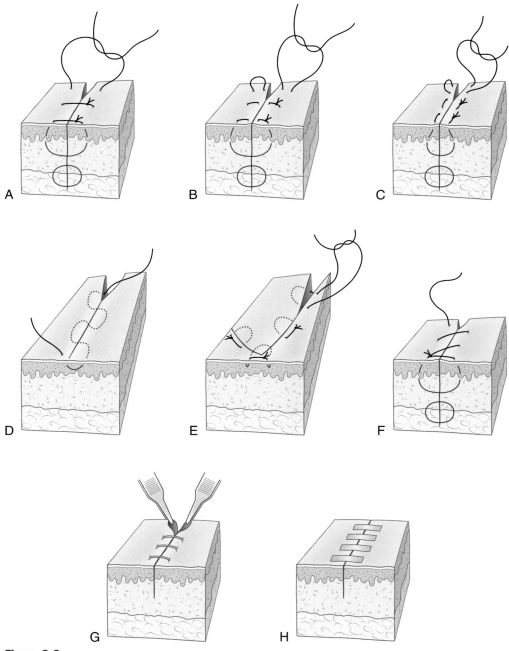

Figure 2-2
Suture techniques. **A,** Simple interrupted. **B,** Vertical mattress. **C,** Horizontal mattress. **D,** Running subcuticular. **E,** Half-buried mattress. **F,** Over-and-over. **G,** Skin staples. **H,** Skin tape (Steri-Strips) and glue. *(From Thorne CH, Beasley RW, Aston SJ, et al: Grabb and Smith's Plastic Surgery, 6th ed. Philadelphia, Lippincott Williams & Wilkins, 2007.)*

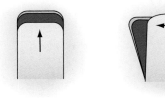

Advancement   Rotation

Figure 2-3
Local flaps. *(From Townsend CM, Beauchamp RD, Evers BM, Mattox KL [eds]: Sabiston Textbook of Surgery: The Biological Basis of Modern Surgical Practice, 18th ed. Philadelphia, Saunders, 2008.)*

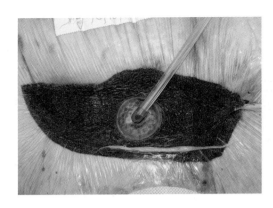

Figure 2-4

Negative pressure–assisted wound closure sponge in place on a wound. *(From Townsend CM, Beauchamp RD, Evers BM, Mattox KL [eds]: Sabiston Textbook of Surgery: The Biological Basis of Modern Surgical Practice, 18th ed. Philadelphia, Saunders, 2008.)*

II. **Wet-to-dry dressings** are commonly used to dress open and contaminated wounds; mechanical debridement of the wound results from removal of dried packing material with adherent devitalized tissue. **Enzymatic agents** (e.g., papain/urea [Accuzyme]) may be used in conjunction with dressings to gently debride fibrinous debris. In addition, application of broad-spectrum **antibacterials** (e.g., silver sulfadiazine) may limit bacterial colonization and promote wound healing.

III. Recently, **VAC dressings** have gained great popularity for the management of open wounds. The VAC dressing has three components: (1) the VAC sponge, which is applied directly to the wound bed; (2) an occlusive dressing, which is applied over the sponge to seal it to the surrounding skin; and (3) a suction pump, which provides regulated negative pressure through the sponge. The VAC has been used extensively to promote granulation tissue formation and wound contraction. A major advantage of the VAC is the need for fewer dressing changes compared with conventional dressings (Fig. 2-4).

SUGGESTED READINGS

Jones KR, Fennie K, Lenihan A: Evidence-based management of chronic wounds. Adv Skin Wound Care 20:591–600, 2007.

Lee CK, Hansen SL: Management of acute wounds. Clin Plast Surg 34:685–696, 2007.

Thorne CH, Beasley RW, Aston SJ, et al: Grabb and Smith's Plastic Surgery, 6th ed. Philadelphia, Lippincott Williams & Wilkins, 2007.

CHAPTER 3

Central Venous Catheterization

Ronald F. Parsons   and   Kristoffel R. Dumon

Case Study

A 68-year-old male undergoes an emergent left hemicolectomy for colonic ischemia. His postoperative course is complicated by a persistent ileus and supplemental oxygen requirement. On the seventh postoperative day, he is transferred to the intensive care unit after he has progressive hypotension, oliguria, and respiratory distress, necessitating intubation. The attending surgeon requests that a triple-lumen central venous catheter be placed to monitor central venous pressures and administer total parenteral nutrition.

BACKGROUND

Central venous catheters (CVCs) are an enormously important tool in clinical medicine; more than 5 million are placed annually in the United States. Notwithstanding, CVCs are associated with a number of complications, including several that are potentially fatal (e.g., pneumothorax and catheter-associated sepsis). Appropriate patient selection and safe insertion techniques are critical in minimizing the risks associated with this common procedure, and they are the focus of this chapter.

Many catheter types are commonly in use. Multilumen catheters allow for concomitant venous pressure monitoring and infusions, or the infusion of multiple products. Larger-lumen catheters (e.g., Cordis, Miami Lakes, FL) allow for more rapid infusion and are, therefore, useful in the resuscitative setting. Moreover, such catheters can serve as conduits for the insertion of multilumen catheters or pulmonary artery catheters. Catheters designed for long-term access, such as **Hickman** (Fig. 3-1A) and **Broviac** catheters, are tunneled under the skin of the chest wall and are equipped with a cuff around which scar tissue forms, holding the catheter in position. **Implantable ports** facilitate long-term, intermittent access (e.g., weekly chemotherapy). These devices have a reservoir that is implanted in a subcutaneous pocket and can be intermittently accessed by needle puncture through the skin (Fig. 3-1B).

In most cases, CVCs are inserted using the **Seldinger technique,** which involves the placement of a wire into the central vein and insertion of a catheter over the wire. Alternatively, a **cut-down** approach may be used, as is commonly the case when inserting an implantable port. Percutaneous approaches to the internal jugular vein (IJ), the subclavian (SC) vein, and the femoral vein; the Seldinger technique; and the cut-down approach to port placement are all discussed in this chapter.

INDICATIONS FOR CENTRAL LINE PLACEMENT

I. **Vascular Access:** CVCs provide durable venous access in patients who have limited peripheral options. The anticipated length of time during which access is

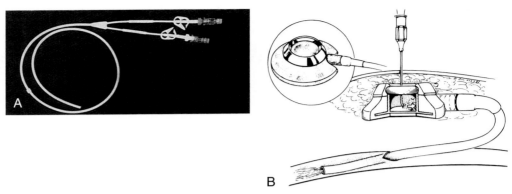

Figure 3-1
Hickman catheter (**A**) and accessed implantable port (**B**). (*A, From Marx J, Hockberger R, Walls R: Rosen's Emergency Medicine: Concepts and Clinical Practice, 6th ed. Philadelphia, Mosby, 2006; **B**, From Hoffman R, Benz E, Shattil S, et al: Hematology: Basic Principles and Practice, 4th ed. Philadelphia, Churchill Livingstone, 2005.*)

required plays a role in the selection of the type of catheter and the insertion site. For example, femoral access is often an appropriate option for short-term emergent access; however, associated risks preclude long-term maintenance. Many vasoactive and chemotherapeutic agents require central administration because peripheral extravasation of pressors or vesicants can result in significant tissue damage. Additionally, peripheral administration of high-osmolarity total parenteral nutrition is associated with complications, including thrombophlebitis and extravasation, and therefore must be administered centrally.

II. **Hemodynamic Monitoring:** Transduction of central venous pressure waveforms through a CVC allows for continuous monitoring of volume status and right heart function.

III. **Plasmapheresis, Hemodialysis, or Continuous Renal Replacement Therapy:** Exchange of blood components requires central venous access in the form of a large-bore catheter.

PREPROCEDURE EVALUATION

I. **History:** A history of deep venous thrombosis, coagulopathy, previous or unsuccessful CVC placement, and previous surgery should be elicited.

II. **Physical Examination:** The patient is examined for evidence of previous CVC placement and signs of central venous occlusion (e.g., upper extremity swelling and superficial venous collaterals).

III. **Laboratory Evaluation:** Thrombocytopenia and coagulopathy are relative contraindications to CVC placement. Optimally, the platelet count and international normalized ratio should be corrected to more than 50,000 and less than 1.5, respectively. In certain circumstances, CVC placement may be necessary with a less optimal coagulation profile.

> What is your patient's platelet count and international normalized ratio?

COMPONENTS OF THE PROCEDURE AND APPLIED ANATOMY

Preprocedure Evaluation

Site selection should be given careful consideration before CVC placement. SC access is associated with low rates of catheter-associated bloodstream infections, but relatively high rates of placement-related complications (e.g., pneumothorax). IJ access is associated with a lower rate of pneumothorax, but a higher rate of infection compared with SC access. Femoral venous catheters are relatively easy to place; however, they are associated with higher rates of thrombosis and infection and should generally be used only for short-term or emergent access.

Patient Positioning and Preparation

I. The patient is placed in the supine position. The sterile preparation is applied at the insertion site. The sterile preparation for IJ and SC catheter placement should include the entire ipsilateral chest wall and neck to allow for access to both sites.

II. IJ and SC catheters should be inserted with the patient in the Trendelenberg position (i.e., the head of the table is tilted down).

III. Before insertion, the catheter is flushed with sterile saline to evacuate intraluminal air.

Internal Jugular Vein Approach

I. The patient's head is rotated 45 degrees away from the planned insertion site (Fig. 3-2).

II. The carotid pulse is palpated and displaced medially with the nondominant hand. A small-gauge **finder** needle is inserted lateral to the carotid pulse at the apex of the triangle formed by the two heads of the sternocleidomastoid muscle and the clavicle, and is advanced toward the ipsilateral nipple. After localization of the IJ with the finder needle (as evidenced by blood return), an introducer needle is inserted along an immediately adjacent path, into the vein.

III. Venous (rather than arterial) catheterization can be confirmed by attaching intravenous extension tubing to the introducer needle and drawing blood into the tubing with a syringe. A column of venous blood readily descends down the intravenous tubing. On the other hand, if the needle is in the carotid artery, the column of blood will continue to ascend through the tubing. In the event that the artery is inadvertently cannulated, the needle should be removed immediately and firm pressure applied at the site.

> **THE COLOR OF THE BLOOD RETURN IS AN UNRELIABLE MARKER FOR VENOUS CATHETER PLACEMENT.**

Subclavian Vein Approach

A rolled towel is placed under the scapulae. Local anesthetic is delivered to the subcutaneous tissues and the periosteum of the clavicle. The introducer needle (i.e., a large-gauge, hollow-bore needle) is attached to a syringe and is inserted 2 to 3 cm inferior to the mid-

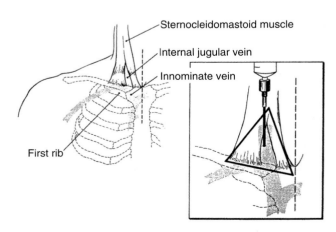

Sternocleidomastoid muscle

Internal jugular vein

Innominate vein

First rib

Figure 3-2

Internal jugular venous anatomy and access. The internal jugular vein is located at the apex of the triangle formed by the two heads of the sternocleidomastoid muscle and the clavicle. The dashed lines demarcate the midline. *(From Roberts JR, Hedges JR: Clinical Procedures in Emergency Medicine, 4th ed. Philadelphia, Saunders, 2004.)*

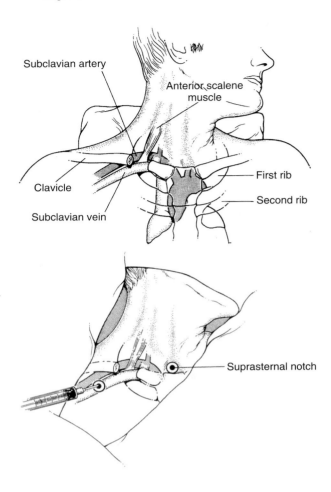

Figure 3-3
Subclavian venous anatomy and access.
The subclavian vein lies directly beneath
the clavicle. The vein is separated from
the subclavian artery by the anterior
scalene muscle (*top*). The subclavian
artery is cannulated beneath the
midportion of the clavicle. On insertion,
the needle is directed toward the
suprasternal notch (*bottom*). *(From Salm
TJV, Cutler BS, Wheeler HB [eds]: Atlas of
Bedside Procedures. Boston, Little, Brown,
1979.)*

point of the clavicle. The needle is advanced under the clavicle toward the sternal notch
until blood return is visualized in the syringe (Fig. 3-3).

Femoral Vein Approach

> The anatomy of the
> femoral triangle is
> summarized by the
> mnemonic NAVEL: from
> lateral to medial, the
> femoral **n**erve, **a**rtery, **v**ein,
> **e**mpty space, and
> **l**ymphatics pass under the
> inguinal ligament.

I. The femoral artery is palpated below the inguinal ligament. If the femoral artery
is not palpable, the point one third of the distance between the pubic tubercle
and the anterior superior iliac crest may serve as a landmark for its location
(Fig. 3-4).
II. An introducer needle is inserted 2 cm below the inguinal ligament and medial to
the femoral artery at a 45-degree angle with the skin. The needle is advanced until
blood return is visualized in the syringe.

Seldinger Technique

> **THE WIRE SHOULD NEVER BE
> ADVANCED WITH THE DILATOR;
> THIS CAN RESULT IN PASSAGE
> OF THE DILATOR THROUGH THE
> VESSEL WALL AND INJURY TO
> ADJACENT STRUCTURES.**

> **THE WIRE SHOULD BE KEPT IN
> SIGHT AT ALL TIMES TO
> PREVENT INTRAVASCULAR
> WIRE LOSS.**

I. After venous cannulation, a wire with a flexible tip (J-wire) is inserted through the
introducer needle into the lumen of the vein. The needle is then withdrawn while
the wire is held in position to maintain venous access. A 5-mm incision is made
in the skin, incorporating the insertion site.
II. A dilator is passed over the wire and into the vein to allow for easy subsequent
insertion of the CVC.
III. The wire is fed through the catheter until it passes out of the catheter port, and
is held in place while the catheter is advanced into the vein. The wire is withdrawn
and the catheter is occluded to prevent air embolism.

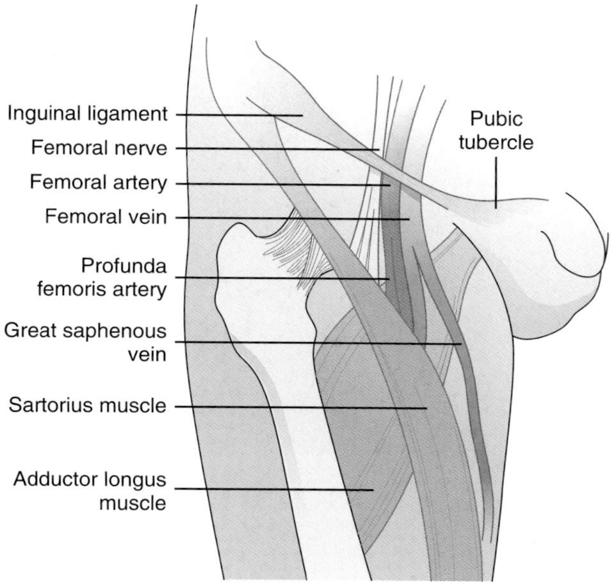
Inguinal ligament
Femoral nerve
Femoral artery
Femoral vein
Profunda femoris artery
Great saphenous vein
Sartorius muscle
Adductor longus muscle
Pubic tubercle

Figure 3-4
Femoral artery and vein anatomy. *(From Dieckmann R, Selbst S: Pediatric Emergency and Critical Care Procedures. St. Louis, Mosby, 1997.)*

Implantable Port Placement

I. An incision is made over the groove between the deltoid and the pectoralis major muscle (the deltopectoral groove) to expose the cephalic vein. The proximal end of the vein is encircled with a suture and the distal end is ligated.
II. A transverse venotomy is made and a plastic vein pick (Fig. 3-5) is inserted into the lumen of the vessel to open the venotomy. The catheter is inserted into the vein through the venotomy and advanced to the cavoatrial junction. Fluoroscopy is used to confirm appropriate location of the catheter tip. The proximal suture is then tied around the cephalic vein firmly enough to secure the catheter in position without occluding it.
III. A subcutaneous pocket large enough to accommodate the port is made in the infraclavicular fossa using blunt dissection.
IV. A noncoring needle (i.e., a Huber needle) is inserted through the skin and the membrane of the port. Any air is withdrawn and the port is flushed with heparinized saline. The skin incision is closed.

Additional Operative Considerations

Ultrasound-Guided Placement: Increasingly, bedside sonography is used to guide IJ catheter placement. In the Trendelenburg position, the IJ is compressible and larger than the carotid artery (Fig. 3-6).

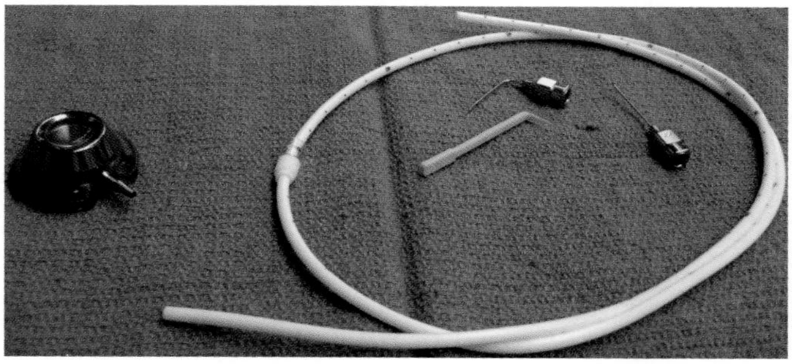

Figure 3-5
Typical implantable port system, including a stainless steel port, catheter, Huber needle, and plastic vein pick.

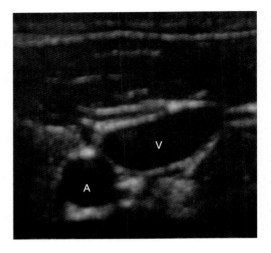

Figure 3-6
Ultrasonography of the right internal jugular vein (V) and right carotid artery (A).

POSTPROCEDURE CONSIDERATIONS

After any attempted SC or IJ CVC insertion, a chest radiograph is obtained to confirm position and identify complications (i.e., pneumothorax).

COMPLICATIONS

I. **Infectious complications,** including site infection, bacteremia, and infection of remote sites (e.g., endocarditis), occur with relative frequency in patients who undergo central venous catheterization. Sterile technique, optimal site selection, and frequent reevaluation of the insertion site may reduce the risk of infection. Routine line changes increase the likelihood of both mechanical and infectious complications and therefore are not recommended.

II. **Technical complications** include arterial catheter placement, hematoma formation, pneumothorax, hemothorax, arrhythmia, and air embolism. **Pneumothorax** is most often associated with SC catheter placement, but may result from IJ cannulation as well. A postoperative chest radiograph should be obtained after attempted SC and IJ catheterization, and postprocedure respiratory distress or hemodynamic instability should raise suspicion for the development of a tension pneumothorax. **Air embolism** results from entry of air into the central venous circulation and subsequent embolization to the pulmonary vasculature. In the presence of a patent foramen ovale, air may also occlude the cerebral circulation and cause an ischemic stroke. Like tension pneumothorax, air embolism may present with dyspnea or hypotension. The incidence of air embolism may be minimized through preventive practices; these include Trendelendurg positioning, limiting the intervals during which an introducer needle and catheter are open to the air, and having the patient perform the Valsalva maneuver or exhale selectively during such intervals.

III. **Thrombotic complications** are most common after femoral vein catheterization and lowest after SC vein catheterization. Thrombosis may occur as early as 1 day after insertion; therefore, catheters should be removed as soon as they are no longer needed.

SUGGESTED READINGS

Graham AS, Ozment C, Tegtmeyer K, Lai S, Braner DA: Central venous catheterization. N Engl J Med 356;e21, 2007.

Kusminsky RE: Complications of central venous catheterization. J Am Coll Surg 204: 681–696, 2007.

Lefor AT, Gomella LG: Bedside procedures. In Mann B, Lefor A, Gomella L (eds): Surgery On Call, 3rd ed. Columbus, OH, McGraw Hill, 2001, pp 342–380.

McGee DC, Gould MK: Preventing complications of central venous catheterization. N Engl J Med 348:1123–1133, 2003.

CHAPTER 4

Inguinal Hernia Repair

Demetri J. Merianos   and   Steven E. Raper

Case Study

A 29-year-old male presents to his primary care physician's office complaining of a bulge in his right groin, which he first noticed 2 weeks earlier. He denies associated pain, nausea, or vomiting. He denies a history of constipation, difficulty with urination, or chronic cough. He recently began a rigorous exercise program involving heavy lifting. Physical examination shows a nontender, reducible right groin mass that protrudes into the right scrotum when the patient coughs.

BACKGROUND

> The processus vaginalis is an outpouching of the peritoneum through which the testicle descends into the scrotum during development.

A hernia is defined as the protrusion of any structure beyond its normal anatomic boundaries. In the case of an inguinal hernia, a peritoneum-lined sac containing abdominal organs (e.g., small intestine or omentum) protrudes through a defect in the inguinal region of the abdominal wall. When a hernia can be replaced within the abdominal wall musculature, it is described as **reducible**; when it cannot, it is described as **incarcerated. Strangulation**, which is caused by compromise of the blood supply to the contents of an incarcerated hernia, is the most serious complication of an untreated hernia.

> Hesselbach's triangle is the space bounded by the lateral border of the rectus abdominis medially, the inguinal ligament inferiorly, and the inferior epigastric vessels laterally. Direct inguinal hernias protrude through this space.

Inguinal hernias are further characterized as either indirect or direct. **Indirect inguinal hernias** enter the inguinal canal through the deep inguinal ring **lateral to the inferior epigastric vessels** and may communicate with the scrotum. **Direct inguinal hernias** protrude directly through the floor of the inguinal canal **medial to the inferior epigastric vessels** through a space known as **Hesselbach's triangle.** The term **pantaloon hernia** describes concomitant direct and indirect hernias. Indirect inguinal hernias are the most common type in both male and female patients and are believed to result from persistent patency of the processus vaginalis. Factors that result in elevation of intra-abdominal pressure (e.g., lifting, straining with urination or defecation, ascites, chronic cough) may contribute to the development of both indirect and direct inguinal hernias.

Approximately 700,000 inguinal hernia repairs are performed annually, making this one of the most common surgical procedures. Historically, surgeons repaired inguinal hernias by directly approximating tissues to reinforce the area of abdominal wall weakness. Over the course of the last two decades, the "tension-free" repair, using prosthetic mesh to repair the hernia defect, has emerged as the preferred technique. More recently, a variety of laparoscopic approaches have gained popularity. The open (anterior) mesh repair is the primary focus of this chapter, but several other approaches are briefly described.

INDICATIONS FOR INGUINAL HERNIA REPAIR

I. **Reducible Hernias:** Traditionally, the presence of an inguinal hernia constituted an indication for its repair. Two major arguments were made in favor of this approach: (1) over time, hernias tend to enlarge and become symptomatic; and (2) the seriousness of complications associated with untreated hernias, namely, incarceration and strangulation, justifies the risks associated with surgical repair.

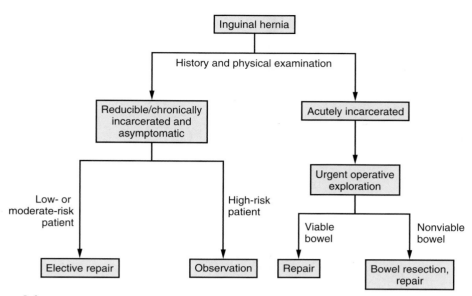

Figure 4-1
Algorithm for the management of reducible versus incarcerated inguinal hernias.

Although many surgeons continue to subscribe to this approach, a role for expectant management of asymptomatic inguinal hernias has emerged, particularly in high-risk patients. Low- to moderate-risk patients are generally offered the option of hernia repair.

II. **Incarcerated Hernias:** Edema of the contents of a hernia, or formation of adhesions to the peritoneum-lined hernia sac, may result in incarceration. Incarceration of a bowel-containing hernia may result in intestinal obstruction and, if left untreated, strangulation and bowel necrosis. Incarceration of a hernia that contains only one sidewall of the bowel may progress to strangulation without signs of obstruction; such hernias are known as **Richter's hernias.** Acutely incarcerated hernias require immediate operative repair. Strangulated, nonviable bowel requires resection at the time of surgery. In contrast, in the absence of pain or obstructive symptoms (e.g., nausea and vomiting), chronically incarcerated hernias may be repaired electively (Fig. 4-1).

> **ACUTE INCARCERATION OF A HERNIA GENERALLY MANDATES URGENT OPERATIVE REPAIR TO PREVENT STRANGULATION.**

PREOPERATIVE EVALUATION

A thorough history and physical examination are nearly always sufficient to make the diagnosis of an inguinal hernia.

I. **History:** Important components of the history include the chronicity of a hernia and the presence of associated symptoms. Additionally, an attempt should be made to elicit a history of straining from constipation, urinary obstruction, or chronic cough; these symptoms sometimes reflect underlying comorbidities necessitating additional evaluation (e.g., colonoscopy or urologic evaluation).

II. **Physical Examination:** Physical examination is performed with the patient supine and standing. The examiner generally places one hand over the inguinal ligament and, if the patient is male, palpates the superficial inguinal ring through the scrotal skin with the other hand. The patient is asked to cough or perform a Valsalva maneuver. Appreciation of a bulge moving from lateral to medial against the examiner's finger suggests an indirect inguinal hernia; a mass that protrudes directly through the abdominal wall suggests a direct hernia. Bilateral examination should be performed to rule out a contralateral hernia. In appropriate patients, a digital rectal examination should be performed to exclude enlargement of the prostate or a rectal mass.

> What predisposing factors may have contributed to hernia formation in your patient?

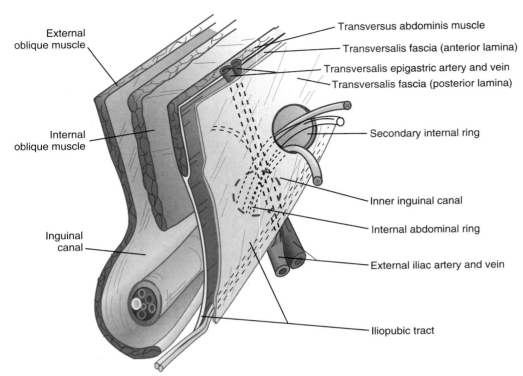

External oblique muscle

Transversus abdominis muscle

Transversalis fascia (anterior lamina)

Transversalis epigastric artery and vein

Transversalis fascia (posterior lamina)

Internal oblique muscle

Secondary internal ring

Inner inguinal canal

Internal abdominal ring

Inguinal canal

External iliac artery and vein

Iliopubic tract

Figure 4-2
The right inguinal canal. The external oblique aponeurosis forms the roof of the inguinal canal. The floor of the canal is formed by the transversalis fascia and the aponeurosis of the transversus abdominis muscle. Superiorly, the canal is bounded by the *conjoint tendon.* Inferiorly, the external oblique aponeurosis folds under itself to form the inguinal ligament. The inferior epigastric vessels course between the transversus abdominis muscle and transversalis fascia. The internal abdominal ring (deep inguinal ring) is an opening in the transversalis fascia and transversus abdominis muscle through which the spermatic cord (or round ligament in females) enters the inguinal canal. The external abdominal ring (superficial inguinal ring) is an opening in the external oblique aponeurosis adjacent to the pubic tubercle through which the cord exits the canal. *(From Read RC: The transversalis and preperitoneal fasciae: A re-evaluation. In Nyhus LM, Condon RE [eds]: Hernia, 4th ed. Philadelphia, Lippincott, 1995, pp 57–63.)*

> The spermatic cord contains cremasteric muscle fibers (derived from the internal oblique muscle), the testicular artery, veins of the pampiniform plexus, the genital branch of the genitofemoral nerve, the vas deferens, lymphatics, and the processus vaginalis.

> Although often referred to as the conjoint tendon, the transversus abdominis and internal oblique aponeuroses, which make up the superior border of the inguinal canal, only fuse to form a true conjoint tendon in a minority of patients.

III. **Imaging.** In rare cases, the diagnosis of a hernia may be aided by ultrasound or cross-sectional imaging (e.g., computed tomography scan or magnetic resonance imaging).

COMPONENTS OF THE PROCEDURE AND APPLIED ANATOMY

See Figure 4-2.

A variation of the procedure described by Lichtenstein, using a mesh patch to reinforce the floor of the inguinal canal and a mesh plug to partially occlude the internal inguinal ring, has become the most common approach to inguinal hernia repair and is described below.

Preoperative Considerations

I. Prophylactic **antibiotics** are often given before hernia repair, particularly in the era of prosthetic mesh repairs.
II. Adequate **anesthesia** can be achieved with regional, spinal, epidural, or general anesthesia.

Patient Positioning and Preparation

I. The patient is placed in the supine position.
II. The sterile preparation should include both inguinal regions and the genitalia, and should extend to the umbilicus superiorly, the midaxillary lines laterally, and the mid-thighs inferiorly.

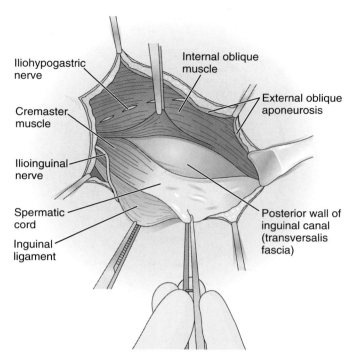

Iliohypogastric nerve

Internal oblique muscle

External oblique aponeurosis

Cremaster muscle

Ilioinguinal nerve

Spermatic cord

Inguinal ligament

Posterior wall of inguinal canal (transversalis fascia)

Figure 4-3
Exposure of the spermatic cord. The spermatic cord is identified and is bluntly dissected free from surrounding structures. (*Adapted from Condon RE, Telford GL: Hernia. In Nora PF [ed]: Operative Surgery: Principles and Techniques, 3rd ed. Philadelphia, Saunders, 1990.*)

Incision and Exposure

I. A 3- to 4-inch incision is made one fingerbreadth above, and parallel to, the inguinal ligament.

II. The incision is carried down through the subcutaneous fat and Scarpa's fascia to the external oblique aponeurosis. The aponeurosis is incised parallel to the direction of its fibers. When encountered, care is taken not to injure the ilioinguinal nerve, which lies directly beneath this layer.

III. The external oblique fascia is bluntly dissected off of the spermatic cord. The cord is then encircled at the level of the pubic tubercle (Fig. 4-3).

High Ligation of the Hernia Sac

I. When present, an indirect hernia sac is usually encountered deep to the cremasteric muscle fibers (which surround the spermatic cord), and anterior and medial (superior) to the cord. To expose the sac, cremasteric fibers are first divided. The hernia sac is then dissected off of the spermatic cord.

II. Direct hernias protruding through the floor of the inguinal canal are likewise dissected free from surrounding structures.

III. The hernia sac is opened (*explored*) to confirm that all hernia contents have been reduced within the peritoneal cavity.

IV. The hernia sac is ligated just above the transversalis fascia (i.e., *high ligation*), and excess sac is excised.

Reconstruction

I. A mesh plug is placed in the internal ring alongside the spermatic cord or Hesselbach's triangle, depending on the type of hernia. The plug is loosely secured to the surrounding tissues and serves to partially occlude the hernia defect.

II. A patch of mesh, sized to cover the floor of the inguinal canal, is sutured to the pubic tubercle medially. The inferior aspect of the mesh is then sutured to the edge of the inguinal ligament (known as the "shelving edge"). The superior aspect of the mesh is sutured to the *conjoint tendon*.

> The inguinal ligament forms a line between the anterior superior iliac spine laterally and the pubic tubercle medially.

> Does the patient have a direct or an indirect inguinal hernia?

> An indirect hernia sac is usually located deep to cremasteric muscle fibers, anterior and medial (superior) to the spermatic cord.

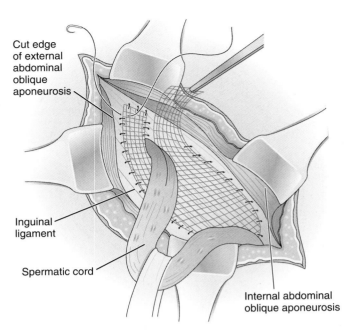

Figure 4-4
Reconstruction with mesh. A mesh patch is sutured to the internal oblique and transversus abdominis aponeuroses superiorly and the shelving edge of the inguinal ligament inferiorly. A slit is cut in the patch laterally to accommodate the spermatic cord. *(Adapted from Knol JA, Eckhauser FE: Inguinal anatomy and abdominal wall hernias. In Greenfield LJ [ed]: Surgery: Scientific Principles and Practice, 2nd ed. Philadelphia, Lippincott, 1997, with permission.)*

III. A slit is cut in the lateral edge of the mesh to accommodate the spermatic cord, which passes through this opening and lies over the mesh patch. The resultant tails of mesh are sutured together laterally around the spermatic cord, recreating the internal ring (Fig. 4-4).

Closure

I. The external oblique aponeurosis is closed over the spermatic cord.
II. The subcutaneous tissues and skin are closed in separate layers.
III. Traction is applied to the ipsilateral testicle at the conclusion of the procedure because this testicle often migrates superiorly secondary to intraoperative traction on the spermatic cord.

> Was traction applied to the testicle on the operative side at the conclusion of the hernia repair?

Other Approaches

I. **Other open approaches** to hernia repair are still occasionally performed. The incision, exposure, and hernia sac ligation as described earlier are common to all of these repairs. They differ from one another mainly in the technique of abdominal wall reconstruction. For example, the **Bassini repair** is performed by suturing the transversus abdominis and internal oblique aponeuroses directly to the shelving edge of the inguinal ligament without mesh (Fig. 4-5). The **McVay repair,** which allows for the repair of inguinal and femoral hernias, involves suturing the transversus abdominis aponeurosis to Cooper's ligament medial to the femoral vein.
II. **Laparoscopic approaches** to hernia repair have gained considerable popularity. Such approaches may be particularly useful for the repair of bilateral or recurrent hernias. There are two basic approaches to laparoscopic hernia repair, the transabdominal preperitoneal (TAPP) repair and the totally extraperitoneal (TEP) repair (Fig. 4-6). Both procedures involve the placement of mesh over the direct and indirect spaces.

> Cooper's ligament, the periosteum and fascia overlying the superior ramus of the pubic bone, forms the posterior border of the femoral canal (through which the femoral vessels pass). Cooper's ligament is an important landmark for both the McVay repair and laparoscopic repairs.

> WHEN PERFORMING LAPAROSCOPIC REPAIR, THE SURGEON MUST BE COGNIZANT OF THE LOCATION OF THE VAS DEFERENS AND SPERMATIC VESSELS TO AVOID INJURY TO THE EXTERNAL ILIAC VESSELS AND FEMORAL NERVE IN THE "TRIANGLE OF DOOM."

POSTOPERATIVE COURSE

Inguinal hernia repairs are generally performed on an outpatient basis. Patients resume a regular diet shortly after surgery and are discharged and prescribed oral pain medications after they urinate successfully. Most surgeons prohibit strenuous activity until approximately 6 weeks after hernia repair.

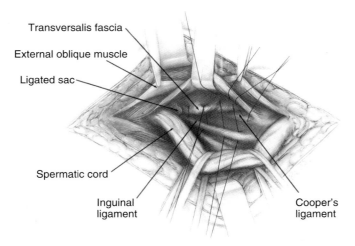

Transversalis fascia
External oblique muscle
Ligated sac
Spermatic cord
Inguinal ligament
Cooper's ligament

Figure 4-5
The Bassini repair. The *conjoint tendon* is sutured to the shelving edge of the inguinal ligament with interrupted sutures. *(From Townsend CM, Beauchamp RD, Evers BM, Mattox KL [eds]: Sabiston Textbook of Surgery: The Biological Basis of Modern Surgical Practice, 16th ed. Philadelphia, Saunders, 2004.)*

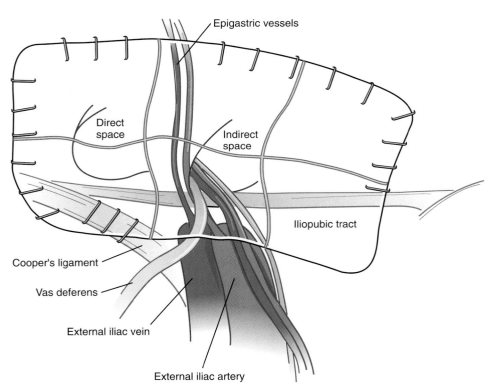

Epigastric vessels
Direct space
Indirect space
Iliopubic tract
Cooper's ligament
Vas deferens
External iliac vein
External iliac artery

Figure 4-6
Totally extraperitoneal repair and preperitoneal anatomy. The spermatic cord structures are seen entering the inguinal canal through the internal ring, lateral to the epigastric vessels (indirect space). The triangular space between the spermatic vessels (*right*) and vas deferens (*left*), known as the "triangle of doom," contains the external iliac vessels and nerve. The totally extraperitoneal repair involves placement of a mesh patch over both direct and indirect spaces after hernia reduction. Mesh is fixed to Cooper's ligament inferiorly and to the rectus musculature and transversus abdominis aponeurosis above the hernia defect. *(From Corbitt J: Laparoscopic transabdominal transperitoneal patch hernia repair. In Ballantyne GH [ed]: Atlas of Laparoscopic Surgery. Philadelphia, Saunders, 2000, p 511.)*

COMPLICATIONS

    I. Postoperative **urinary retention,** believed to be secondary to both anesthesia and manipulation of pelvic nerves, is common after inguinal hernia repair. It is almost always self-limited, but may require temporary bladder catheterization.

    II. Approximately 5% of patients experience **chronic pain** after inguinal hernia repair. Chronic pain may be related to nerve entrapment. The most commonly injured nerves are the ilioinguinal and the genitofemoral. Both nerves are routinely encountered during open inguinal hernia repairs. Division of these nerves may result in numbness. Some surgeons advocate transection of these structures when they are encountered to avoid entrapment, which may result in chronic pain. Analgesics and local anesthetic nerve blocks are sometimes helpful in treating chronic pain syndromes. Occasionally, if nerve entrapment is suspected and symptoms are severe, reoperation and neurectomy (excision of a segment of nerve) are indicated.

III. Rates of hernia **recurrence** are generally reported as less than 1%. Recurrent inguinal hernias are most commonly direct hernias at the medial aspect of the previous repair, near the pubic tubercle. Recurrences may be repaired using an open (anterior) approach. However, increasingly, laparoscopic approaches are used in this setting to avoid dissection through scar tissue.

IV. **Infection** rates of less than 1% are reported after inguinal hernia repair. When surgical site infections involve underlying mesh prostheses, mesh removal is frequently necessary.

V. **Ischemic Orchitis:** Compromise of the venous drainage of the testicle, typically from thrombosis of the small vessels of the pampiniform plexus, may result in testicular congestion, pain, swelling, and subsequent atrophy. Symptoms may persist for a period of several weeks and, rarely, orchiectomy is indicated.

VI. **Injury to intra-abdominal organs** and the vas deferens are rare but serious complications of inguinal hernia repair. Such injuries may be more common during the repair of large hernias, which can displace the vas deferens, making its identification challenging. The presence of a *sliding hernia*, in which part of a hernia sac is composed of intra-abdominal viscera (e.g., the bladder or colon), can also increase the likelihood of injuries.

SUGGESTED READINGS

Eubanks WS: Hernias. In Townsend CM, Beauchamp RD, Evers BM, Mattox KL (eds): Sabiston Textbook of Surgery: The Biological Basis of Modern Surgical Practice, 16th ed. Philadelphia, Saunders, 2001, pp 783–801.

Fitzgibbons RJ Jr, Giobbie-Hurder A, Gibbs JO, et al: Watchful waiting versus repair of inguinal hernia in minimally symptomatic men. JAMA 295:285–292, 2006.

Malangoni MA, Gagliardi RJ: Hernias. In Townsend CM, Beauchamp RD, Evers BM, Mattox KL (eds): Sabiston Textbook of Surgery: The Biological Basis of Modern Surgical Practice, 17th ed. Philadelphia, Saunders, 2004, pp 1199–1218.

Neumayer L, Giobbie-Hurder A, Jonasson O, et al: Open mesh versus laparoscopic mesh repair of inguinal hernia. N Engl J Med 350:1819–1827, 2004.

CHAPTER 5

Ventral Herniorrhaphy

Joshua Fosnot and Matt L. Kirkland III

Case Study

A 67-year-old male with a history of a laparotomy presents with a complaint of a "large bulge" in the midline of his abdomen. He has always had mild discomfort over his incision; however, this bulge has been getting larger over the past year and now causes significant discomfort with activity. On examination, he has a large nontender reducible incisional hernia. A large midline fascial defect is appreciable. He denies any episodes of abdominal distention, nausea, or vomiting.

BACKGROUND

A variety of abdominal wall hernias (ventral hernias) are commonly treated by the general surgeon (Fig. 5-1). **Umbilical hernias** are common in young children; most close by 2 years of age, and repair is rarely considered before 5 years of age. Umbilical hernias in adults are most commonly acquired and typically develop in patients with elevated intra-abdominal pressure (e.g., from obesity, pregnancy, or ascites). **Epigastric hernias** are found in the midline, superior to the umbilicus, and are often small and multiple. Pain may result from incarceration of properitoneal fat. **Spigelian hernias** result from herniation at the lateral border of the rectus sheath (linea semilunaris). A bulge is rarely apparent because these hernias usually dissect behind the external oblique aponeurosis. **Incisional hernias** are a common complication of abdominal surgery, occurring after up to 10% of abdominal wall closures. Technical error (e.g., excessive tension on the abdominal closure and inadequate approximation of the fascial edges) is the major etiology. Factors that result in increased intra-abdominal pressure (e.g., obesity, pregnancy, and ascites) and compromise wound healing (e.g., malnutrition and immunosuppression) may be contributory.

> Spigelian hernias should be repaired because of the high associated risk of incarceration.

The repair of all abdominal wall hernias involves reduction, closure of the fascial defect, and in many cases, reinforcement with a mesh prosthesis. Primary closure (without mesh) may be considered for defects smaller than 4 cm in diameter. Primary closure of larger defects is prone to failure, relating to the degree of tension on the repair, and should be avoided.

INDICATIONS FOR VENTRAL HERNIA REPAIR

I. **Reducible Hernias:** Ventral hernias are associated with a small risk of incarceration (i.e., entrapment of the contents of a hernia within the fascial defect). Generally, small hernias are more likely to become incarcerated than are larger hernias. In patients without significant comorbidity, ventral hernias may be repaired electively to minimize this risk, to alleviate associated symptoms (e.g., discomfort), or to improve cosmesis. A role for observation of asymptomatic and minimally symptomatic hernias has emerged in patients with significant comorbidity and those willing to accept the small risk of incarceration.

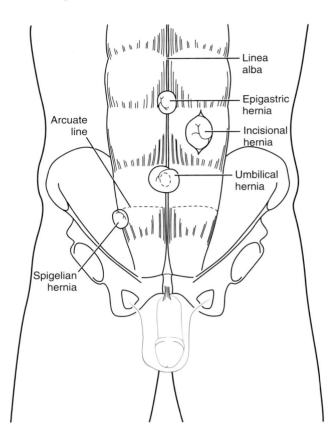

Figure 5-1
Different types of ventral hernias. *(From Roberts JR, Hedges JR, Chanmugam AS, et al [eds]: Clinical Procedures in Emergency Medicine, 4th ed. Philadelphia, Saunders, 2004.)*

II. **Incarceration:** Incarceration of bowel within a hernia may result in intestinal obstruction or compromise of the blood supply to the hernia contents (i.e., strangulation). Acute incarceration generally mandates urgent surgical intervention. In the absence of associated symptoms, chronically incarcerated ventral hernias may be managed expectantly.

PREOPERATIVE EVALUATION

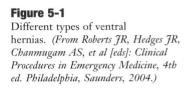

Does your patient have symptoms consistent with intestinal obstruction?

Rectus diastasis is thinning of the linea alba and lateralization of the rectus muscles without a fascial defect.

I. **History:** Symptoms suggesting incarceration or intestinal obstruction (e.g., abdominal pain, nausea, vomiting, and constipation) and factors that may contribute to abdominal wall herniation (e.g., chronic cough, constipation, or previous abdominal surgery) should be elicited.
II. **Physical Examination:** The goals of the physical examination are: (1) to determine the size of the hernia defect, (2) to distinguish a true hernia from a diastasis, and (3) to distinguish a reducible hernia from an incarcerated hernia. In the patient with an acutely incarcerated hernia, signs consistent with strangulation should be elicited (e.g., focal abdominal tenderness or peritonitis).
III. **Imaging:** In the setting of an incarcerated ventral hernia, **plain abdominal radiographs** may show dilated bowel or air–fluid levels consistent with intestinal obstruction. Ventral hernias are often better assessed with a **CT scan,** which may help to characterize the contents of the hernia (e.g., bowel vs. fat), localize and delineate the degree of bowel obstruction in the setting of incarceration, or identify signs consistent with strangulation (e.g., bowel wall edema).
IV. **Laboratory Studies:** In the patient with an incarcerated hernia, leukocytosis and elevated lactate levels should raise concern for bowel strangulation. Importantly, these signs are typically late findings and may reflect irreversible ischemia.

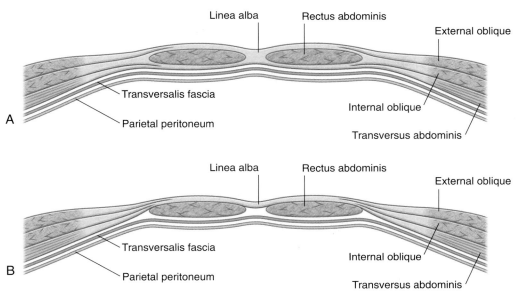

Figure 5-2
Anatomy of the anterior abdominal wall. **A,** Transverse section through the rectus sheath above the arcuate line. The external oblique and internal oblique aponeuroses contribute to the anterior sheath. The internal oblique and transversus abdominis aponeuroses contribute to the posterior sheath. **B,** Below the arcuate line (halfway between the umbilicus and pubis), there is no posterior rectus sheath. *(From Drake RL, Vogl W, Mitchell AWM: Gray's Anatomy for Students. Philadelphia, Churchill Livingstone, 2005.)*

COMPONENTS OF THE PROCEDURE AND APPLIED ANATOMY

Ventral hernias may be repaired using a variety of approaches. Factors that influence the choice of approach include the size of the defect, the integrity of the abdominal wall fascia surrounding the hernia, and surgeon preference (Fig. 5-2).

Patient Positioning and Preparation

   I. The patient is placed in the supine position with the arms extended.
  II. The sterile preparation is applied to the abdominal wall and should reflect the size of the hernia. For large hernias, the preparation typically extends to the nipple line superiorly, the pubis inferiorly, and the midaxillary lines laterally.

Preoperative Considerations

   I. Prophylactic antibiotics are indicated before elective repairs with mesh. The chosen antibiotic should have efficacy against skin flora (i.e., gram-positive organisms) and should be administered within 1 hour prior to incision.
  II. A urinary catheter should be inserted before repairs anticipated to last longer than 3 hours or for laparoscopic repairs.
 III. Nasogastric tube placement is often indicated before large ventral hernia repairs and laparoscopic repairs, which sometimes require extensive bowel manipulation or lysis of intra-abdominal adhesions.

Operative Repair

   I. **Types of Mesh:** Most current approaches to ventral hernia repair involve placement of a mesh prosthesis. A variety of mesh types are available; each has distinct advantages and disadvantages.
     A. **Permanent synthetic:** Polypropylene (Prolene), high-density polyethylene (Marlex), and coated PTFE (Gore-tex) are commonly used permanent syn-

thetic mesh products. They are designed to serve as permanent structural components of the hernia repair and are incorporated into scar tissue over time. Because of associated risks of intra-abdominal adhesion and fistula formation, placement of uncoated mesh adjacent to the bowel should be avoided. The use of permanent mesh is contraindicated for the repair of acutely incarcerated or strangulated hernias because bacteria translocation resulting from bowel stasis, distention, and ischemia can lead to mesh infection. Similarly, infected mesh should not be replaced with a new permanent mesh prosthesis during reoperative hernia operations.

B. **Bioprosthetic:** Bioprosthetic mesh made out of materials such as collagen, porcine gut submucosa, or cadaveric dermis is increasingly being used. Bioprosthetics are more resistant to infection and are sometimes used despite contamination.

C. **Nonpermanent synthetic:** Nonpermanent synthetic mesh products, such as polyglactin (Vicryl), are sometimes used to reinforce hernia repairs in the setting of contamination. Alternatively, such products may be used as a temporary barrier against evisceration when the fascia cannot be approximated or when a wound is contaminated.

II. **Open Primary Repair:** Primary repair involves closure of the fascial defect without prosthetic mesh. This approach is generally reserved for cases in which the fascial defect is small (e.g., epigastric and umbilical hernias).

A. An incision is made to allow for complete exposure of the defect. Umbilical hernia repairs are often performed through a curvilinear horizontal or midline vertical incision. Epigastric hernias are usually repaired through a vertical midline incision.

B. The subcutaneous tissues are dissected to expose the hernia sac.

C. The fascia is exposed circumferentially. In the case of an umbilical hernia, the hernia sac is divided from the umbilical stalk, avoiding injury to the umbilical skin.

D. The hernia contents and sac are reduced into the abdomen.

E. The sac is bluntly freed from the posterior surface of the abdominal fascia around the defect.

F. The fascial edges are reapproximated with interrupted sutures.

G. The subcutaneous tissue is closed over the repair to eliminate dead space, and the skin is closed.

III. **Open Repair with Mesh Implant:** In cases in which there is a large fascial defect, most surgeons elect to bolster the repair with mesh. Mesh may be secured anterior to the fascia (onlay), posterior to the fascia (inlay), or posterior to the rectus muscle within the rectus sheath (retrorectus). The retrorectus repair avoids potential pitfalls associated with onlay (e.g., mesh infection) and inlay (e.g., adhesion formation and fistula), but requires more extensive dissection and is generally more time consuming.

A. Onlay mesh repair

1. The first five steps proceed as described for primary repair (A–E).

2. A piece of mesh is cut large enough to allow for ample overlap of mesh with the fascial edges.

3. Several heavy nonabsorbable "U" stitches are placed through the mesh, into the fascia, and back through the mesh circumferentially around the defect. The sutures are left untied.

4. The fascia is reapproximated with interrupted sutures, as in primary closure.

5. The sutures through the mesh are tied down to fix the mesh to the anterior rectus sheath over the primary closure.

6. The subcutaneous tissue is closed over the repair to eliminate dead space, and the skin is closed.

B. Inlay mesh repair

1. The first five steps proceed as described for primary repair (A–E).

2. A piece of mesh is cut large enough to allow for ample overlap of mesh with the fascial edges.

3. Several nonabsorbable sutures are used to affix the mesh to the posterior surface of the fascia. Sutures are thrown through the fascia and then through the mesh and are brought back out through the fascia circumferentially around the fascial defect. The sutures are left untied. If possible, peritoneum is preserved to prevent subsequent adhesion formation between bowel and mesh.

4. The fascia is reapproximated with interrupted sutures, as in primary closure.

5. The sutures through the mesh are tied down, fixing the mesh to the posterior rectus sheath behind the primary closure.

6. The subcutaneous tissue is closed over the repair to eliminate dead space, and the skin is closed.

C. Retrorectus repair (Fig. 5-3)

1. The first five steps proceed as described for primary repair (A–E).

2. Adhesions are cleared from the undersurface of the abdominal wall.

3. The rectus sheath on each side of the fascial defect is divided. This incision is extended vertically along the length of the rectus sheath. The rectus muscle is dissected off of the posterior sheath bilaterally.

4. The posterior rectus sheath is then closed in the midline with a running suture.

5. A piece of mesh is cut large enough to allow for ample overlap of mesh with the edges of the anterior rectus sheath.

6. The mesh is sutured into place behind the rectus muscles circumferentially around the defect.

7. The anterior rectus fascia is reapproximated with interrupted sutures.

8. The subcutaneous tissue is closed over the repair to eliminate dead space, and the skin is closed.

D. Laparoscopic ventral hernia repair

1. Port placement is highly variable. Initially, port placement may be in the subxiphoid midline or along either costal margin at the anterior axillary line, where there are least likely to be adhesions to bowel. The port must be placed far enough from the fascial defect to allow for adequate visualization

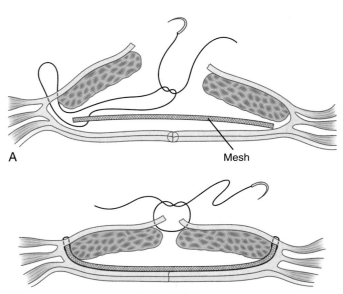

A

Mesh

B

Anterior fascial closure

Figure 5-3
Retrorectus repair. **A,** Mesh is placed in front of the posterior sheath and behind the rectus muscle. The mesh is anchored in place with interrupted sutures. **B,** The anterior sheath is closed. *(From Berry MF, Paisley S, Low DW, Rosato EF: Repair of large complex recurrent incisional hernias with retromuscular mesh and panniculectomy. Am J Surg 194: 99–204, 2007.)*

of the hernia on insertion of the laparoscope. Because most patients have had previous surgery, an "open" technique for port insertion is generally preferred. Additional ports are placed as needed.

2. Adhesions to the anterior abdominal wall are lysed using a combination of sharp and blunt dissection.

3. Gentle traction is placed on the hernia contents to reduce the hernia.

4. The mesh prosthesis is cut to size outside of the abdomen. The piece of mesh should be large enough to allow for 5-cm margins of overlap with the fascia in all directions. Four sutures are placed equidistant from each other around the perimeter of the mesh and are left untied. The mesh is marked for orientation, rolled into a cylinder, and inserted through the largest port. The mesh is unrolled in the abdomen and oriented for fixation.

5. Small incisions are made in four quadrants 5 cm beyond the perimeter of the hernia defect, corresponding to the sutures placed through the mesh. A suture-passing instrument is inserted through the fascia underlying each incision at two points several millimeters apart. With each pass, one end of the suture is retrieved and brought out through the corresponding incision. The two tails of each suture are then tied to fix the mesh behind the fascial defect. A tacker is used to fix the mesh to the anterior abdominal wall at multiple points between the sutures.

6. All ports are removed, the fascia at the camera port site is closed, and the skin incisions are closed.

> The fascial defect is not closed in the laparoscopic approach.

Additional Operative Considerations

Drain Placement: Repairs of larger ventral hernias often involve creation of extensive subcutaneous skin flaps. Disruption of dermal lymphatics and the large resultant potential space lead to seroma formation. Placement of subcutaneous drains at the conclusion of the repair may limit fluid accumulation.

POSTOPERATIVE COURSE

The postoperative course is dictated, in part, by the size of the hernia. Many small epigastric and umbilical hernias can be repaired on an outpatient basis. After larger hernia repairs, patients typically require admission for pain management. Despite the *minimally invasive* moniker, laparoscopic approaches to hernia repair often result in significant pain. If extensive adhesiolysis is necessary, the return of bowel function may be delayed for several days. If drains are placed, they are maintained until their output is minimal. The use of an abdominal binder may minimize seroma formation. Most surgeons recommend that patients limit rigorous exercise for the first 6 weeks after surgery.

COMPLICATIONS

I. **Seromas** are common after repairs of larger hernias involving the creation of subcutaneous flaps; drain placement is indicated in such cases. Seroma formation often complicates laparoscopic repairs as well. Reabsorbtion occurs over time, and intervention is usually unnecessary.

II. **Surgical site infections** are of particular concern after mesh hernia repairs and sometimes mandate reoperation and mesh removal.

III. **Recurrence** may result from technical error (e.g., excessive tension on the repair or inadequate mesh coverage). Factors that increase intra-abdominal pressure (e.g., obesity and ascites) or compromise wound healing (e.g., immunosuppression and malnutrition) may predispose to recurrence.

IV. The **repair of very large ventral hernias,** in which a significant portion of the abdominal contents is contained within the hernia sac (i.e., loss of domain), is associated with a unique set of complications. Replacement of the hernia contents within the abdominal cavity may result in greatly elevated intra-abdominal pressures. **Abdominal compartment syndrome,** characterized by cardiovascular compromise secondary to decreased venous return, elevated peak airway pressures, and end-organ hypoperfusion (e.g., renal failure and visceral ischemia), may ensue. Reoperation and release of the abdominal closure is required if abdominal compartment syndrome is suspected.

SUGGESTED READINGS

Berry MF, Paisley S, Low DW, Rosato EF: Repair of large complex recurrent incisional hernias with retromuscular mesh and panniculectomy. Am J Surg 194:199–204, 2007.

Malangoni MA, Gagliardi RJ. Hernias. In Townsend CM, Beauchamp RD, Evers BM, Mattox KL (eds): Sabiston Textbook of Surgery: The Biological Basis of Modern Surgical Practice, 17th ed. Philadelphia, Saunders, 2004, pp 1199–1218.

Esophagectomy

Ibrahim Abdullah   and   Ernest F. Rosato

Case Study

A 65-year-old male reports a 5-month history of weight loss, difficulty swallowing solid food, and progressive discomfort in the region of the midsternum. He denies cough or other respiratory symptoms. He reports a history of long-standing intermittent heartburn and has used both alcohol and cigarettes in the past. On physical examination, he appears thin. No abdominal masses are palpable. A computed tomography (CT) scan of the chest and abdomen and a barium swallow show a mass in the lower portion of his esophagus. An upper endoscopy confirms the presence of a mass at 35 to 38 cm. Biopsy specimens show adenocarcinoma with Barrett's epithelium background changes. Endoscopic ultrasound shows tumor extending into the muscularis without obvious lymph node enlargement. A positron emission tomography (PET) scan does not show any evidence of distant metastatic disease.

BACKGROUND

The esophagus extends from the hypopharynx to the stomach. The cervical esophagus begins at the cricopharyngeus muscle and is approximately 5 cm in length. The thoracic esophagus, measured from the level of the first thoracic vertebra, is typically 20 to 25 cm in length. The blood supply to the esophagus is segmental and arises from the inferior thyroid arteries proximally and the left gastric artery distally. The aortic esophageal and bronchial arteries supply the mid-esophagus. The lymphatic drainage of the esophagus is extensive. Mucosal and submucosal lymphatics communicate along the entire length of the muscular esophagus; because of this, tumors of the esophagus have a tendency to spread longitudinally. Moreover, esophageal lymphatics drain to multiple regional beds and drainage may proceed in either a proximal or a distal direction. Lesions of the upper and middle thirds of the esophagus most often drain to the hilar, periesophageal, and supraclavicular nodes, whereas lesions of the distal third drain to the lesser curvature, left gastric, and celiac nodes. Notwithstanding, positive celiac nodes are found in up to 10% of metastatic tumors of the upper esophagus and distal esophageal tumors may drain to the hilar and supraclavicular nodes.

Endoscopic localization of esophageal tumors is measured in relation to the central incisors. Typically, the cervical esophagus begins at approximately 15 cm and the gastro-esophageal junction is located at approximately 40 cm.

INDICATIONS FOR RESECTION

I. **Esophageal Malignancies**

  A. The overwhelming majority of esophageal resections are performed for the treatment of carcinoma or premalignant lesions. The incidence of esophageal cancer varies greatly with geography; incidences are particularly high in China and South Africa. Esophageal carcinoma in the United States occurs more frequently in African Americans than in whites. The incidence of **adenocarcinoma,** however, has been rapidly increasing among middle-aged white men;

it has now surpassed **squamous cell cancer** as the most prevalent histologic subtype of esophageal cancer in the United States. Alcohol and cigarette use are risk factors for both histologic subtypes. Approximately 15% of esophageal cancers occur in the upper one third, with the remainder occurring in the middle and lower thirds of the esophagus.

B. Staging of primary esophageal tumors is usually best achieved with the combination of CT, endoscopic ultrasound (EUS), and PET. CT is used to assess tumor invasion of local structures and identify distant metastatic disease. EUS (which can be combined with fine-needle aspiration) and PET are used to assess the regional lymph nodes. PET is probably the most sensitive modality for identifying distant metastases as well, assuming that the primary tumor is fluorine-18 fluorodeoxyglucose (FDG) avid. Carcinoma of the esophagus can spread widely. If a suspicious subcutaneous mass is found, biopsy should be performed. Neurologic symptoms should be evaluated using magnetic resonance imaging examination of the brain, and bone symptoms should be evaluated by bone scan.

C. The primary modalities for the treatment of esophageal cancers are surgery and chemoradiation therapy. Low survival rates with single-modality therapy, however, have prompted fairly uniform application of multimodality therapy, often consisting of neoadjuvant chemoradiation therapy and surgical resection of residual local disease. Surgery (either alone for very early disease or in combination with chemoradiation therapy for more advanced disease) provides potentially curative therapy. Importantly, surgical therapy may also provide significant palliation for dysphagia and local disease control so that oral intake may be maintained, even in patients who ultimately succumb to metastatic disease. In patients with clearly unresectable disease, palliative therapy without surgery should be the goal of treatment (Fig. 6-1).

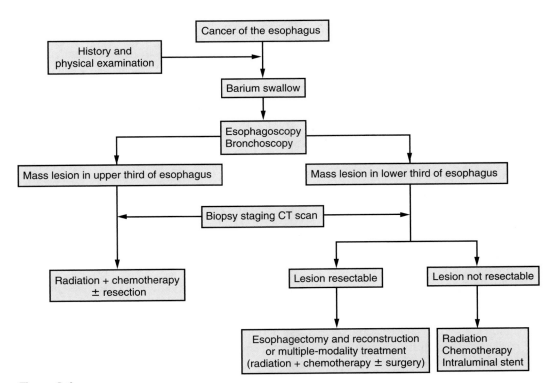

Figure 6-1

Evaluation and treatment of esophageal cancer. *(Adapted from Townsend CM, Beauchamp RD, Evers BM, Mattox KL [eds]: Sabiston Textbook of Surgery: The Biological Basis of Modern Surgical Practice, 17th ed. Philadelphia, Saunders, 2004.)*

II. **Other Indications**
   A. **Barrett's esophagus** describes the replacement of the esophageal squamous epithelium with sheets of columnar cells. The presence of Barrett's esophagus is associated with severe gastroesophageal reflux disease and incompetence of the lower sphincter, which allows for prolonged exposure of the esophageal mucosa to acid. Barrett's epithelium requires regular endoscopic surveillance with biopsies because it represents the first step toward dysplasia, a precursor to adenocarcinoma of the esophagus. Once Barrett's epithelium has developed, the symptoms of heartburn may be somewhat ameliorated because the columnar epithelium is less sensitive to acid reflux. Close endoscopic surveillance is still required, however, even if symptoms have resolved or an antireflux procedure has been undertaken because neither of these guarantees subsistence of reflux or the return to normal mucosa. The presence of **high-grade dysplasia** or carcinoma on surveillance biopsy is an indication for esophageal resection. More recently, endoscopic therapies for dysplasia, Barrett's epithelium, and early focal esophageal carcinoma have been explored. In skilled hands, these may displace resection for the treatment of early cases; however, long-term outcomes after such approaches have yet to be determined.
   B. **Caustic injury of the esophagus** does not usually require immediate resection except in the rare case in which perforation occurs. Caustic burns, however, may result in stricture formation and contribute to the development of carcinoma; these may ultimately require esophagectomy for management.
   C. **Esophageal perforation** is most commonly spontaneous (Boerhaave's syndrome) or a complication of instrumentation (e.g., endoscopy). Esophageal perforation represents a surgical emergency; if untreated, severe mediastinitis may ensue. Surgical options include primary repair with drainage and esophagectomy.
   D. **Collagen vascular disorders,** such as scleroderma, may result in significant esophageal atony, reflux esophagitis, and stricture formation. Patients with late-stage disease may require esophagectomy.
   E. **Achalasia** is a functional disorder of the esophagus involving the destruction of Auerbach's intermyenteric plexus. Patients typically have dysphagia that progresses over years. The esophageal dysfunction of achalasia is characterized by lack of coordinated peristalsis as well as nonrelaxation of the lower esophageal sphincter. These, in turn, lead to stasis and progressive esophageal dilation. Treatment may consist of endoscopic dilation of the lower esophageal sphincter or surgical esophagomyotomy. Because the stasis of achalasia favors the development of squamous cell carcinoma, long-term endoscopic surveillance is required, even after successful treatment. The persistent risk of carcinoma despite these therapies probably reflects imperfect relief of obstruction. In the absence of esophageal cancer, esophagectomy may be considered in patients with symptomatic megaesophagus or after failure of esophagomyotomy.

PREOPERATIVE EVALUATION

Although mortality rates have declined, particularly at high-volume centers, esophageal resection continues to be associated with significant morbidity, particularly in older patients and those with comorbidities. The preoperative evaluation should identify significant comorbidities that may increase perioperative risk. Pulmonary function studies, an electrocardiogram, and an echocardiogram should be performed. Cardiac catheterization and revascularization should be performed when appropriate. Smoking cessation and avoidance of alcohol should be encouraged. Patients who lost significant weight before surgery should receive preoperative nutritional support and reversal of malnutrition should be documented. On occasion, this may require enteral feedings via a feeding tube or intravenous parenteral nutrition. Oral hygiene should be optimized before surgery

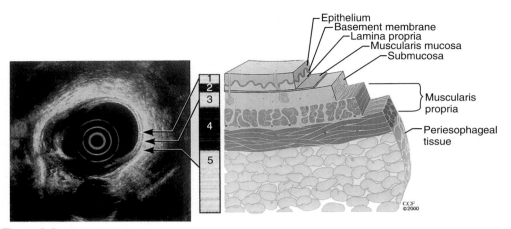

Epithelium
Basement membrane
Lamina propria
Muscularis mucosa
Submucosa
Muscularis propria
Periesophageal tissue

Figure 6-2
Endoscopic ultrasonographic image demonstrating the layers of the esophageal wall. *(From Pearson FG, Cooper JD, Deslauriers J, et al [eds]: Esophageal Surgery. Philadelphia, Churchill Livingstone, 2002.)*

to lessen the risk of severe infection in the event of a leak from the cervical anastomosis.

I. **History and Physical Examination:** Dysphagia and weight loss are the hallmarks of esophageal carcinoma and mandate a thorough evaluation. A history of gastro-esophageal reflux disease, previous endoscopy, alcohol and tobacco use, and weight loss should be elicited. Specific symptoms suggesting advanced disease include hoarseness (sometimes indicative of recurrent nerve invasion) and cough or hemoptysis (sometimes indicative of a tracheoesophageal fistula).

II. **Studies**

A. **Esophagoscopy** allows for visualization of the entire esophagus. Brush cytology with biopsy is obtained when appropriate. **EUS** may be used to improve the sensitivity of esophagoscopy, particularly when brush cytology or biopsy is not diagnostic. EUS is also used to stage esophageal carcinoma and allows for an assessment of the depth of invasion of the tumor and involvement of regional lymph nodes (Fig. 6-2).

B. **Barium swallow** provides detailed imaging of the mucosal contour of the esophagus and serves as an important adjunct to esophagoscopy in the evaluation of symptoms and the characterization and localization of esophageal lesions.

C. **CT** of the chest and upper abdomen is routine in the preoperative evaluation of esophageal cancer and allows identification of metastatic disease and tumor invasion into adjacent structures.

D. **PET** is increasingly included in the preoperative evaluation of esophageal cancers. Because of the increased uptake of FDG by tumor cells, PET is more sensitive than conventional imaging modalities (e.g., CT) in detecting metastatic disease.

COMPONENTS OF THE PROCEDURE AND APPLIED ANATOMY

Approaches to Esophagectomy

All approaches to esophagectomy include resection of the diseased segment of esophagus and restoration of gastrointestinal continuity. Generally, resections for cancer require disease-free margins of at least 5 cm. A variety of approaches may be used, including Ivor-Lewis, performed through a right thoracotomy and an abdominal incision; en bloc, performed through a left thoracoabdominal incision; and transhiatal, performed through abdominal and left cervical incisions and discussed later. Clinical outcomes after esophagectomy are more clearly related to the stage of the disease than to the choice of operation.

I. **Ivor-Lewis esophagectomy** is most often used for midthoracic tumors and allows for preparation of the conduit through an abdominal incision and dissection of the esophageal tumor and anastomosis in the chest under direct visualization.

II. **En bloc esophagectomy** may be used for distal tumors and, like the Ivor-Lewis approach, allows for nodal dissection and dissection of tumor from adherent pleura under direct visualization. A disadvantage of this approach is the limited proximal resection margin it affords because the anastomosis must be performed distal to the aortic arch.

III. Lesions involving the lower third of the esophagus are ideally suited to resection via **transhiatal esophagectomy** (described later), which allows for local regional nodal dissection and resection of the primary tumor under direct vision via the abdominal incision. Upper esophageal and pharyngeal cancers can be removed via the transhiatal approach as well; in such cases, the abdominal portion of the operation consists of removal of the distal normal esophagus and preparation of a stomach conduit. Restoration of gastrointestinal continuity is achieved through an anastomosis of the cervical esophagus to a conduit. This represents a theoretical advantage of the transhiatal approach over approaches that involve the creation of thoracic anastomoses because a leak in the neck is generally better tolerated than one in the chest.

IV. **Minimally invasive esophagectomy** usually involves mobilization of the esophagus through right thoracoscopy or laparoscopy and dissection of the most proximal esophagus and anastomosis through an open cervical incision. The operation can be safely performed in the hands of surgeons who are skilled in minimally invasive procedures, but significant benefits over the standard approach have yet to be demonstrated.

Choice of a Conduit

The stomach is the preferred conduit because of the relative ease with which it can be mobilized and the reliable blood supply. Additionally, the use of the stomach requires only a single anastomosis. Colonic interposition is the preferred approach in cases in which a gastric conduit is not feasible (e.g., after a previous gastric resection). Importantly, the use of colonic interposition requires three anastomoses: a coloesophagostomy, a colojejunostomy, and a colocolostomy.

Preoperative Considerations

I. **Prophylactic antibiotics** should be administered before skin incision and should cover mouth flora. When esophageal obstruction has been significant, agents that provide broader-spectrum coverage as well as antifungal agents should be used.

II. Given the length of the procedure and the risk of intraoperative blood loss, a urinary catheter should be placed to decompress the bladder and facilitate intraoperative monitoring of volume status.

III. An **epidural catheter** should be placed preoperatively, particularly in patients with a thoracic incision, to facilitate postoperative pain management.

IV. A **nasogastric tube** should be inserted preoperatively and is replaced after creation of the anastomosis. Postoperatively, the tube is maintained until adequate gastric emptying is confirmed, as judged by the amount of effluent as well as the nature of the fluid (i.e., bilious vs. nonbilious).

V. An **arterial catheter** is inserted to allow for continuous blood pressure monitoring.

Patient Positioning and Preparation

I. The patient is placed in the supine position, with the head turned toward the right.

II. The sterile preparation is applied to the entire abdominal wall, anterior chest, and left side of the neck.

Diagnostic Laparoscopy and Incision

A diagnostic laparoscopy may be performed before open abdominal exploration to exclude distant metastatic disease. If metastases are identified, a large incision can be avoided. If no distant metastases are identified during laparoscopy, an upper midline incision is made.

Exposure and Creation of the Gastric Conduit

I. The greater omentum is divided to release the stomach from its connection to the colon. Care is taken to preserve the right gastroepiploic vessel, which traverses the omentum parallel to the greater curvature of the stomach and will serve as the major blood supply to the gastric conduit (Fig. 6-3).

II. The stomach is freed from the spleen by dividing the gastrosplenic ligament, which contains the short gastric vessels. The vessels are ligated as far from the gastric wall as possible to preserve intramural collaterals.

III. The right gastric artery is identified and ligated just distal to the angularis incisura.

IV. The stomach is reflected cephalad. The left gastric artery is identified and ligated near its take-off from the celiac axis (Fig. 6-4).

V. The stomach is divided along a line beginning at the lesser curvature and ending at the fundus, ensuring a distal tumor margin of 5 cm or more (Fig. 6-5).

VI. Left gastric artery lymph nodes are dissected for removal with the specimen.

VII. A pyloroplasty is performed by making a longitudinal incision through the pylorus, which is then closed transversely. Mobilization of the duodenum is usually not necessary and does not provide significant additional stomach length. If stomach

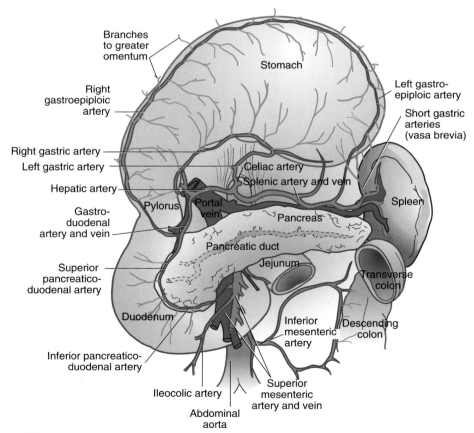

Figure 6-3

Blood supply to the stomach. *(From Zuidema G: Shackelford's Surgery of the Alimentary Tract, 4th ed. Philadelphia, Saunders, 1995.)*

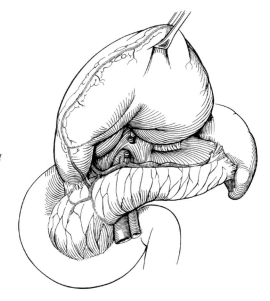

Figure 6-4
Mobilization of the stomach and ligation of the left gastric artery. *(From Cameron JL [ed]: Current Surgical Therapy, 8th ed. Philadelphia, Mosby, 2004.)*

> Pyloroplasty is performed to improve gastric emptying, which is impaired in approximately 15% of patients after esophagectomy.

length is insufficient to allow a tension-free anastomosis with the cervical esophagus, a right thoracic incision and creation of an anastomosis in the upper right chest should be considered (Fig. 6-6).

Mobilization of the Esophagus and Anastomosis

I. The diaphragmatic hiatus is widened using manual retractors to allow for dissection of the distal esophagus.
II. The esophagus is separated from the crux under direct vision. If necessary, the fibers of the crux can be divided anteriorly to provide wider access to the lower mediastinum. Mobilization of the esophagus under direct visualization can gener-

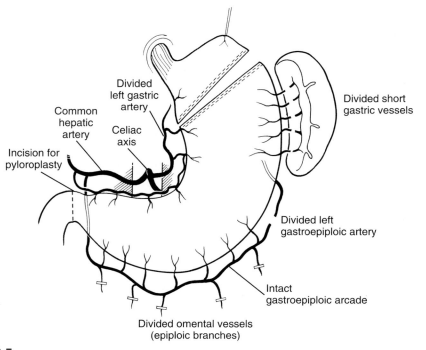

Figure 6-5
Preparation of the gastric conduit. *(From Khatri VP, Asensio JA: Operative Surgery Manual. Philadelphia, Saunders, 2003.)*

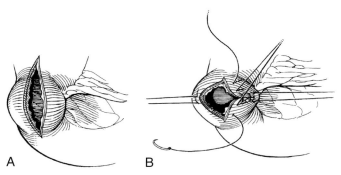

Figure 6-6
Pyloroplasty. **A,** A longitudinal incision is made through the pylorus. **B,** The incision is closed transversely. *(From Cameron JL [ed]: Current Surgical Therapy, 8th ed. Philadelphia, Mosby, 2004.)*

ally be carried out up to the level of the inferior pulmonary vein and frequently to the level of the carina (Fig. 6-7).

III. A left neck incision is made parallel to the sternocleidomastoid muscle. The omohyoid muscle is divided in its midportion. The esophagus is identified medial to the carotid sheath. The recurrent laryngeal nerve is identified in the tracheoesophageal groove and left in situ.

IV. The esophagus is freed from surrounding tissues circumferentially. Blunt dissection is then carried out through the hiatus and neck incision to complete mobilization of the esophagus.

V. Mobilization of the esophagus is frequently associated with hypotension secondary to displacement of the heart or compression of the vena cava. Mediastinal dissection should be interrupted as frequently as is necessary to avoid prolonged hypotension.

VI. A stapler is used to transect the cervical esophagus. A large Penrose drain is sutured to the transected esophagus and is delivered into the abdomen through the posterior mediastinum as the esophagus is removed through the hiatus.

VII. A Penrose drain is attached to the gastric conduit, which is then delivered through the posterior mediastinum to the neck with gentle traction.

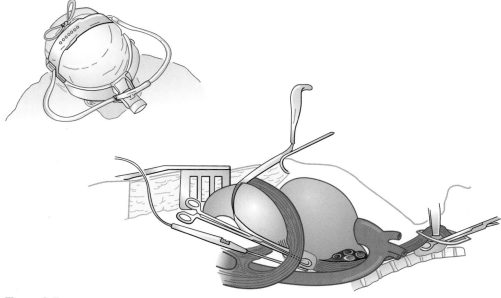

Figure 6-7
Mobilization of the esophagus. *(From Townsend CM, Beauchamp RD, Evers BM, Mattox KL [eds]: Sabiston Textbook of Surgery: The Biological Basis of Modern Surgical Practice, 17th ed. Philadelphia, Saunders, 2004.)*

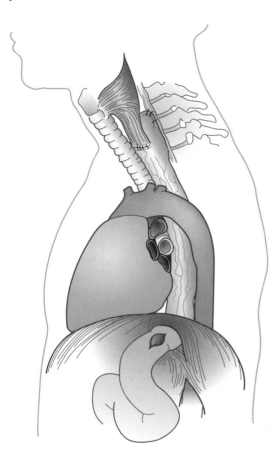

Figure 6-8
Transhiatal esophagectomy. (*Adapted from Orringer MB, Sloan H: Esophagectomy without thoracotomy. J Thorac Cardiovasc Surg 76:643–654, 1978.*)

VIII. A single-layer anastomosis between the proximal cervical esophagus and the gastric conduit is created using absorbable sutures (Fig. 6-8).

IX. A feeding jejunostomy tube is placed approximately 20 to 30 cm distal to the ligament of Treitz.

X. A closed-suction drain is placed in proximity to the cervical anastomosis.

XI. The abdominal and cervical incisions are closed.

POSTOPERATIVE COURSE

After esophagectomy, patients are monitored in an intensive care setting. Continuous electrocardiographic monitoring, aggressive chest and physical therapy, and head elevation are initiated in the early postoperative period. Jejunal tube feedings are typically started within 24 hours of surgery. Output from the cervical drain is monitored on a daily basis to assess the quantity and character of drainage. Between the fifth and seventh postoperative days, a swallow study with water-soluble contrast followed by barium is obtained to assess the integrity of the anastomosis. If the anastomosis appears to be intact and drainage is not excessive, the nasogastric tube is removed and the patient is given a clear liquid diet and advanced to soft food as tolerated. The cervical drain is removed after the patient has resumed oral intake if drainage remains minimal.

COMPLICATIONS

I. **Pulmonary complications,** including atelectasis and pneumonia, are frequent after esophagectomy. Aggressive pain control, chest physiotherapy, and pulmonary toilet are essential components of postoperative management and may lessen the incidence of these complications.

II. **Cardiac arrhythmias** (e.g., atrial fibrillation) are likewise common after esophagectomy, as with many intrathoracic procedures.

III. **Cervical anastomotic leak** is more likely when the anastomosis is under tension or when the blood supply to the conduit is tenuous. Some surgeons advocate routine evaluation of the anastomosis with a swallow study before removal of the nasogastric tube. If adequately drained, most anastomotic leaks will heal. Larger leaks may be complicated by a cervical or mediastinal abscess and require reopening of the left neck incision and antibiotic therapy.

IV. **Recurrent laryngeal nerve injuries** are most often traction-related. Patients may complain of hoarseness and may aspirate thin liquids. Most injuries of this type resolve over a period of 2 to 3 months.

V. **Chylothorax** may result from injury to the thoracic duct during right-sided esophageal dissection. The diagnosis is suggested by the development of a pleural effusion in the right side of the chest and may be confirmed by measurement of elevated triglycerides and protein in the pleural fluid. Drainage with serial thoracenteses or placement of a chest tube and bowel rest may allow for resolution of the chyle leak. If the drainage does not subsist, an operation to ligate the thoracic duct or placement of a pleuroperitoneal shunt may be necessary. Angiographic occlusion of the thoracic duct is a preferable approach in centers where this technique is available.

SUGGESTED READINGS

Casson AG: Thoracic approaches to esophagectomy. In Kaiser LR, Kron IL, Spray TL, et al (eds): Mastery of Cardiothoracic Surgery. Philadelphia, Lippincott Williams & Wilkins, 1998, pp 141–150.

Cope C, Salem R, Kaiser LR: Management of chylothorax by percutaneous catheterization and embolization of the thoracic duct: prospective trial. J Vasc Interv Radiol 10:1248–1254, 1999.

Inculet RI: Transhiatal esophagectomy. In Kaiser LR, Kron IL, Spray TL, et al [eds]: Mastery of Cardiothoracic Surgery. Philadelphia, Lippincott Williams & Wilkins, 1998, pp 134–140.

Zwischenberger JB, Savage C, Bhutani MS: Esophagus. In Townsend CM, Beauchamp RD, Evers BM, Mattox KL (eds): Sabiston Textbook of Surgery: The Biological Basis of Modern Surgical Practice, 17th ed. Philadelphia, Saunders, 2004, pp 1091–1150.

Laparoscopic Nissen Fundoplication and Heller Myotomy

Michael E. Friscia and Jo Buyske

LAPAROSCOPIC NISSEN FUNDOPLICATION

Case Study

A 38-year-old female is referred for management of gastroesophageal reflux. She reports a 10-year history of severe substernal postprandial chest pain. Calcium carbonate tablets and diet modification do little to improve these symptoms. She is currently taking a proton pump inhibitor, which provides moderate control of her symptoms. She denies dysphagia or weight loss. On recent esophagoscopy, orange patches interspersed between normal-appearing mucosa were noted in the distal esophagus. Biopsy confirmed the diagnosis of Barrett's esophagus without dysplasia.

BACKGROUND

Some degree of reflux from the stomach into the esophagus is normal, particularly after meals, and is easily cleared by esophageal peristalsis. The high-pressure zone created by the lower esophageal sphincter (LES), diaphragmatic contraction at the esophageal hiatus during periods of increased abdominal pressure (e.g., coughing and bending), and the intra-abdominal positive pressure exerted on the distal esophagus serve to impede reflux. In contrast, migration of the distal esophagus and LES into the chest, as in a **hiatal hernia,** transient relaxation of the LES, and inhibitors of LES contraction, including caffeine, smoking, and alcohol, may exacerbate reflux. Repetitive injury of the esophageal mucosa by gastric acid results in gastroesophageal reflux disease (GERD) characterized by chronic symptoms (e.g., substernal chest pain and regurgitation) and, sometimes, complications such as Barrett's esophagus and stricture formation.

Surgical therapy for the treatment of GERD is a relatively recent innovation. Indeed, the gastric fundoplication operations still performed today were introduced in the 1950s by Nissen, Belsey, and others. The application of minimally invasive techniques has led to more rapid recovery and reduced morbidity after antireflux surgery. As a result, the indications for surgery have broadened despite the availability of relatively effective medical therapies. In most cases, the antireflux operation of choice is the Nissen fundoplication, which involves a 360-degree wrap of the fundus of the stomach around the distal esophagus. In selected circumstances (e.g., when esophageal motility is markedly abnormal), a partial wrap may be preferable. Laparoscopic Nissen fundoplication is the focus of the first part of this chapter.

INDICATIONS FOR SURGERY

There are few absolute indications for antireflux surgery. A number of relative indications have emerged and must be weighed against associated risks.

I. **Intractability of symptoms** despite maximal medical therapy with proton pump inhibitors and H_2 receptor blockers is the most common indication for surgery. Although the presence of typical primary symptoms (e.g., heartburn) is generally predictive of good outcomes after antireflux surgery, patients with **pulmonary manifestations** attributable to GERD (e.g., cough, pharyngitis, and recurrent pneumonia) may benefit from surgery as well, assuming other etiologies have been excluded. Patient age is an important factor in identifying appropriate surgical candidates; the benefits of surgery over lifelong proton pump inhibitor therapy are greatest in younger patients with severe disease. When patients receive no benefit from proton pump inhibition, diagnoses other than GERD should be considered. In general, such patients benefit little from antireflux surgery.

> Are your patient's symptoms controlled with proton pump inhibitors?

II. **Peptic strictures** are areas of fibrotic narrowing in the distal esophagus. Patients typically present with dysphagia and obstruction. The presence of a stricture suggests severe, repetitive esophageal injury from acid exposure. After evaluation, including endoscopy and biopsy to exclude malignancy, consideration should be given to antireflux surgery to reduce esophageal acid exposure and promote healing. Strictures are sometimes accompanied by a shortened esophagus. In such cases, fundoplication should be performed with an esophageal lengthening procedure (e.g., Collis gastroplasty).

III. **Barrett's esophagus,** columnar metaplasia of the distal esophagus, is a premalignant condition that predisposes to the development of esophageal adenocarcinoma. Delayed progression or even regression of Barrett's esophagus has been documented after antireflux surgery. However, whether surgery influences the subsequent risk of esophageal cancer remains controversial. Barrett's esophagus with high-grade dysplasia is associated with undiagnosed esophageal adenocarcinoma in 38% to 72% of cases and should be treated with a resection (i.e., esophagectomy) rather than antireflux surgery.

PREOPERATIVE EVALUATION

I. **History:** The timing and chronicity of symptoms, modifying factors, and the effect of reflux symptoms on the patient's lifestyle should be elicited. Response to acid suppression medications should be determined and is predictive of outcome after fundoplication.

II. **Upper gastrointestinal fluoroscopy with barium** allows for the diagnosis of a shortened esophagus, hiatal hernia, or mass, which may influence the surgical approach (e.g., the addition of an esophageal lengthening procedure).

III. **Esophagogastroduodenoscopy** allows for an assessment of the degree of esophageal injury. Specifically, esophagitis can be graded, and the presence of Barrett's esophagus, dysplasia, and neoplasm can be identified.

IV. **Twenty-four–hour pH monitoring** is the gold standard for documentation of acid reflux into the distal esophagus. After the patient undergoes a 1-week hiatus from acid suppression therapy, pH probes are passed through the nose into the stomach, the distal esophagus above the LES, and the upper esophagus. Symptoms that correlate with episodes of acidification of the distal esophagus are more likely to improve with antireflux surgery.

V. **Esophageal manometry** provides information about the function of the LES and contractile properties of the esophageal body. Patients with abnormal peristalsis of the esophageal body will likely experience dysphagia when a 360-degree fundoplication is used and are better served by a partial fundoplication.

COMPONENTS OF THE PROCEDURE AND APPLIED ANATOMY
See Figure 7-1.

I. **Preoperative Considerations**
  A. Prophylactic antibiotics to cover gram-positive and enteric organisms are administered within 1 hour before skin incision.
  B. An orogastric tube is inserted to decompress the stomach.
  C. A urinary catheter is inserted to decompress the bladder and to facilitate intraoperative assessment of volume status.

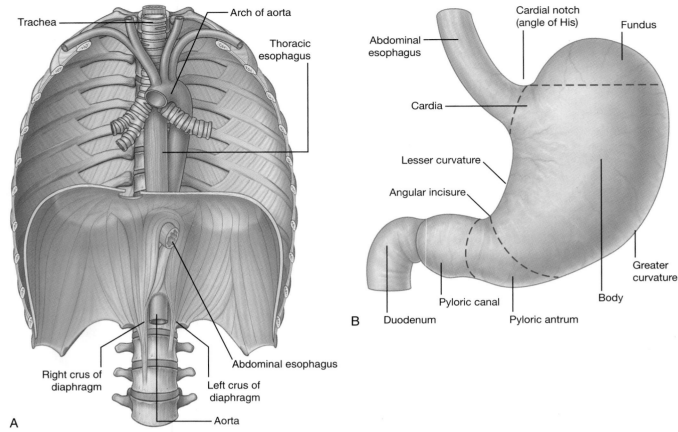

Figure 7-1
Anatomy of the esophagus (**A**) and stomach (**B**). *(From Drake RL, Vogl W, Mitchell AWM: Gray's Anatomy for Students. Philadelphia, Churchill Livingstone, 2005.)*

II. **Patient Position and Preparation**

  A. The patient is placed in the modified lithotomy or split-leg position, allowing the operating surgeon to stand between the patient's legs. The table is placed in the reverse Trendelenburg position (i.e., the bottom of the table tilted down) so that intra-abdominal fat falls away from the esophageal hiatus. The video monitor is positioned at the patient's head so that the surgeon's body, the instruments, and the video screen form a straight line, to optimize the surgeon's spatial orientation.

  B. The sterile preparation is applied and should extend to the nipples superiorly, the pubis inferiorly, and the midaxillary lines laterally.

III. **Port Placement**

  A. A 10-mm port is placed 15 cm inferior to the xiphoid process (Fig. 7-2), just to the left of the midline. Either an open technique or a Veress needle technique may be used to access the peritoneal cavity; however, the former should always be used if the patient has had previous abdominal surgery. After port insertion, pneumoperitoneum is established with insufflation of CO_2.

  B. Four additional ports (see Fig. 7-2) are placed under laparoscopic visualization. The left and right subcostal ports, placed in the midclavicular lines, function as the primary operative ports and correspond to the surgeon's left and right hands, respectively. A lateral right subcostal port is placed to allow for the insertion of a self-retaining liver retractor, and a lateral left subcostal port provides access through which an assistant can retract.

IV. **Exposure**

  A. A liver retractor is inserted through the right lateral port and positioned to elevate the left lateral segment of the liver, exposing the esophageal hiatus.

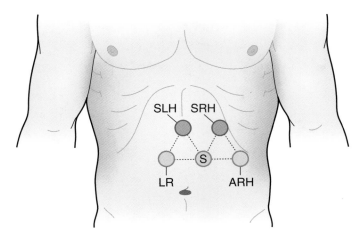

Figure 7-2

Port placement for laparoscopic Nissen fundoplication. The port for the laparoscope is positioned 15 cm inferior to the xiphoid process. Subcostal surgeon's right (SRH) and left (SLH) hand working ports are positioned superiorly. Lateral ports are for the liver retractor (LR), and the assistant's right hand (ARH). S, laparoscope. *(From Townsend CM, Beauchamp RD, Evers BM, Mattox KL [eds]: Sabiston Textbook of Surgery: The Biological Basis of Modern Surgical Practice, 17th ed. Philadelphia, Saunders, 2004.)*

B. The avascular portion of the gastrohepatic ligament (pars flaccida) is divided, exposing the right crus of the diaphragm. Care is taken to avoid injury to the hepatic branch of the vagus nerve or a replaced left hepatic artery arising from the left gastric artery.

C. The phrenoesophageal ligament is incised and attachments to the esophagus are swept down toward the gastroesophageal (GE) junction to allow for visualization of the left and right crura (Fig. 7-3). The anterior vagus nerve is identified and preserved.

D. Posterior attachments to the esophagus are dissected bluntly. The posterior vagus nerve is identified behind the esophagus and is preserved. Once the distal esophagus has been fully mobilized, it is encircled with a rubber drain (*Penrose drain*).

E. The short gastric vessels are divided from the mid-greater curvature to the angle of His to allow for mobilization of the fundus of the stomach and fundoplication (Fig. 7-4).

V. **Crural Closure and Fundoplication**

A. The right and left crura are approximated through placement of interrupted sutures to recreate a snug hiatus around the distal esophagus (Fig. 7-5).

> DIVISION OF THE HEPATIC BRANCH OF THE VAGUS NERVE CAN LEAD TO GALLBLADDER STASIS AND GALLSTONE FORMATION.

> WHEN PLACING SUTURES IN THE CRURA, CARE MUST BE TAKEN TO AVOID INJURY TO THE AORTA, WHICH LIES IMMEDIATELY DORSAL TO THE ESOPHAGEAL HIATUS.

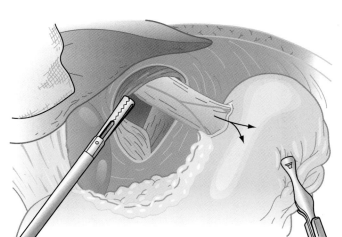

Figure 7-3

Exposure of the right and left crura and mobilization of the esophagus. *(From Townsend CM, Beauchamp RD, Evers BM, Mattox KL [eds]: Sabiston Textbook of Surgery: The Biological Basis of Modern Surgical Practice, 17th ed. Philadelphia, Saunders, 2004.)*

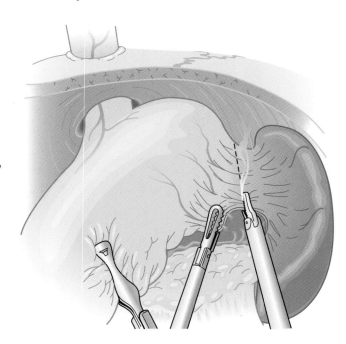

Figure 7-4
Division of the short gastric vessels along the line of transection (*dashed line*). *(From Townsend CM, Beauchamp RD, Evers BM, Mattox KL [eds]: Sabiston Textbook of Surgery: The Biological Basis of Modern Surgical Practice, 17th ed. Philadelphia, Saunders, 2004.)*

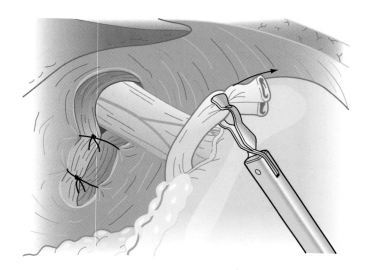

Figure 7-5
Crural closure. The crura are reapproximated with interrupted sutures. Retracting the esophagus to the left enhances exposure. *(From Townsend CM, Beauchamp RD, Evers BM, Mattox KL [eds]: Sabiston Textbook of Surgery: The Biological Basis of Modern Surgical Practice, 17th ed. Philadelphia, Saunders, 2004.)*

B. The posterior fundus is passed posterior to the esophagus and retracted toward the patient's right. A bougie (a flexible tube used to dilate the esophagus) is placed in the esophagus and a loose, 360-degree wrap is created around 2 to 3 cm of distal esophagus and secured with several interrupted permanent sutures (Fig. 7-6).

C. The bougie is removed and a nasogastric tube is inserted under laparoscopic visualization.

D. Fascial defects from ports greater than 5 mm in diameter are closed. All skin incisions are closed.

POSTOPERATIVE COURSE

A nasogastric tube is left in place overnight. Antiemetics are used liberally to prevent retching or vomiting, which can disrupt the wrap or crural repair. On the first postoperative day, the nasogastric tube is removed and a liquid diet is initiated. Patients may be advanced to a soft solid diet as tolerated but are instructed to avoid bread, meat, and raw

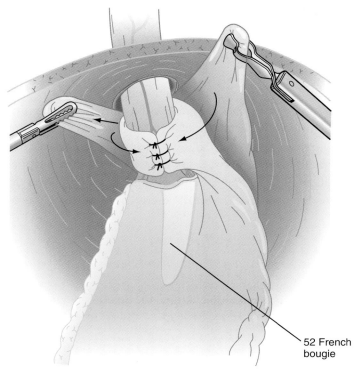

Figure 7-6
Fundoplication. The fundus is wrapped around the distal esophagus loosely enough to allow for passage of a 52 French bougie. *(From Townsend CM, Beauchamp RD, Evers BM, Mattox KL [eds]: Sabiston Textbook of Surgery: The Biological Basis of Modern Surgical Practice, 17th ed. Philadelphia, Saunders, 2004.)*

vegetables until after the first postoperative visit. In the absence of dysphagia, the diet can then be liberalized.

COMPLICATIONS

   I. **Immediate complications** include **esophageal or gastric perforation, pneumothorax,** and **splenic or liver trauma.** Hollow viscus perforations are repaired intraoperatively if recognized. Delayed recognition of such injuries often results in significant morbidity. Early postoperative fevers, tachycardia, tachypnea, or abdominal tenderness should prompt evaluation with a gastrograffin swallow, and surgical exploration should be considered. Likewise, splenic or liver injuries are addressed intraoperatively when recognized and often require surgical exploration when diagnosed postoperatively. Pneumothorax usually results from passage of insufflated CO_2 into the pleural space and resolves without intervention.
  II. **Early complications** include **bloating** (30%) and **dysphagia** (20%). Bloating results from an inability to reflux gas past the wrap or gastric dysfunction from vagal irritation and can be exacerbated by ileus. Dysphagia in the early postoperative period is generally due to edema of the distal esophagus and, in most cases, is self-limited. Persistent dysphagia, however, may reflect an overly tight wrap and sometimes necessitates surgical revision.
 III. The most important **late complication** of fundoplication is recurrent symptomatic reflux. Although this may occur in the absence of a technical failure, the wrap should be evaluated with upper gastrointestinal fluoroscopy with barium. Reasons for failure include **recurrent hiatal herniation** resulting in an intrathoracic wrap, **breakdown of the fundoplication,** and herniation of the stomach cephalad to the wrap. All of these are best addressed with surgery, particularly when associated with symptoms.

LAPAROSCOPIC HELLER MYOTOMY

Case Study

A 45-year-old male with a history of a 10-pound weight loss over the previous 6 months presents for evaluation. He describes progressive difficulty swallowing over several years and intermittent regurgitation of foul-smelling undigested food. Additionally, he notes that he has always been a "slow eater," and he often walks after meals to "help the food go down." He appears thin, but otherwise, findings on physical examination are unremarkable. A barium swallow shows a dilated esophagus that tapers distally at the GE junction. Subsequent esophageal manometry reveals aperistalsis and an elevated LES resting pressure.

BACKGROUND

Achalasia is a rare disorder characterized by esophageal aperistalsis, high resting LES pressures, and failure of LES relaxation. Although the etiology of achalasia is unknown and is likely multifactorial, the pathogenesis involves loss of inhibitory ganglion cells in the esophageal body and LES. Typical symptoms include dysphagia and regurgitation; however, the onset of symptoms is often insidious. Early in the disease course, dysphagia is more pronounced with liquids than with solids. Patients with achalasia often eat slowly and contort their bodies to propel food through the esophagus. Ultimately, as esophageal dysfunction progresses, food cannot transit through the LES and is regurgitated. Malnutrition, weight loss, and recurrent pulmonary complications, such as pneumonia, bronchiectasis, and lung abscess, may ensue.

> Squamous cell carcinoma of the esophagus is associated with longstanding achalasia.

Surgical intervention should be considered for all patients with achalasia; however, two effective nonsurgical therapies are available: pneumatic dilation and botulinum toxin injection. **Pneumatic dilation** involves passage of a balloon dilator to the level of the LES and disruption of the muscular fibers of the LES through balloon inflation under endoscopic guidance. The vast majority of patients experience symptomatic relief after balloon dilation, but it is frequently short-lived. Additionally, pneumatic dilation is associated with a 5% risk of esophageal perforation. **Botulinum toxin** inhibits acetylcholine release from the excitatory neurons in the LES, thereby reducing the resting pressure. Injection of botulinum toxin in the area of the LES results in symptomatic relief in the majority of patients, but like pneumatic dilation, this therapy is often transient. Generally, patients at lower surgical risk should be offered surgical myotomy or pneumatic dilation. Patients at high surgical risk should be offered botulinum toxin injection and medical therapies (e.g., calcium channel blockers) aimed at reducing LES pressure (Fig. 7-7).

INDICATIONS FOR SURGERY

The most durable method of reducing resting LES pressure in patients with achalasia is surgical esophagomyotomy. The procedure can be approached through the chest or abdomen. The transabdominal laparoscopic approach is most frequently used.

PREOPERATIVE EVALUATION

I. **History and Physical Examination:** Patients with achalasia typically report a history of progressive dysphagia to both solids and liquids as well as regurgitation. Weight loss is a late finding and indicates severe esophageal dysfunction. When pain is a prominent symptom, other diagnoses (e.g., esophageal spasm syndromes) should be considered. The presence of cervical adenopathy on physical examination suggests esophageal or GE junction neoplasia rather than achalasia in the patient with progressive dysphagia.

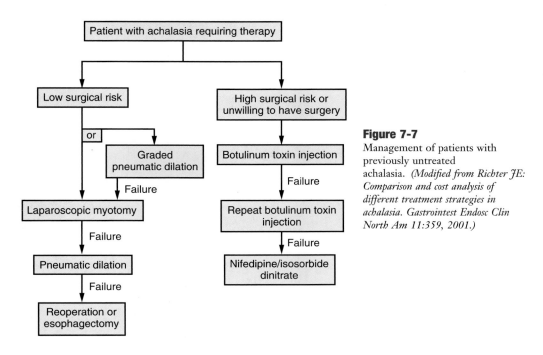

Figure 7-7
Management of patients with previously untreated achalasia. *(Modified from Richter JE: Comparison and cost analysis of different treatment strategies in achalasia. Gastrointest Endosc Clin North Am 11:359, 2001.)*

II. **Upper gastrointestinal fluoroscopy with barium** allows for the identification of mass lesions, dilation, tortuosity (*sigmoid esophagus*), air–fluid levels, strictures, or tapering of the esophagus (Fig. 7-8). Esophageal aperistalsis, failure of LES relaxation, and abnormal progression of the food bolus may also be noted.

III. **Esophageal manometry** is required to confirm the diagnosis of achalasia and exclude other esophageal motility disorders associated with a similar constellation of symptoms, such as scleroderma and diffuse esophageal spasm. Manometric findings associated with achalasia include a resting LES pressure of greater than 45 mm Hg, aperistalsis, and failure of LES relaxation during swallowing (Fig. 7-9). The latter finding in particular distinguishes achalasia from other disorders that lead to aperistalsis of the esophageal body (e.g., scleroderma).

IV. **Upper endoscopy** is performed to exclude GE junction tumors, which may produce similar findings on manometry and barium studies to achalasia (*pseudo-achalasia*). Several other rare infiltrative processes can also result in pseudoachalasia and can be distinguished by histology. The presence of squamous cell carcinoma of the esophagus must also be excluded by endoscopy before esophagomyotomy, particularly in older patients with achalasia.

COMPONENTS OF THE PROCEDURE AND APPLIED ANATOMY

I. As noted in the "Indications for Surgery" section, the transabdominal laparoscopic approach to Heller myotomy is most frequently used today. Alternatively, Heller myotomy can be performed through a left thoracotomy. The latter approach has particular advantages in patients who have undergone extensive intra-abdominal surgery. Patients with achalasia are particularly vulnerable to reflux because the aperistaltic esophagus does not effectively clear gastric acid. Because Heller myotomy obliterates the antireflux barrier of the LES, most surgeons combine this operation with a fundoplication. A 360-degree fundoplication may result in functional obstruction of the esophagus in the patient with achalasia; a posterior 270-degree (Toupet) fundoplication is generally the preferred approach. Alternatively, an anterior 180-degree (Dor) fundoplication may be performed but provides less of a barrier against reflux. Preoperative considerations, patient positioning and preparation, port placement, and initial exposure proceed as described in the section on Nissen fundoplication.

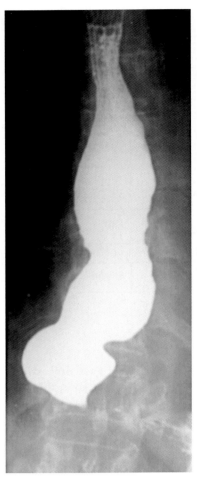

Figure 7-8
Radiographic appearance of the esophagus in a patient with achalasia. A barium esophagogram reveals a dilated esophagus ending in a so-called *pointed bird's beak* at the nonrelaxing lower esophageal sphincter. *(From Feldman M, Friedman LS, Brandt JL [eds]: Sleisenger and Fordtran's Gastrointestinal and Liver Disease, 8th ed. Philadelphia, Saunders, 2006.)*

Figure 7-9
Manometric findings recorded from the lower esophageal sphincter (LES) and the esophagus 3, 8, and 13 cm proximal to the LES in two patients with achalasia. Tracings at the different locations within the esophageal body are largely identical suggesting aperistalsis. The LES does not relax appropriately in response to a wet swallow (WS). *(From Feldman M, Friedman LS, Brandt JL [eds]: Sleisenger and Fordtran's Gastrointestinal and Liver Disease, 8th ed. Philadelphia, Saunders, 2006.)*

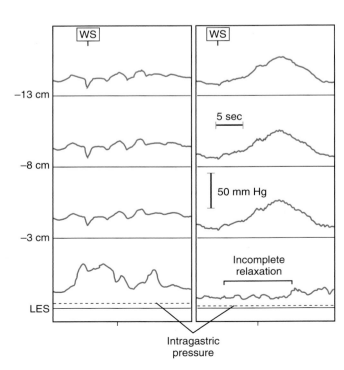

II. **Myotomy**

   A. After mobilization of the distal esophagus, a point just proximal to the GE junction, on the anterior surface of the esophagus, to the left of the anterior vagus nerve, is chosen for the myotomy. Fibers of the outer longitudinal muscle layer of muscle are dissected, exposing the circular muscle fibers. These inner fibers are gently lifted away from the underlying mucosa and divided. The myotomy is extended 5 to 6 cm proximal to the GE junction and then across the GE junction and onto the stomach for 1 to 2 cm.

   B. The mucosa along the length of the myotomy is inspected for injuries that, if identified, are immediately repaired. Mucosal injuries that are not initially apparent can be identified by instilling dilute methylene blue dye through the gastric tube while gently occluding the gastric lumen with a dissector. In the presence of a perforation, the blue dye will extravasate into the peritoneal cavity.

III. **Crural Repair and Fundoplication**

   A. The right and left crura are approximated through placement of interrupted sutures to recreate a snug hiatus around the distal esophagus.

   B. Posterior (**Toupet**) fundoplication is performed by delivering the fundus of the stomach behind the esophagus from left to right. The fundus is secured to the diaphragmatic crura and the free edges of the myotomy on both sides with interrupted sutures. This buttresses the GE junction posteriorly and helps to maintain the myotomy.

   C. Anterior (**Dor**) fundoplication is performed by wrapping the fundus around the anterior esophagus, directly over the myotomy and exposed mucosa. As in the Toupet fundoplication, the fundus is secured to the edges of the myotomy and crura. Dor fundoplication can be used to reinforce a mucosal repair if a perforation resulted from the dissection.

   D. Fascial defects from ports larger than 5 mm in diameter are closed. All skin incisions are closed.

> An anterior fundoplication should be performed after repair of a mucosal injury.

POSTOPERATIVE COURSE

The nasogastric tube is left in place overnight. On the first postoperative day, a barium swallow is performed to exclude a perforation. If the findings are normal, the nasogastric tube is removed and the patient's diet is advanced slowly to thickened liquids. Patients are typically discharged on the second or third postoperative day. In the absence of dysphagia, the patient's diet may be liberalized after the first postoperative visit (typically 2 weeks after surgery). Routine endoscopic surveillance is recommended for all patients with achalasia because of the associated increased incidence of esophageal cancer.

COMPLICATIONS

   I. **Immediate complications** include **esophageal or gastric perforation, pneumothorax,** and **splenic or liver trauma** (see discussion in the section on Nissen fundoplication). The incidence of esophageal perforation is higher during Heller myotomy.

  II. **Late complications** of Heller myotomy include dysphagia and gastroesophageal reflux.

   A. **Dysphagia** that persists beyond 2 weeks after surgery should prompt investigation with a barium swallow and endoscopy. Causes of persistent dysphagia include incomplete myotomy and an overly tight fundoplication. The former may be addressed with pneumatic dilation or reoperation, whereas the latter usually requires reoperation. A very small percentage of patients still have a poor quality of life despite myotomy. This is often a result of poor esophageal motility from long-standing, progressive disease. In these patients, an esophagectomy with gastric pull-up or colonic interposition may be considered as a last option. Onset of dysphagia after a symptom-free period should raise concern for the development of an esophageal malignancy, peptic stricture, or paraesophageal hernia.

B. **Gastroesophageal reflux,** both symptomatic and asymptomatic, is common after myotomy. Symptoms are usually well controlled with pharmacologic acid suppression. Dietary modification and sleeping at a 45-degree angle to enhance nighttime emptying of the esophagus may also improve symptoms.

SUGGESTED READINGS

Bonavina L: Minimally invasive surgery for esophageal achalasia. World J Gastroenterol 12: 5921–5925, 2006.

Christian DJ, Buyske J: Current status of antireflux surgery. Surg Clin North Am 85:931–947, 2005.

Oelschlager BK, Eubanks TR, Pellegrini CA: Hiatal hernia and gastroesophageal reflux disease. In Townsend CM, Beauchamp RD, Evers BM, Mattox KL (eds): Sabiston Textbook of Surgery: The Biological Basis of Modern Surgical Practice, 17th ed. Philadelphia, Saunders, 2004, pp 1151–1168.

Zwischenberger JB, Savage C, Bhutani MS: Esophagus. In Townsend CM, Beauchamp RD, Evers BM, Mattox KL (eds): Sabiston Textbook of Surgery: The Biological Basis of Modern Surgical Practice, 17th ed. Philadelphia, Saunders, 2004, pp 1091–1150.

CHAPTER 8

Gastrectomy

Andrew S. Newman and Francis R. Spitz

Case Study

A 62-year-old black male presents to his primary care provider complaining of vague abdominal cramping and generalized fatigue. He has lost 20 pounds over the last 3 months because of poor appetite. He denies fever, nausea, or vomiting. He was started on proton pump inhibitor therapy 4 months earlier, after being diagnosed with a gastric ulcer by endoscopy.

He appears thin, with slight temporalis wasting bilaterally. His sclera are anicteric and his skin is warm and dry. His abdomen is soft, nondistended, and slightly tender to palpation in the midepigastrium, with no appreciable masses. Results of laboratory studies are remarkable only for a hemoglobin level of 8.7 g/dL.

Repeat endoscopy shows a nonhealing ulcer. Biopsy of the rim of the ulcer reveals adenocarcinoma.

BACKGROUND

The stomach may be divided into four anatomic regions: the cardia, fundus, body, and antrum. The stomach derives its blood supply from four main arterial trunks: the right and left gastric arteries along the lesser curvature and the right and left gastroepiploic arteries along the greater curvature. Additional blood supply is provided by the short gastric arteries (Fig. 8-1). Given this extensive collateral vascular network, the stomach may remain viable after ligation of multiple main feeding vessels. Venous and lymphatic drainage, in general, follows the arterial supply.

INDICATIONS FOR GASTRECTOMY

The two most common indications for partial or total gastrectomy are malignancy and peptic ulcer disease (PUD).

I. **Adenocarcinoma:** Adenocarcinoma accounts for 95% of gastric malignancies and is the 14th most common cancer and the 8th leading cause of cancer-related death in the United States.
  A. Gastric adenocarcinoma typically presents with nonspecific symptoms, and the diagnosis may be delayed until the disease is relatively advanced. In the absence of metastatic disease, surgical resection is indicated. Gastric adenocarcinoma frequently spreads intramurally, and the extent of disease may be masked by normal-appearing gastric mucosa; thus, resection should include 6-cm margins. Because of the high morbidity rate associated with proximal partial gastric resections, proximal tumors and midbody tumors are usually treated with total or near-total gastrectomy. In patients with distal lesions, subtotal gastrectomy is an acceptable alternative approach if appropriate margins can be obtained; otherwise, total gastrectomy is required.

Risk factors for gastric adenocarcinoma include cigarette smoking, a history of partial gastrectomy, chronic inflammation of the stomach (atrophic gastritis, pernicious anemia), *H. pylori* infection, and a diet high in salt and smoked foods.

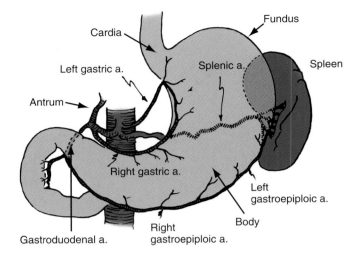

Figure 8-1
Anatomy and arterial supply of the stomach. (*Adapted from Wein AJ [ed]: Campbell-Walsh Urology, 9th ed. Philadelphia, Saunders, 2007.*)

> Regardless of the extent of nodal dissection, at least 15 nodes should be harvested.

    B. The role of extended lymphadenectomy for gastric adenocarcinoma is controversial. A **D1 dissection** includes removal of perigastric nodes only; a **D2 dissection** includes removal of regional lymph nodes along the celiac axis (left gastric, common hepatic, and splenic arteries). A **D3 dissection** includes removal of additional regional nodes within the porta hepatis and next to the aorta. Numerous prospective randomized clinical trials have failed to demonstrate an improvement in 5-year survival rates with more extensive dissections. In the United States, most surgeons advocate a limited (D1 or D2) nodal dissection, harvesting at least 15 nodes for pathologic evaluation. Although once routinely performed during resection for gastric cancer, splenectomy is associated with higher perioperative morbidity and mortality rates and is no longer recommended unless there is direct invasion of the spleen or splenic hilum.

  II. **Other Gastric Malignancies**

    A. **Gastric lymphoma** is the second most common malignancy of the stomach. Treatment regimens vary; however, most gastric lymphomas are initially treated with chemoradiation therapy. Mucosal-associated lymphatic tissue tumors are low-grade lymphomas and are associated with *Helicobacter pylori* infection. Treatment aimed at eradication of the bacteria often results in tumor regression. Surgical resection of lymphomas is reserved for tumors refractory to other therapies and cases with complications, including perforation and bleeding. If indicated, the goal of resection is to obtain circumferential negative margins.

    B. **Gastrointestinal stromal tumors (GISTs)** are mesenchymal tumors. GISTs may arise throughout the gastrointestinal (GI) tract, although the stomach is the most common site. Surgical resection with wide negative margins remains the primary treatment modality; however, encouraging results have been achieved with imatinib (Gleevec), a tyrosine kinase inhibitor, for the treatment of metastases and as an adjuvant to resection for high-risk tumors (as defined by necrosis, mitosis, and size).

    C. **Gastric carcinoids** are rare and account for only 0.5% of all gastric tumors. Multiple gastric carcinoid tumors may be associated with enterochromaffin-like cell hyperplasia, chronic atrophic gastritis, and pernicious anemia, and have a low risk of malignancy. Solitary gastric carcinoid tumors have higher malignant potential. Resection is the mainstay of treatment.

  III. **Peptic Ulcer Disease:** PUD results from an imbalance between physiologic acid secretion and mucosal defense mechanisms and causes erosion of either the gastric or the duodenal wall. Advances in our understanding of the pathophysiology of PUD (specifically, the implications of *H. pylori* infection of the gastric mucosa) as well as the development of proton pump inhibitors for the management of acid

TABLE 8-1 Johnson Classification of Gastric Ulcers

Johnson Classification	Location	Acid Hypersecretion
Type I	Lesser curve	No
Type II	Lesser curve and duodenum	Yes
Type III	Prepyloric	Yes
Type IV	Proximal lesser curve near gastroesophageal junction	No

hypersecretion have made elective surgery for the treatment of PUD uncommon. Initial treatment of PUD includes lifestyle modification (e.g., avoidance of tobacco, alcohol, and nonsteroidal anti-inflammatory drugs) and a pharmacologic regimen that includes an H_2 receptor antagonist or proton pump inhibitor and antibiotic therapy for *H. pylori* infection.

A. Indications for surgery include emergent complications of PUD (e.g., obstruction and perforation) and bleeding refractory to endoscopic intervention. Rarely, failure of medical therapy and concern about malignancy constitute additional indications. The location of the ulcer dictates the surgical approach. The modified Johnson classification categorizes gastric ulcers according to their location. Acid hypersecretion is believed to play a role in types II and III ulcers only (Table 8-1 and Fig. 8-2). Surgical therapy for these types of ulcers is therefore aimed not only at resection of the ulcer, but also at acid reduction. Treatment of types I and IV gastric ulcers, on the other hand, involves resection of the ulcer only (Fig. 8-3).

B. Patients with free perforation or hemorrhage are often systemically ill and hemodynamically unstable. A focused surgical approach is appropriate in such settings; perforated ulcers are typically patched with omentum (i.e., Graham patch) and bleeding vessels are oversewn. In the stable patient, optimal treatment for a bleeding or perforated gastric ulcer includes resection (distal gastrectomy or antrectomy). Proximal ulcers are treated with wedge resection.

> Where in the stomach is the gastric ulcer located?

PREOPERATIVE EVALUATION

The evaluation of a patient before partial or total gastrectomy should include a thorough history, review of systems, and physical examination, with attention directed toward the patient's comorbidities, previous surgeries, and nutritional status. Physical examination may reveal a palpable abdominal mass, or less commonly, evidence of metastatic disease (e.g., Virchow's node, Sister Mary Joseph's node, Krukenberg's tumor, or Blummer's shelf).

I. **Laboratory testing** should include a complete blood count, blood chemistry, liver function tests, coagulation studies, and blood type and screen in anticipation of surgical blood loss. Patients are often anemic as a result of chronic blood loss within the GI tract. Elevated liver function tests may reflect the presence of hepatic metastases.

II. **Esophagogastroduodenoscopy** is required for the diagnosis and localization of gastric malignancies and PUD. **Endoscopic ultrasound** can be used to assess depth of tumor invasion and nodal involvement.

III. **Barium swallow** may provide additional information about the size and location of a gastric lesion. It is especially useful in the evaluation of large tumors that preclude passage of an endoscope.

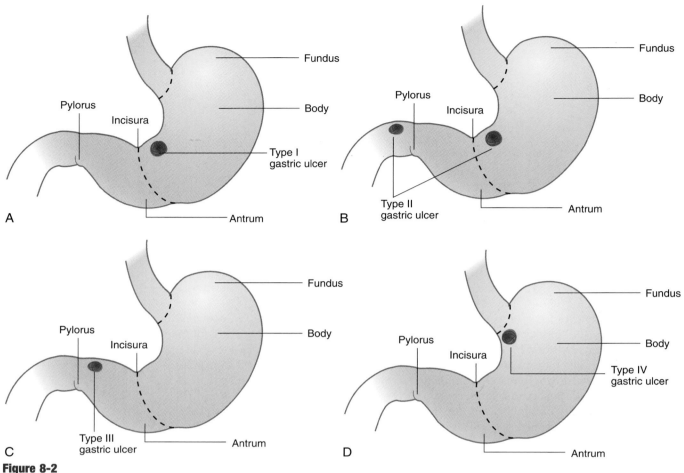

Figure 8-2
Gastric ulcers types I to IV. **A,** Type I. **B,** Type II. **C,** Type III. **D,** Type IV. *(From Townsend CM, Beauchamp RD, Evers BM, Mattox KL [eds]: Sabiston Textbook of Surgery: The Biological Basis of Modern Surgical Practice, 18th ed. Philadelphia, Saunders, 2008.)*

IV. **Computed tomography (CT) of the abdomen and pelvis** may identify visceral metastases or malignant ascites, either of which render the disease unresectable. CT is sensitive in detecting liver metastases larger than 5 mm, but may miss smaller lesions. Additionally, CT does not reliably detect peritoneal metastases and is inferior to endoscopic ultrasound in assessing nodal disease.

V. **Laparoscopy** is often performed before gastrectomy and is used to identify liver and peritoneal metastases that may have been missed with CT.

COMPONENTS OF THE OPERATION AND APPLIED ANATOMY

Total gastrectomy is described below. Unique features of partial resections (Fig. 8-4), including reconstructive options, are discussed in the subsequent section on additional operative considerations.

Patient Positioning and Preparation

I. The patient is placed in the supine position with the arms extended at 90 degrees.

II. The sterile preparation should extend to the nipples superiorly, the inguinal regions inferiorly, and the midaxillary lines laterally.

III. Resection of tumors of the proximal or gastroesophageal junction sometimes necessitates a thoracoabdominal incision or a thoracotomy. These approaches

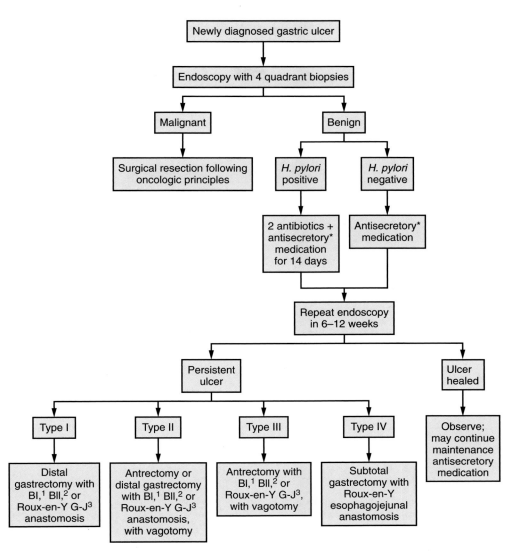

Figure 8-3
Treatment algorithm for newly diagnosed gastric ulcers.

require positioning on a pneumatic beanbag and intubation with a double-lumen endotracheal tube.

Preoperative Considerations

I. **Antibiotics** are administered within 1 hour before the skin incision.
II. A **urinary catheter** is inserted to decompress the bladder and facilitate resuscitative monitoring.
III. A **nasogastric tube (NGT)** is inserted into the stomach for decompression.
IV. Placement of an **epidural catheter** should be considered for postoperative analgesia.

Incision

I. Gastrectomy is performed through an upper midline abdominal or a bilateral subcostal incision.

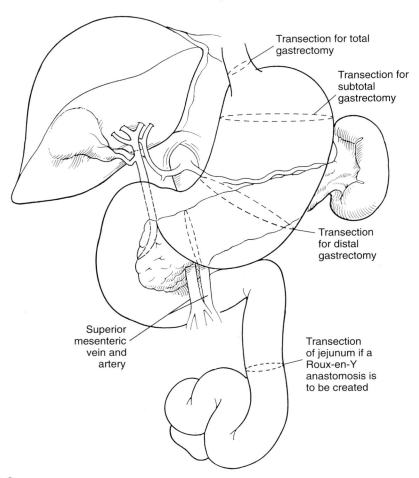

Figure 8-4
The levels of transection of the stomach for total, subtotal, or distal gastrectomy. *(From Khatri VP, Asensio JA: Operative Surgery Manual. Philadelphia, Saunders, 2003.)*

II. A left thoracoabdominal incision provides excellent exposure of the gastroesophageal junction and distal esophagus and may facilitate resection of proximal tumors.

Exposure and Dissection: Total Gastrectomy

I. After the abdomen is entered, the greater omentum is retracted upward and dissected away from the transverse colon to enter the lesser sac (Fig. 8-5).
II. The left gastroepiploic vessels are ligated along the greater curve of the stomach, and the short gastric arteries are ligated within the gastrosplenic ligament (Fig. 8-6).
III. The stomach is retracted cephalad, exposing the aorta and celiac trunk. The celiac lymph tissue is dissected up toward the stomach, starting at the superior border of the pancreas.
IV. The left gastric artery is identified and is ligated near its origin from the celiac trunk (Fig. 8-7).
V. The pylorus is mobilized, and branches of the right gastroepiploic vessels are identified inferiorly and ligated. Similarly, the right gastric artery is identified as it courses superior to the pylorus and is divided (Fig. 8-8).

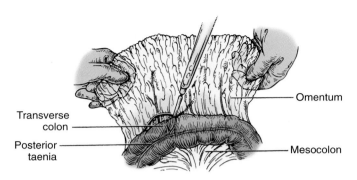

Figure 8-5
Cephalad retraction of the greater omentum allows access to the avascular plane above the transverse colon. *(From Yeo C: Shackelford's Surgery of the Alimentary Tract, 6th ed. Philadelphia, Saunders, 2007.)*

Transverse colon

Posterior taenia

Omentum

Mesocolon

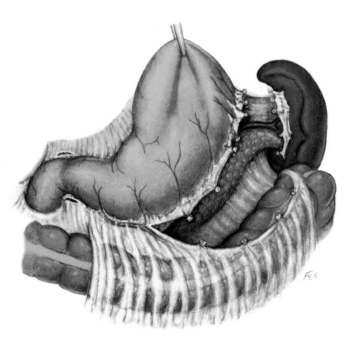

Figure 8-6
Dissection along the greater curvature includes omentectomy and ligation of the left gastroepiploic and short gastric arteries. *(From Yeo C: Shackelford's Surgery of the Alimentary Tract, 6th ed. Philadelphia, Saunders, 2007.)*

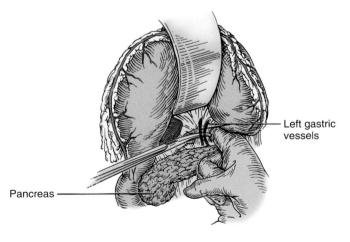

Figure 8-7
Cephalad retraction of the stomach allows for identification and ligation of the left gastric artery near its origin off the celiac trunk. *(From Yeo C: Shackelford's Surgery of the Alimentary Tract, 6th ed. Philadelphia, Saunders, 2007.)*

Left gastric vessels

Pancreas

VI. The duodenum is mobilized by sharply dissecting its lateral retroperitoneal and posterior pancreatic attachments.

VII. The first portion of the duodenum is divided approximately 2 to 3 cm distal to the pylorus using a thoracoabdominal stapler, leaving a closed duodenal stump.

VIII. The gastrohepatic ligament is divided near the liver, and the left hepatic lobe is retracted laterally, exposing the esophagus.

ALWAYS CONFIRM THE POSITION OF THE NASOGASTRIC TUBE BEFORE DUODENAL OR GASTRIC DIVISION.

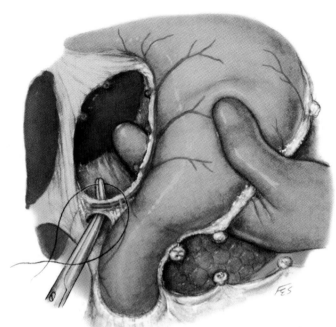

Figure 8-8
After mobilization of the pylorus and ligation of the right gastroepiploic vessels, the right gastric artery is identified superior to the pylorus and is ligated. *(From Yeo C: Shackelford's Surgery of the Alimentary Tract, 6th ed. Philadelphia, Saunders, 2007.)*

IX. An incision is made in the peritoneum overlying the esophagus and is extended laterally onto the diaphragm above the fundus of the stomach. Small vessels in this area are ligated individually.

X. If necessary, the posterior aspect of the esophagus is dissected to allow for additional mobilization. The esophagus is then sharply divided.

Reconstruction: Roux-en-Y Anastomosis

I. A loop of jejunum is mobilized to allow for subsequent esophagojejunostomy without tension.

II. After an appropriate jejunal transection point is identified, an opening in the mesentery is created immediately adjacent to the bowel. A gastrointestinal anastomosis surgical stapler is placed around the bowel, with the lower jaw inserted through the mesenteric opening. The stapler is fired, leaving two closed ends of transected bowel.

III. The distal end of transected jejunum is brought up to the esophagus. The jejunal limb can be placed in an antecolic (i.e., in front of the transverse colon) or retrocolic (i.e., behind the transverse colon through a defect in the mesocolon) position.

IV. An end-to-side anastomosis between the esophagus and the distal segment of jejunum is performed.

V. The proximal segment of transected jejunum is anastomosed to the jejunum 45 to 50 cm beyond the newly created esophagojejunal junction (Fig. 8-9).

Additional Operative Considerations

I. **Partial Gastrectomy:** Partial gastrectomy may be indicated for the treatment of distal tumors or benign gastric ulcer disease. The initial dissection required for a subtotal gastrectomy is similar to that described for total gastrectomy. Of note, during partial gastrectomy, only the most distal short gastric arteries are ligated because the proximal short gastric vessels serve as the blood supply to the gastric remnant.

II. **Reconstruction:** After total gastrectomy, GI continuity is most often reestablished with a Roux-en-Y esophagojejunostomy (as described in the previous

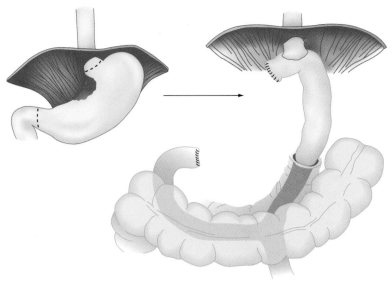

Figure 8-9
Total gastrectomy with Roux-en-Y esophagojejunal reconstruction. *(From Townsend CM, Beauchamp RD, Evers BM, Mattox KL [eds]: Sabiston Textbook of Surgery: The Biological Basis of Modern Surgical Practice, 18th ed. Philadelphia, Saunders, 2008.)*

section). After partial gastrectomy, however, multiple reconstructive options exist. A Billroth I reconstruction involves anastomosis of the distal stomach to the proximal divided duodenum (Fig. 8-10). An alternative is a Billroth II reconstruction, in which a loop of jejunum is mobilized and anastomosed to the gastric remnant (Fig. 8-11).

III. **Vagotomy:** In patients undergoing a gastric resection for refractory type II or III gastric ulcers, a **truncal vagotomy** may be performed to reduce acid secretion.

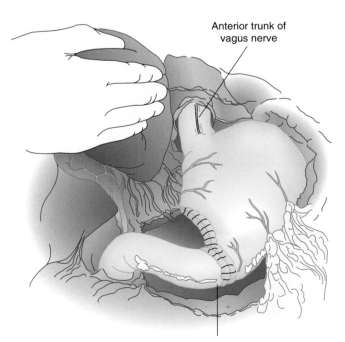

Anterior trunk of vagus nerve

Billroth I gastroduodenal anastomosis completed

Figure 8-10
Partial gastrectomy with Billroth I reconstruction. *(From Dempsey D, Pathak A: Antrectomy. Op Tech Gen Surg 5:86–100, 2003.)*

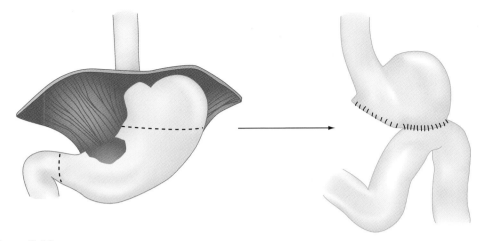

Figure 8-11
Partial gastrectomy with Billroth II reconstruction. *(From Townsend CM, Beauchamp RD, Evers BM, Mattox KL [eds]: Sabiston Textbook of Surgery: The Biological Basis of Modern Surgical Practice, 18th ed. Philadelphia, Saunders, 2008.)*

This procedure involves the ligation of the left and right vagus nerves above the take-off of the hepatic and celiac branches just proximal to the gastroesophageal junction (Fig. 8-12A). **Selective vagotomy,** which preserves the hepatic and celiac branches of the vagal nerves (Fig. 8-12B), has few advantages over standard truncal vagotomy and is rarely performed. Both of these approaches may compromise gastric emptying and are typically performed in combination with a distal gastrectomy or pyloroplasty. **Highly selective vagotomy,** or parietal cell vagotomy, involves the selective ligation of only those vagal branches supplying the parietal, acid-producing cells; because innervation to the antrum and pylorus is preserved, this procedure has less effect on gastric emptying than does truncal vagotomy. When performed with a distal gastrectomy or antrectomy, the highly selective approach has little advantage over truncal vagotomy (Fig. 8-12C).

IV. **Splenectomy:** Clinical trials have shown a significant increase in perioperative morbidity when splenectomy is performed with gastrectomy for malignancy. The spleen should be removed only if there is evidence of direct tumor invasion of the splenic hilum or parenchyma.

V. **Frozen Sections:** The diffuse intramural growth pattern of gastric adenocarcinoma makes it difficult to assess resection margins clinically. Intraoperative frozen sections are routinely obtained to ensure negative margins.

VI. **Enteral Access:** Many surgeons advocate routine insertion of a tube jejunostomy after total gastrectomy to facilitate the administration of postoperative nutritional support.

VII. **Drainage:** Placement of a closed-suction drain in the resection bed may facilitate surveillance for an anastomotic leak in the postoperative period and is advocated by some surgeons.

POSTOPERATIVE CARE

Patients are monitored and resuscitated in the intensive care unit during the initial postoperative period. If a feeding jejunostomy was placed, enteral feeding is initiated within 24 hours after surgery and continued until the patient's nutritional goals are met through oral intake. The NGT is removed with the return of bowel function. The use of routine upper GI tract contrast studies before NGT removal and the initiation of oral intake is advocated by some surgeons. Oral intake is generally started after NGT removal. Small frequent meals are recommended initially. Within months, patients are typically able to tolerate larger amounts of food.

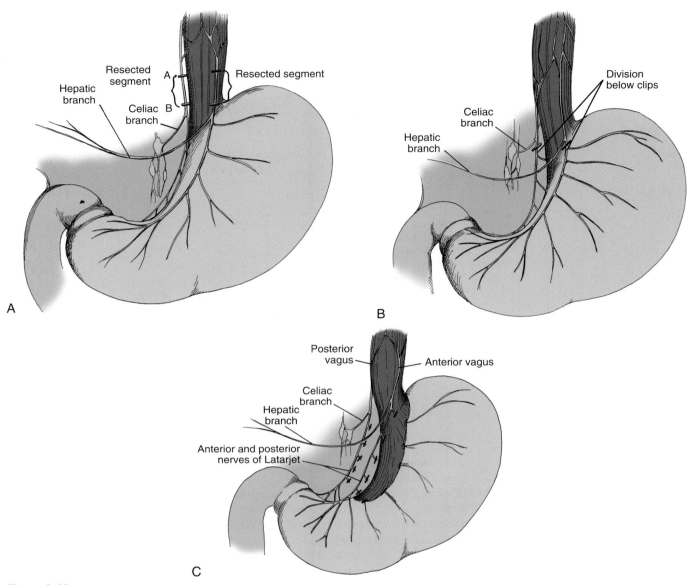

Figure 8-12
Vagotomy for the treatment of type II or III gastric ulcers. Clips indicate the level of nerve division. **A,** Truncal vagotomy. **B,** Selective vagotomy. **C,** Highly selective vagotomy. *(From Yeo C: Shackelford's Surgery of the Alimentary Tract, 6th ed. Philadelphia, Saunders, 2007.)*

EARLY COMPLICATIONS

I. **Anastomotic Leak:** A leak may develop at any newly constructed anastamoses or from the divided duodenal stump. Leaks usually present between the fifth and seventh postoperative days and may be heralded by fever, abdominal pain, leukocytosis, and enteric or bilous drainage. An upper GI contrast study or CT scan may be used to confirm the diagnosis. Duodenal stump leaks generally require prompt re-exploration. Anastomotic leaks may sometimes be managed with bowel rest, intravenous antibiotics, and observation, assuming that the patient is stable without signs of peritonitis. If a fluid collection is present, percutaneous drainage is indicated. Clinical deterioration after nonoperative management of an anastomotic leak mandates surgical exploration.

II. **Hemorrhage:** Postoperative bleeding may be extraluminal or intraluminal. Intraluminal bleeding can present with upper (hematemesis) or lower (hematochezia) GI bleeding. Endoscopy can be used to both diagnose and treat

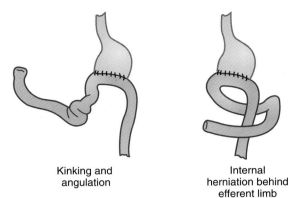

Kinking and angulation

Internal herniation behind efferent limb

Figure 8-13
Causes of mechanical afferent loop obstruction. *(From Townsend CM, Beauchamp RD, Evers BM, Mattox KL [eds]: Sabiston Textbook of Surgery: The Biological Basis of Modern Surgical Practice, 18th ed. Philadelphia, Saunders, 2008.)*

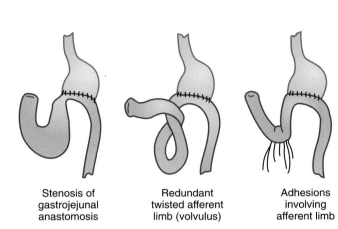

Stenosis of gastrojejunal anastomosis

Redundant twisted afferent limb (volvulus)

Adhesions involving afferent limb

anastomotic bleeding. Rarely, reoperation is required to control postoperative hemorrhage.

III. **Obstruction: Afferent limb obstruction** refers to obstruction of the bowel proximal to the gastrojejunostomy after a Billroth II anastomosis and classically presents with pain and bilious emesis (Fig. 8-13). Initial treatment typically involves endoscopic decompression and placement of an NGT. The majority of these obstructions are functional in etiology. Mechanical obstruction or refractory functional obstruction requires reoperation. The latter may be treated with conversion of the Billroth II reconstruction to a Roux-en-Y anastomosis. **Gastric outlet obstruction** after distal gastrectomy is typically functional in nature and resolves with temporary nasogastric decompression and promotility agents.

LATE COMPLICATIONS

I. **Dumping syndrome** refers to a constellation of symptoms (fatigue, lightheadedness, flushing, diaphoresis) followed by cramping and diarrhea that occur after eating a meal. "Early" dumping syndrome occurs approximately 30 minutes after eating and is caused by dysregulation of GI hormone secretion. Treatment involves dietary modification (avoidance of hyperosmolar liquids and fiber supplementation) and octreotide. "Late" dumping occurs approximately 2 hours after a meal and is caused by hyperinsulinemia that results in hypoglycemia. Administration of sugar is generally sufficient treatment.

II. **Bile reflux gastritis** occurs after a partial gastrectomy with Billroth I or II reconstruction. Patients may present with pain, nausea, and bilious emesis. Severely symptomatic patients may require reoperation and conversion of the Billroth I or II reconstruction to a Roux-en-Y gastrojejunal reconstruction.

III. **Metabolic abnormalities** may result from gastric resection. Resection of the proximal stomach and parietal cell mass results in decreased intrinsic factor secretion and vitamin B_{12} deficiency; this may manifest with megaloblastic anemia. The achlorhydria associated with partial gastrectomy may also result in bacterial overgrowth, malabsorption of nutrients and vitamins, and diarrhea. After Billroth II reconstruction in particular, inadequate mixing of digestive enzymes, and ingested fats may lead to fat and calcium malabsorption, steatorrhea, and osteopenia.

IV. Partial gastrectomy has been associated with a risk of subsequent **gastric remnant cancer.** Achlorhydria, enterogastric reflux, bacterial overgrowth, and *H. pylori* infection may be contributory factors.

SUGGESTED READING

Robinson EK, Mercer DW: Stomach. In Townsend CM, Beauchamp RD, Evers BM, Mattox KL [eds]: Sabiston Textbook of Surgery: The Biological Basis of Modern Surgical Practice, 18th ed. Philadelphia, Saunders, 2008, pp 1265–1321.

Gastric Bypass

Robert T. Lewis   and   Noel N. Williams

Case Study

A 42-year-old female presents to a surgeon's office requesting a gastric bypass operation. She weighs 290 pounds and is 5 feet 4 inches tall (body mass index, 49.8). She reports a history of hypercholesterolemia, hypertriglyceridemia, degenerative joint disease, gastroesophogeal reflux disease, hypertension, and obstructive sleep apnea requiring the use of a continuous positive airway pressure (CPAP) machine at night. She has been overweight since childhood and has attempted multiple diet programs throughout her life, many with good short-term results; however, she has repeatedly regained the lost weight. She is unable to exercise consistently because of joint pain.

Her physical examination is significant for central obesity and mild hypertension. Her fasting serum glucose level is 110 mg/dL, consistent with prediabetes.

> Body mass index (BMI) = weight (kg)/height (m)^2

BACKGROUND

Obesity is the most prevalent health problem in developed countries worldwide. More than 60% of all Americans are **overweight,** more than 30% are **obese,** and more than 4% are **severely obese.** Obesity and associated comorbidities cost the United States more than $150 billion annually and are responsible for more than 280,000 annual deaths. The rate of childhood and teenage obesity has nearly doubled in less than a decade, resulting in the earlier onset of associated comorbidities. **Bariatric surgery** is the only treatment for morbid obesity with proven efficacy and results in the loss of 50% to 70% of excess weight in nearly all individuals. In contrast, dietary modification results in long-term weight loss in fewer than 3% of patients. Perhaps more importantly, bariatric surgery is associated with decreased mortality rates and improved control or resolution of diabetes, hypertension, hyperlipidemia, and obstructive sleep apnea in a majority of patients. The most common bariatric procedures performed in the United States are the **Roux-en-Y gastric bypass** (RYGB) and the **adjustable gastric band.** The RYGB works through two mechanisms: (1) gastric restriction and (2) reduction of the functional absorptive capacity of the small bowel. The gastric band works through the former mechanism only.

> Overweight: Body mass index (BMI) = 25–30
> Obese: BMI > 30
> Severely obese: BMI > 40 or patient > 100 lb above ideal weight

INDICATIONS FOR SURGERY

Obesity: The specific indications for bariatric surgery continue to evolve. The National Institutes of Health issued a consensus statement in 1991 that established guidelines for identifying patients for whom the benefits of surgery outweigh the associated risks (Box 9-1). Importantly, patients weighing more than 600 pounds exceed the maximum weight capacity of many operating tables and may require staged therapy (including dietary modification) before a definitive surgery.

> **BOX 9-1 National Institutes of Health Eligibility Criteria for Weight Loss Surgery**
>
> - Body mass index (BMI) > 40 or BMI > 35 with comorbid conditions
> - Failed medical therapy
> - Informed in detail about the procedure and its risks
> - Motivated and psychiatrically stable
> - Able to tolerate surgery with acceptable medical risk
>
> Data from Buchwald H: Consensus Conference Panel: Consensus conference statement: Bariatric surgery for morbid obesity: Health implications for patients, health professionals, and third-party payers. Surg Obes Relat Dis 1:371–381, 2005.

PREOPERATIVE EVALUATION

A thorough preoperative assessment aimed at identifying modifiable risk factors is mandatory before bariatric surgery.

I. **Cardiovascular:** A preoperative electrocardiogram should be obtained for men older than 40 years, women older than 50 years, or patients with known coronary artery disease, diabetes mellitus, hypertension, obstructive sleep apnea, or arrhythmias. Patients with multiple cardiac risk factors should also undergo stress testing when possible. Unfortunately, this is not always feasible because most patients cannot tolerate even moderate exercise and thallium stress testing is inaccurate in patients with a BMI of more than 30. When available, transesophageal dobutamine stress echocardiogram is often the optimal study. In patients found to be at moderate or high cardiovascular risk, perioperative β-blockade may be recommended, although no study has yet demonstrated a benefit in this population.

II. **Pulmonary:** Between 40% and 80% of patients undergoing bariatric surgery have obstructive sleep apnea. Generally, patients should undergo preoperative sleep studies. If obstructive sleep apnea is shown, 4 weeks of CPAP or bilevel positive airway pressure (biPAP) is required before surgery. Long-standing OSA or reactive airway disease (also associated with obesity) can lead to pulmonary hypertension, which substantially increases operative risk. Systolic pulmonary artery pressures of greater than 50 mm Hg are a contraindication to surgery.

III. **Psychiatric:** More than 50% of candidates for bariatric surgery take psychotropic medication, most often for depression. The presence of inadequately treated psychiatric conditions has been correlated with inadequate weight loss and dissatisfaction after surgery. A structured interview with a psychologist or psychiatrist using a validated questionnaire, such as the Weight and Lifestyle Inventory or the Beck Depression Inventory, is recommended.

IV. **Gastrointestinal:** Nonalcoholic steatohepatitis (NASH) and cirrhosis are present in 40% and 2% of the severely obese population, respectively. Hepatic compromise is a contraindication to surgery, and liver function tests should, therefore, be obtained for all surgical candidates. Because of the high rate of postoperative cholelithiasis, some surgeons advocate screening for gallstones with a right upper quadrant ultrasound and, if the study is positive, removal of the gallbladder at the time of bariatric surgery.

V. **Educational:** Bariatric surgery results in the loss of 60% of excess body weight in most individuals, but requires extensive lifestyle changes postoperatively. Many patients have unrealistic expectations and require preoperative education. Postoperative referral to a support group may also be beneficial.

Does your patient have obesity-related comorbidities?

COMPONENTS OF THE PROCEDURE AND APPLIED ANATOMY

Preoperative Considerations

I. **Sequential compression devices** should be applied before the induction of anesthesia to prevent deep vein thrombosis (DVT). Some centers advocate preoperative treatment with subcutaneous heparin as well.

II. More than 50% of obese patients have gastroesophageal reflux disease. Supine positioning increases intra-abdominal pressure and the risk of aspiration during intubation. Intubation with the head of the table elevated at 15 degrees to 20 degrees is often preferred to decrease this risk.

III. Prophylactic **antibiotics** are administered before skin incision.

IV. A **urinary catheter** is placed to allow for continuous urine output monitoring.

V. A **nasogastric tube** is inserted to decompress the stomach.

Patient Positioning and Preparation

I. The patient is placed in the supine position with the arms extended. Pressure points are padded to prevent necrosis. Additionally, buttresses are constructed under the arms to minimize the amount of traction placed on the torso and to decrease the risk of **brachial plexopathies.**

II. The sterile preparation should extend to the nipples superiorly, to the pubis inferiorly, and to the posterior axillary lines laterally.

> **ALL PRESSURE POINTS SHOULD BE PADDED TO AVOID PRESSURE NECROSIS.**

Roux-en-Y Gastric Bypass

Roux-en-Y gastric bypass (Fig. 9-1) has three major components: (1) construction of the gastric pouch, (2) division of the small bowel and creation of the Roux limb, and (3) creation of an anastomosis between the gastric pouch and jejunum (gastrojejunostomy). Approaches to gastric bypass include: (1) laparoscopic, (2) hand-assisted laparoscopic, and (3) open. Specific techniques related to port placement and incisions for each approach

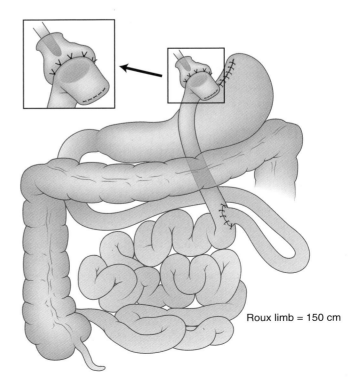

Figure 9-1
Roux-en-Y gastric bypass. *(From Kendrick ML, Dakin GF: Surgical approaches to obesity. Mayo Clin Proc 81[10 Suppl]:S18–S24, 2006.)*

Roux limb = 150 cm

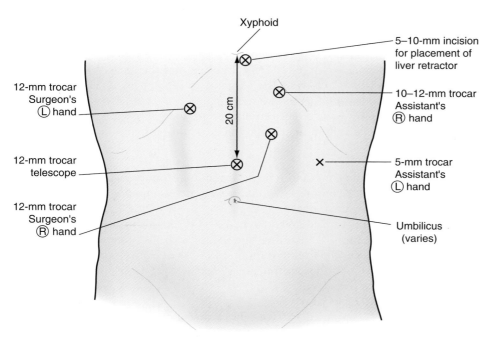

Figure 9-2
Trocar placement for laparoscopic Roux-en-Y gastric bypass. *(From Townsend CM, Beauchamp RD, Evers BM, Mattox KL [eds]: Sabiston Textbook of Surgery: The Biological Basis of Modern Surgical Practice, 17th ed. Philadelphia, Saunders, 2004.)*

are discussed first, followed by a discussion of the components of the procedure common to all three.

I. **Laparoscopic Approach:** Six ports are required for gastric bypass, including a camera port, two ports for the primary surgeon, a port for a liver retractor, and two ports for the assistant (Fig. 9-2).

A. The midline supraumbilical port is typically placed first. A blind (Veress needle) approach or an open (Hassan) approach may be used. The former is contra-indicated in patients who have had previous abdominal surgery.

1. Blind technique

a. The skin is incised. A Veress needle, which has a retractable cutting tip as well as a channel that allows for insufflation, is inserted through the incision, abdominal fascia, and peritoneum.

b. CO_2 is insufflated to distend the abdomen.

2. Open technique

a. The skin is incised. The subcutaneous tissue is dissected to expose the linea alba.

b. The fascia is grasped and opened under direct vision. The peritoneum is visualized and opened under direct vision.

c. A port is placed into the incision using a blunt-tipped trocar.

d. CO_2 is insufflated to distend the abdomen.

B. The remaining ports are inserted under laparoscopic visualization.

II. **Hand Assist:** A hand port can replace one of the surgeon's instrument ports (typi-cally, the left-sided port) to allow for increased intracorporeal needle control and a faster operative time.

A. The first port is inserted as described under "Laparoscopic Approach," and CO_2 is insufflated into the abdomen.

B. A left-sided vertical paramedical incision (i.e., an incision adjacent to the midline) is made. The incision should be just large enough to accommodate the surgeon's hand.

C. The subcutaneous tissues are divided to expose the rectus fascia. The anterior rectus sheath, rectus muscle, posterior rectus sheath, and peritoneum are sequentially opened.

D. A laparoscopic system (GelPort) is inserted into the incision; this functions as a one-way valve, allowing the surgeon to place a hand into the abdomen without the loss of pneumoperitoneum.

E. The remaining ports are placed under laparsocopic visualization. A static liver retractor port is often unnecessary because the surgeon's hand can retract the liver.

III. **Open**

A. An upper midline incision is made, extending from the xiphoid process toward the umbilicus. Generous incisions are sometimes required to allow for adequate exposure in severely obese patients.

B. The incision is carried down to the fascia through the fat.

C. The midline raphe is identified and incised sharply, preferably near the top of the incision over the liver to minimize the risk of inadvertent injury to abdominal viscera. Once the peritoneum is opened, the fascia is lifted up and the incision is extended.

IV. **Exposure and Dissection**

A. The liver is examined for signs of cirrhosis or fatty replacement indicative of NASH. The gallbladder is inspected for the presence of gallstones or sludge.

B. The mobility of the small bowel is assessed and the ligament of Treitz is identified.

V. **Construction of the Biliopancreatic Limb:** The jejunum is divided approximately 40 cm distal to the ligament of Treitz. The specific length of the resultant limb is less important than is the mobility of the bowel at the site of division. The distal bowel must reach the stomach without tension to allow for subsequent construction of an end-to-side gastrojejuostomy.

VI. **Construction of the Jejunojejunostomy and Roux Limb**

A. A side-to-side anastomosis is created between the proximal end of the divided jejunum and the jejunum 120 to 150 cm beyond the stapled division (Fig. 9-3).

B. The length of the resulting bypassed limb directly influences the degree of malabsorption after surgery. Some surgeons vary the length of the bypassed limb based on BMI (e.g., creating longer limbs in larger patients).

VII. **Construction of the Gastric Pouch and Gastrojejunostomy**

A. The patient is placed in the steep Trendelenburg position, allowing the small bowel and omentum to fall away from the diaphragmatic hiatus.

B. The left lobe of the liver is retracted laterally to expose the stomach.

C. The stomach is grasped and retracted toward the feet to expose the gastroesophageal junction.

D. The pars flaccida, the avascular portion of the gastrohepatic ligament, is identified and divided to expose the lesser sac.

E. Dissection is carried posteriorly around the back wall of the stomach toward the spleen.

F. Once the stomach has been adequately mobilized, a stapler is used to partition the gastric pouch from the remainder of the stomach. Typically, the staple line extends from the angle of His to the midportion of the lesser curve. The nasogastric tube is withdrawn into the esophagus during the creation of the pouch.

G. The Roux limb is brought up to the stomach either anterior or posterior to the transverse colon. If it is brought up posteriorly (i.e., retrocolic), a defect is created in the transverse colon mesentery through which the limb is passed.

H. A hole is made in the anterior wall of the gastric pouch, and an anastomosis is created between the gastric pouch and the distal end of the divided small bowel.

> Carbohydrates and protein are primarily absorbed in the duodenum and the first 100 cm of the jejunum.

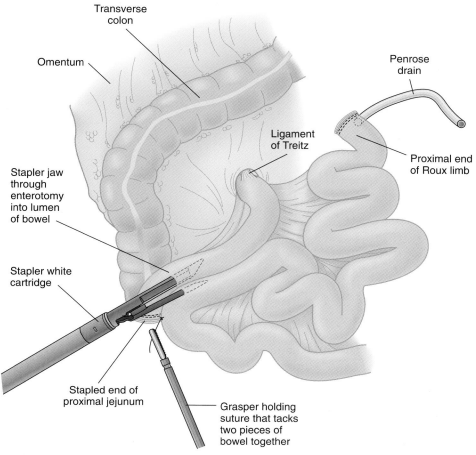

Figure 9-3
Side-to-side jejunojejunostomy. *(From Townsend CM, Beauchamp RD, Evers BM, Mattox KL [eds]: Sabiston Textbook of Surgery: The Biological Basis of Modern Surgical Practice, 17th ed. Philadelphia, Saunders, 2004.)*

VIII. **Testing of the Anastomosis and Closure**
   A. Once the procedure is complete and hemostasis is confirmed, the gastrojejunostomy may be inspected endoscopically. Any apparent leaks are repaired with interrupted stitches.
   B. All port site incisions greater than 1 cm in length are closed in two layers, approximating the fascia and skin. All skin incisions are closed with absorbable subcutaneous sutures.

Laparoscopic Adjustable Gastric Band

The laparoscopic adjustable gastric band has gained popularity in recent years as an alternative to RYGBP (Fig. 9-4). The band can be placed laparoscopically, with or without a hand port.
   I. **Exposure and Dissection**
      A. The liver is retracted to expose the stomach and esophageal hiatus.
      B. The gastrohepatic ligament is identified and the pars flaccida is divided.
      C. A tunnel is bluntly created along the posterior aspect of the stomach, beginning 5 cm below the gastroeophoageal junction on the lesser curve and continuing toward the superior pole of the spleen.
   II. **Placement of the Band**
      A. The band is inserted into the abdomen, pulled through the retrogastric tunnel, and locked into place around the stomach.

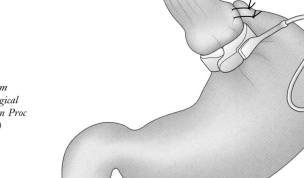

Figure 9-4
A diagram of the completed adjustable gastric band. *(From Kendrick ML, Dakin GF: Surgical approaches to obesity. Mayo Clin Proc 81[10 Suppl]:S18–S24, 2006.)*

    B. Several interrupted sutures between the stomach above and below the band are placed to fix the band in position.

III. **Placement of the Subcutaneous Port**

    A. The band tubing is threaded out through one of the port sites and attached to a reservoir.

    B. The skin incision at the chosen port site is lengthened to allow for dissection down to the fascia. A subcutaneous pocket is created to accommodate the reservoir, which is secured to the fascia at several points.

IV. **Testing the Band and Closure**

    A. The system is de-aired by aspirating with an empty syringe. Saline is then injected into the reservoir to fill the band.

    B. The laparoscope and ports are removed, and the skin is closed with absorbable suture.

POSTOPERATIVE COURSE

Obesity-related comorbidities are managed aggressively in the perioperative period (e.g., patients with sleep apnea are encouraged to use BiPAP or CPAP machines). Postoperative continuous end-tidal CO_2 monitoring allows for early detection of respiratory acidosis and is increasingly used as an adjunct to postoperative care in the obese population. Prolonged postoperative maintenance of a nasogastric tube is generally unnecessary, and patients may be advanced to a liquid diet on the first postoperative day and a modified diet thereafter, consisting of small portions of soft and pureed foods. Early ambulation is encouraged.

COMPLICATIONS

I. **Short-Term Complications**

    A. **Inadvertent bowel injuries** most often occur during entry into the abdomen. Recognized injuries should be repaired immediately. Unrecognized enterotomies and **anastomotic leaks**, more common from the gastrojejunostomy than from the jejunojejunostomy, may present in the early postoperative period with nonspecific signs, including tachycardia, leukocytosis, and fever. If not promptly addressed, such complications can rapidly progress to peritonitis and sepsis. Suspicion of a leak or unrecognized enterotomy should prompt an aggressive evaluation (which may include a CT scan or swallow study) or operative re-exploration.

B. **Pulmonary embolism** (PE) is the most common cause of postoperative death after bariatric surgery. Many centers administer high-dose subcutaneous heparin immediately before surgery and encourage early ambulation after surgery, in an effort to reduce the incidence of perioperative DVT and subsequent PE. Signs associated with PE (e.g., tachycardia, pleuritic pain, shortness of breath, and right-sided heart strain by ECG) must be promptly evaluated. CT scanning of the chest with intravenous contrast is the preferred study, but may not be feasible because most CT equipment will not accommodate the severely obese patient; V-Q scanning is an alternative. Once a PE is diagnosed, intensive care unit–level care, systemic anticoagulation with intravenous heparin, and when appropriate, early elective reintubation are important components of management.

II. **Long-Term Complications**
   A. **Strictures** are most common at the gastrojejunostomy anastomosis and have an incidence of 2% to 14%. Strictures are believed to result from ischemia or subclinical anastomotic leaks, with resultant inflammation. Strictures most often develop 1 to 3 months after surgery and are typically associated with progressive epigastric pain and dysphagia within 10 minutes of eating. Diagnosis may be confirmed with an upper gastrointestinal barium swallow. Treatment consists of endoscopic dilation.
   B. **Marginal ulcers** are erosions adjacent to an anastomosis. After gastric bypass, marginal ulcers most commonly develop at the gastrojejunostomy anastomosis. Tension on the anastomosis, ischemia, *Helicobacter pylori* infection, smoking, and nonsteroidal anti-inflammatory drug (NSAID) use may all play contributory roles in the pathogenesis of marginal ulceration. Patients typically present 1 to 3 months after surgery with epigastric pain unrelated to eating, occult gastrointestinal bleeding, or dysphagia. Diagnosis may be confirmed with an upper endoscopy. Treatment consists of eradication of *H. pylori infection*, smoking and NSAID cessation, and the use of proton pump inhibitors. If ulcerations are severe, reoperation and revision of the anastomosis is sometimes necessary.
   C. **Internal hernias** complicate 1% to 3% of open cases and 3% to 4% of laparoscopic cases and may develop a year or more after surgery. Weight loss increases mesenteric laxity, allowing for herniation of the small bowel through postsurgical mesenteric defects. Herniation can occur: (1) behind the Roux limb (Peterson's space), (2) through the mesocolonic tunnel, or (3) through the mesenteric defect adjacent to the jejunojejunostomy. Patients may present with symptoms consistent with small bowel obstruction. Treatment consists of reoperation, reduction of the hernia, resection of necrotic bowel, and closure of the hernia defect.
   D. **Malnutrition** is common after bariatric surgery, justifying close postoperative monitoring and nutritional counseling. Patients must modify their eating habits to maintain adequate protein intake and should be prescribed vitamin supplementation.
   E. **Gallbladder disease** develops in 50% to 70% of patients after bariatric surgery. Rapid weight loss results in biliary sludge and stone formation.

III. **Band-Specific Complications**
   A. **Slipped band position** results from prolapse of the greater curvature of the stomach through the band. Prolapsed tissue may become edematous and incarcerate, leading to symptoms including nocturnal reflux, dysphagia, vomiting, and pain, which may radiate to the shoulder secondary to diaphragmatic irritation. The diagnosis may be confirmed with an abdominal radiograph that shows migration of the band along the greater curvature. Treatment consists of reoperation and replacement of the band.
   B. **Band erosion** through the stomach wall is typically a later complication of band placement. The most common presentation of band erosion is a port site infection caused by enteric bacteria tracking along the band and catheter.

Diagnosis may be confirmed by upper endoscopy, and treatment consists of band removal. A feeding jejunostomy may be placed to allow for enteral nutritional support during healing.

SUGGESTED READINGS

Adams TD, Gress RE, Smith SC, et al: Long-term mortality after gastric bypass surgery. N Engl J Med 357:753–761, 2007.

Buchwald H, Avidor Y, Braunwald E, et al: Bariatric surgery: a systematic review and meta-analysis. JAMA 292:1724–1737, 2004.

Kendrick ML, Dakin GF: Surgical approaches to obesity. Mayo Clin Proc 81(10 Suppl):S18–S24, 2006.

Malinowski SS: Nutritional and metabolic complications of bariatric surgery. Am J Med Sci 331:219–225, 2006.

Schirmer BD: Morbid obesity. In Townsend CM, Beauchamp RD, Evers BM, Mattox KL (eds): Sabiston Textbook of Surgery: The Biological Basis of Modern Surgical Practice, 17th ed. Philadelphia, Saunders, 2004, pp 357–399.

CHAPTER 10

Enteral Access Procedures

Benjamin Herdrich   and   Jon B. Morris

Case Study

A 63-year-old male with an extensive smoking history presents to his physician complaining of 2 months of increasing hoarseness and difficulty swallowing. Workup, including laryngoscopy, reveals a large pharyngeal tumor. Plans are made for radical surgical resection, including partial pharyngectomy. The patient is referred to a general surgeon for placement of a feeding tube at the time of his operation in anticipation of postoperative difficulty tolerating oral intake.

BACKGROUND

Nutritional support is an essential component of the treatment of critically and chronically ill patients. Patients who cannot meet their own nutritional needs through oral intake can be supported with **parenteral** (intravenous) or **enteral** (gastrointestinal tract) feeding. Parenteral feeding is an effective means of providing nutritional support to those patients who cannot be fed enterally and provides lifesaving therapy for patients with limited gastrointestinal tract absorptive capacity. The shortcomings of parenteral nutrition, however, have become increasingly evident as experience with this approach has grown; these include high rates of catheter-related, infectious, and metabolic complications as well as liver dysfunction. In contrast, enteral feeding is associated with fewer complications, is less expensive, and is not dependent on central venous access.

A number of options for enteral access exist; each has unique advantages and disadvantages. These include nasoenteric tubes, gastrostomy tubes, and jejunostomy tubes. **Nasoenteric tubes,** which include large-bore nasogastric tubes and small-bore nasoenteric tubes, can be placed at the bedside without the need for surgery and provide safe, short-term enteral access. Nasoenteric tubes are associated with several complications, including errors in tube placement (e.g., intracranial or intrabronchial intubations), sinusitis, nasal synechiae, and nasal alar necrosis. Surgically placed **gastrostomy tubes (G-tubes)** provide more durable, long-term enteral access and can be used for feeding or gastric decompression. In appropriate patients, they may be placed percutaneously with endoscopic assistance, obviating the need for larger open incisions. **Jejunostomy tubes (J-tubes)** are indicated in patients with contraindications to gastrostomy tube placement (e.g., patients undergoing a transhiatal esophagectomy) and patients with severe reflux or delayed gastric emptying. A variety of laparoscopic approaches to tube gastrostomy and jejunsotomy are in use, increasing the options further. This chapter focuses on the most common enteral access procedures: **percutaneous endoscopic gastrostomy (PEG)** tube placement and open approaches to tube gastrostomy and tube jejunostomy.

> **CORRECT PLACEMENT OF NASOENTERIC TUBES SHOULD BE CONFIRMED RADIOGRAPHICALLY BEFORE THE INITIATION OF ENTERIC FEEDING.**

INDICATIONS FOR SURGERY

I. **Nutritional Support:** Enteral access is required when patients' oral intake is insufficient to meet their nutritional needs. Nutritional support should be considered if: (1) a patient has been without nutrition for 5 to 7 days; (2) the duration of the condition is expected to exceed 10 days; or (3) the patient is malnourished. Enteral nutritional support is only feasible in patients with sufficient small bowel absorptive capacity. Patients who do not meet this requirement (e.g., patients with short gut syndrome) require parenteral nutrition.

II. **Prophylactic Enteral Access:** Patients with upper-airway or foregut cancers who undergo extensive surgical resection and adjuvant radiation and chemotherapy often have difficulty maintaining adequate caloric intake during the treatment period. In anticipation of this, many of these patients undergo either gastrostomy or jejunostomy placement at the time of surgical resection.

III. **Decompression:** Patients who cannot tolerate gastric feeding because of severe reflux, gastric atony, or inoperable bowel obstruction (e.g., patients with metastatic cancer) may benefit from G-tube placement for gastric decompression.

PREOPERATIVE EVALUATION

I. **History:** The preoperative history should allow for a determination of the amount of time enteral access will be needed and whether gastric or jejunal feeding is preferable. A history of feeding intolerance should be elicited in patients already being fed through a nasoenteric tube; patients who are not tolerating gastric feeding through a nasogastric tube may be better served by a J-tube (Fig. 10-1).

II. **Laboratory Testing:** Laboratory testing should include a complete blood count, electrolytes, and coagulation studies. Thrombocytopenia and coagulopathies should be corrected before enteral access procedures.

COMPONENTS OF THE PROCEDURE AND APPLIED ANATOMY

Preoperative Considerations

I. Prophylactic antibiotics to cover gram-positive organisms should be given within 1 hour before the procedure.

II. G-tubes and J-tubes are placed under general anesthesia. PEG tubes can be placed with intravenous sedation and local anesthetics.

Positioning and Preparation

I. The patient is placed in the supine position with the arms extended. The head of the bed is elevated.

II. The surgical preparation should extend to the nipples superiorly, the pubic symphysis inferiorly, and the midaxillary lines laterally.

PEG Tube

I. Placement of a PEG tube is best accomplished by two surgeons, one operating the endoscope and the other positioned next to the patient's abdomen.

II. **Passing the Endoscope**
   A. The endoscope is lubricated and passed through the pharynx and esophagus, into the stomach.
   B. The stomach is insufflated with air.

III. **Choosing the Gastrostomy Site**
   A. The ideal site for gastrostomy placement is identified by palpation, transillumination, and needle aspiration. The site is typically two fingerbreadths below the costal margin, just to the left of the midline.
   B. Potential sites for tube insertion are palpated with a single finger. The impression of the finger on the stomach wall is noted by the endoscopist. Inability to appreciate this impression suggests interposition of other organs, such as the colon or liver, between the stomach and the abdominal wall (Fig. 10-2).
   C. Once an appropriate site is identified using palpation, the room lights are dimmed. Transillumination of the abdominal wall with endoscopic light can

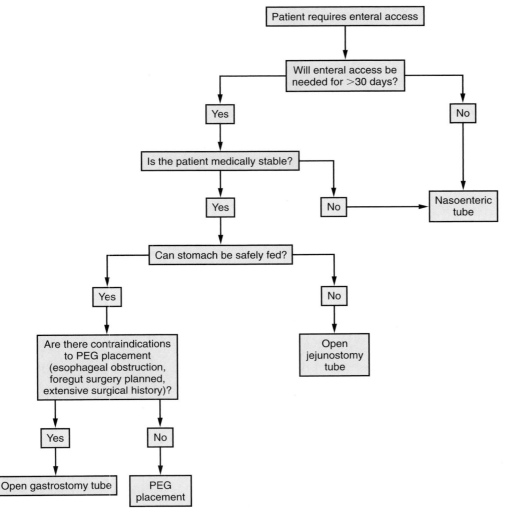

Figure 10-1
Preoperative evaluation for enteral access.

be appreciated in most patients unless colon or liver is interposed between the stomach and the abdominal wall.

D. The presence of bowel interposed between the abdominal wall and the stomach can also be excluded by inserting a 21-gauge needle attached to a syringe partially filled with saline at the site while aspirating. If bubbles are noted in the syringe before the needle is seen entering the stomach by the endoscopist, a different site should be identified.

E. If a safe site cannot be identified, tube gastrostomy should be performed through an open incision.

IV. **Accessing the Stomach**
A. A 14-gauge angiocatheter is inserted into the stomach under endoscopic visualization.
B. A wire is passed through the catheter into the stomach.
C. A snare is threaded through the endoscope and used to grasp the wire.
D. The endoscope is withdrawn with the snare and wire, and one end of the wire is pulled out of the patient's mouth.

V. **Tube Placement**
A. The distal end of the PEG tube is attached to the end of the wire that has been pulled through the patient's mouth.

PALPATION, TRANSILLUMINATION, AND NEEDLE ASPIRATION AT THE PROPOSED INSERTION SITE MINIMIZE THE RISK OF LIVER OR COLON INJURY.

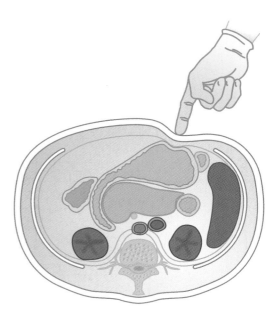

Figure 10-2
During PEG tube placement, the proposed gastrostomy site is palpated. The impression of the finger on the stomach wall is noted by the endoscopist. *(From Yeo C: Shackelford's Surgery of the Alimentary Tract, 6th ed. Philadelphia, Saunders, 2007.)*

> **STOMACH WALL NECROSIS MAY RESULT IF THE SELF-RETAINING BAR AND BUMPER ARE BROUGHT TOO CLOSE TOGETHER AROUND THE INTERPOSED ABDOMINAL AND STOMACH WALLS.**

    B. The proximal end of the PEG tube (the bumper) is grasped with the endoscopist's snare (still threaded through the endoscope).

    C. The wire is withdrawn through the abdominal wall, thus pulling the PEG tube through the esophagus, into the stomach, and out the anterior abdominal wall. The endoscopist follows the tube into the stomach.

    D. The endoscopist opens the snare when the bumper is in place, within the stomach, and the gastrostomy site is inspected to ensure hemostasis.

    E. A self-retaining bar is threaded over the distal end of the PEG tube to secure it at the skin. Care is taken not to advance the bar too far; by applying gentle traction on the PEG tube, the physician should easily be able to lift the bar 1 cm off the skin and rotate it 360 degrees (Fig. 10-3).

    F. Air is suctioned out of the stomach. The endoscope is removed.

Open Tube Gastrostomy

    I. **Incision:** Open G-tube placement is performed through an upper midline incision, 6 to 8 cm in length. Alternatively, a left paramedian incision can be used.

    II. **Insertion of the Gastrostomy Tube**
        A. The stomach is identified and grasped with an instrument.
        B. The site for the gastrostomy tube is chosen, typically in the midportion of the stomach, closer to the greater curvature. Two concentric purse-string sutures are placed at the proposed site.
        C. A gastrotomy (an opening in the stomach) is made at the center of the purse-string sutures, and the tube is inserted into the stomach (Fig. 10-4).
        D. The inner and outer purse-string sutures are tied down, invaginating the stomach wall around the gastrostomy tube.

    III. **Securing the Stomach to the Anterior Abdominal Wall**
        A. The distal end of the tube is brought out through a stab incision in the anterior abdominal wall left of the midline.
        B. The stomach surrounding the tube is sutured to the anterior abdominal wall around the exit site (Fig. 10-5).

    IV. **Closure of the Wound**
        A. The fascia and the skin are closed.
        B. The gastrostomy tube is secured to the abdominal wall with either a self-retaining bar or sutures.

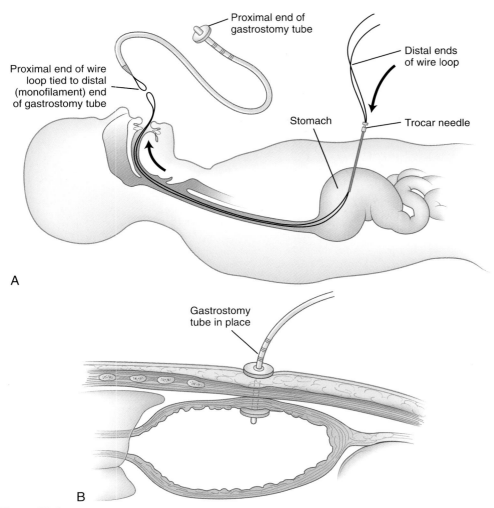

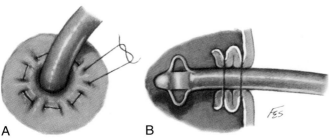

Figure 10-3

A, The gastrostomy tube is pulled through the mouth and esophagus, into the stomach, and out the abdominal wall. **B,** An inner plastic bumper and an outer self-retaining bar are approximated to hold the tube in place. *(From Sabiston DC Jr [ed]: Atlas of General Surgery. Philadelphia, Saunders, 1994.)*

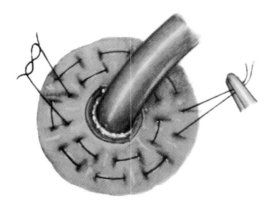

Figure 10-4

During placement of a gastrostomy tube, two purse-string sutures are placed around the proposed site. The tube is placed through an enterotomy in the center of those sutures. *(From Yeo C: Shackelford's Surgery of the Alimentary Tract, 6th ed. Philadelphia, Saunders, 2007.)*

Figure 10-5

A and **B,** The purse-string sutures are tied down and invaginate the gastric wall around the gastrostomy tube. *(From Yeo C: Shackelford's Surgery of the Alimentary Tract, 6th ed. Philadelphia, Saunders, 2007.)*

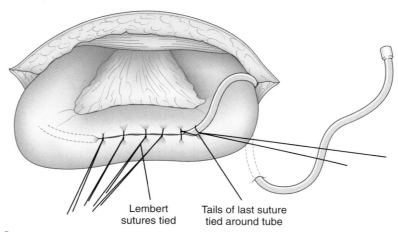

Lembert
sutures tied

Tails of last suture
tied around tube

Figure 10-6
Seromuscular sutures create a serosal tunnel for the jejunostomy tube. *(From Sabiston DC Jr [ed]: Atlas of General Surgery. Philadelphia, Saunders, 1994.)*

Open Tube Jejunostomy

  I. **Incision:** Open J-tube placement is performed through an upper midline incision, 6 to 8 cm in length. Alternatively, a paramedian incision can be used.
 II. **Insertion of the Jejunostomy Tube**
     A. The transverse colon is retracted cephalad, and the ligament of Treitz is identified.
     B. A site for insertion of the J-tube, typically 30 to 40 cm distal to the ligament, where the mesentery is mobile enough to allow the small bowel to reach the abdominal wall, is identified.
     C. A single purse-string suture is placed at the chosen site, and an enterotomy is made in the center of the purse string.
     D. The J-tube is inserted through the enterotomy and passed approximately 10 cm distally. The purse string is tied.
III. **Creation of a Serosal Tunnel:** Beginning at the insertion site and extending proximally, the jejunal serosa is closed over the tube with four to six interrupted sutures (Fig. 10-6).
 IV. **Securing the Jejunum to the Anterior Abdominal Wall**
     A. The end of the tube is brought out through a stab incision to the left of the midline.
     B. The jejunum around the J-tube is sutured to the anterior abdominal wall in multiple locations.
  V. **Wound Closure:** The fascia and skin are closed. The J-tube is sutured to the skin.

> CARE MUST BE TAKEN TO AVOID NARROWING THE LUMEN OF THE JEJUNUM BECAUSE DOING SO MAY CAUSE AN OBSTRUCTION.

> NEWLY PLACED ENTERAL TUBES SHOULD BE SECURED WITH A BULKY DRESSING TO PREVENT EARLY TUBE DISLODGEMENT.

> Benign pneumoperitoneum is common immediately after PEG tube placement and does not require further workup unless the patient has peritonitis or other concerning findings.

> MINIMIZE ASPIRATION BY CHECKING RESIDUAL VOLUMES AND ELEVATING THE HEAD OF THE BED BEFORE THE ADMINISTRATION OF FEEDING.

POSTOPERATIVE COURSE

During recovery from anesthesia, enteral tubes are attached to drainage bags or capped. The latter approach is often preferable, particularly during patient transport, to avoid early tube dislodgement. Patients requiring immediate enteral nutrition can usually begin enteral feeding on the first postoperative day. G-tube feeding is typically administered in intermittent boluses. Residual gastric volumes should be checked before each bolus. If residual volumes exceed 200 mL, feedings should be held until gastric emptying improves. In contrast, J-tube feeding is usually administered as a continuous infusion. Enteral tubes should be flushed at least once a day or after each feeding to avoid clogging.

After enteral tube placement, formation of an epithelialized tract requires approximately 6 weeks. Gastrostomy and jejunostomy tubes should not be removed or replaced before this time.

COMPLICATIONS

I. **Wound complications** are common after enteral tube placement. Even mild **drainage** of enteral contents around a gastrostomy tube or jejunostomy tube may lead to skin **excoriation.** Antacid therapy can help to make the draining enteral contents less irritating. However, in severe cases, tube feeds may need to be held or the tube may need to be removed to allow for healing. The pressure exerted by the tube on the abdominal wall can also result in **skin ulceration.** If severe, the tube may need to be removed to allow for wound healing. It is usually counterproductive to replace the tube with a larger one because this enlarges the defect and causes continued erosion.

> UPSIZING A TUBE TO TREAT DRAINAGE IS RARELY EFFECTIVE AND MAY CAUSE ABDOMINAL WALL EROSION.

II. Although rare, fungal and bacterial skin **infections** sometimes develop around the tube site. Such infections usually respond to topical antifungal agents and systemic antibiotic therapy.

III. **Bleeding** after PEG tube placement may result from trauma during passage of the tube through the stomach and abdominal wall. Bleeding is usually self-limited and in some cases can be controlled by transiently tightening the self-retaining bar. Pressure should be released once the bleeding has stopped to avoid pressure necrosis of the gastric wall. Rarely, bleeding requires operative exploration.

IV. Mechanical **obstruction** must be distinguished from postoperative ileus in all patients who cannot tolerate feeding after an enteral access procedure; computed tomography scanning with contrast administered through the tube is frequently a useful study in this regard. Mechanical obstruction can be caused by proximal or distal migration of the tube, volvulus of the jejunum around the point of fixation to the abdominal wall, or adhesions. If the tube has migrated, repositioning it is often sufficient treatment. Other causes of mechanical obstruction typically require reoperation.

V. **Injury to other organs,** including the liver and bowel, can occur during PEG tube placement. If recognized at the time of the procedure, such injuries are immediately repaired. Unrecognized colonic injuries can result in fistula formation between the stomach and colon and may present with feeding intolerance or diarrhea. If the diagnosis of a gastrocolic fistula is made, operative repair is indicated.

VI. **Diarrhea** is often associated with enteral feeding. Mild antidiarrheal agents (i.e., bismuth subsalicylate [Kaopectate]) and bulking agents (i.e., psyllium) may provide symptomatic improvement. Decreasing the feeding rate or bolus volume and switching formulations (e.g., isotonic, low-fat, lactose-free) may also help to relieve symptoms if other causes have been ruled out. Antimotility agents can be used only if infection has been ruled out.

VII. **Dislodgement** of a PEG tube in the postoperative period (i.e., <2 weeks after placement) may result in free spillage of gastric contents into the peritoneal cavity and generally necessitates immediate operative exploration and repair of the gastrotomy. Surgical approaches to tube placement that involve approximation of the bowel or stomach to the anterior abdominal wall safeguard against spillage of enteric contents into the peritoneal cavity. Patients may be observed without immediate intervention in the event that such tubes are dislodged in the early postprocedure period. Tubes dislodged 6 weeks or more after placement can usually be replaced through the tract, which is well epithelialized by this time. Radiographic confirmation of appropriate positioning is recommended before reinitiation of tube feeding.

VIII. **Metastases** at the abdominal insertion site have been reported after PEG tube placement in patients with cancers of the head, neck, or esophagus.

SUGGESTED READINGS

Gorman R, Nance ML, Morris JB: Enteral feeding techniques. In Torosian MH [ed]: Nutrition for the Hospitalized Patient: Basic Science and Principles of Practice. New York: CRC Press, 1995, pp 329–351.

Mullen JL, Morris JB, Yu JC: Enterostomies. In Daly JM, Cady B (eds): Atlas of Surgical Oncology. Philadelphia: Mosby-Year Book, 1993, pp 19–37.

Tapia J, Murguia R, Garcia G, et al: Jejunostomy: techniques, indications, and complications. World J Surg 23:596–602, 1999.

Weltz CR, Morris JB, Mullen JL: Surgical jejunostomy in aspiration risk patients. Ann Surg 215:140–145, 1992.

CHAPTER 11

Small Bowel Resection

Dale Han   and   Alan Schuricht

Case Study

A 65-year-old male presents to the emergency room complaining of crampy abdominal pain, nausea, and bilious vomiting that began 24 hours earlier. He has not had a bowel movement or passed flatus since the onset of symptoms. He underwent a right hemicolectomy 1 year earlier for colon cancer. He has no other significant medical history.

He is tachycardic. His abdomen is markedly distended, but minimally tender. Laboratory study findings are significant for a mild hypokalemic, hypochloremic metabolic alkalosis.

Supine and upright abdominal radiographs show dilated loops of small bowel, air–fluid levels, and minimal air in the colon, consistent with a small bowel obstruction. A computed tomography (CT) scan of the abdomen and pelvis shows dilated loops of small bowel and a point of transition to collapsed bowel in the right lower quadrant (Fig. 11-1).

BACKGROUND

The small intestine, the portion of the gastrointestinal (GI) tract located between the stomach and the ileocecal valve, is composed of three sections: the duodenum, jejunum, and ileum. The partially retroperitoneal duodenum is approximately 20 cm long and ends at the ligament of Treitz, a band of muscle that extends from the right crus of the diaphragm. Beyond the ligament of Treitz are the jejunum and ileum, which are attached to the retroperitoneum by a mesentery oriented obliquely from left to right and terminating at the cecum.

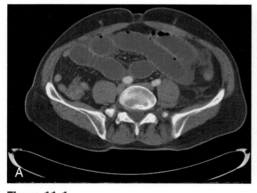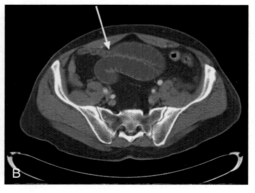

Figure 11-1
Computed tomography scan of the abdomen and pelvis. **A,** Multiple loops of small intestine are dilated, consistent with small bowel obstruction. **B,** There is a transition point (*arrow*) between dilated proximal small bowel and collapsed distal small bowel.

Digestion and absorption are the primary roles of the small intestine. Exocrine secretions from the liver and pancreas are delivered to the duodenum via the ampulla of Vater, and nutrients are absorbed through the small bowel mucosa. The small bowel is also the largest endocrine organ in the body and secretes numerous hormones that regulate both GI motility and pancreatic and gallbladder exocrine function. Finally, the small bowel protects the body from pathogens in the GI tract through a variety of mechanisms, including the secretion of mucin, peristalsis, and antigen sampling in lymphoid tissues (e.g., Peyer's patches).

A wide range of disease processes affect the small bowel, including embryologic defects (e.g., malrotation and intestinal atresia), inflammatory diseases (e.g., Crohn's disease), vascular diseases (e.g., mesenteric ischemia), and neoplasia. The surgical management of such processes may require the resection of small bowel, the topic of this chapter.

INDICATIONS FOR SMALL BOWEL RESECTION

I. **Small Bowel Obstruction**

A. Postoperative **adhesions** are the most common cause of small bowel obstruction. Other etiologies include **hernias** (e.g., inguinal and femoral), **volvulus, intussusception, benign and malignant tumors, Crohn's disease, gallstone ileus, foreign bodies, parasites, bezoars,** and **radiation enteritis.** Bowel obstructions are classified as **complete** or **partial.** This distinction is often inferred from the severity of clinical symptoms and radiographic findings (e.g., absence of colonic air on abdominal radiograph). Patients with a bowel obstruction typically present with nausea and vomiting, diffuse abdominal pain, abdominal distention, and obstipation. Dehydration may result from vomiting and GI fluid secretion into obstructed bowel. A potential endpoint of many obstructive processes is bowel ischemia. This may result from compromise of the vascular supply to the small bowel in an **incarcerated** hernia (**strangulation**) or from progressive distention of obstructed bowel, leading to increased wall pressure, obstruction of venous outflow, and subsequent arterial compromise.

B. The initial management of a small bowel obstruction includes nasogastric tube (NGT) decompression and fluid resuscitation. Small bowel obstructions resulting from adhesions are more likely to resolve without surgical management than are obstructions from other causes. Focal or worsening abdominal tenderness, signs of peritonitis, fever, hemodynamic instability, leukocytosis, and lactic acidosis, suggesting bowel compromise, require urgent operative exploration. In addition, patients with complete obstructions and those without a history of abdominal surgery are more likely to require early operative intervention. Operative management is primarily aimed at relieving the obstruction, which may require lysis of adhesions, hernia repair, or bowel resection.

II. **Perforation** may result from bowel necrosis as a result of a number of processes, including small bowel obstruction and **acute mesenteric ischemia.** Alternatively, perforation may occur without preceding necrosis of the small bowel wall (e.g., perforated small bowel tumors, perforated duodenal ulcers, and Crohn's disease). Patients typically present with fever, hemodynamic instability, and focal or generalized peritonitis. With few exceptions, bowel perforations mandate immediate surgical exploration and resection of perforated segments.

III. **Bleeding** from the small bowel may be caused by small bowel tumors or by **Meckel's diverticulum.** In the latter case, bleeding is usually caused by exposure of the surrounding small bowel mucosa to secretions from ectopic gastric mucosa within the diverticulum. Small bowel **arteriovenous malformations** and **hemangiomas** are two additional sources of small bowel bleeding.

IV. A **fistula** is defined as an abnormal connection between two epithelialized surfaces. Some examples of small bowel fistulas include enterocutaneous fistulas (fistula between bowel and skin) and fistulas between the small bowel and the urinary tract

> Has your patient had previous abdominal surgery?

or vagina. Small bowel fistulas may result from iatrogenic bowel injuries during surgery or an anastomotic leak after bowel resection. Additionally, cancer, Crohn's disease, infection, and radiation may all lead to fistula formation. Initial treatment of a small bowel fistula usually consists of bowel rest and total parenteral nutrition (TPN) to decrease fistula output and optimize nutrition. In some patients, this treatment leads to closure of the fistula tract. However, in patients in whom conservative management is unsuccessful, surgery is performed to excise the fistula tract and resect involved segments of bowel.

V. **Small bowel tumors** may be benign (e.g., adenomas, lipomas, hamartomas, and leiomyomas) or malignant (e.g., adenocarcinomas, carcinoids, leiomyosarcomas, and lymphomas). When a benign or malignant small bowel tumor is diagnosed, segmental resection is performed to relieve symptoms or prevent progression. If a small bowel mass is suspicious for malignancy, it should be resected with wide margins and sampling of the regional mesenteric lymph nodes.

> FRIEND is a mnemonic for factors that cause and maintain the patency of fistulae: **f**oreign body, **r**adiation, **i**nfection/ **i**nflammatory bowel disease, **e**pithelialization, **n**eoplasm, and **d**istal obstruction.

PREOPERATIVE EVALUATION

The preoperative evaluation for a small bowel resection frequently includes:

I. **Laboratory Studies:** Before a small bowel resection, a **complete blood count** and a **chemistry panel** are usually obtained. Leukocytosis may reflect an ongoing inflammatory or infectious process (e.g., Crohn's disease). In the setting of a small bowel obstruction, leukocytosis is a concerning finding and is sometimes indicative of bowel ischemia or perforation. Electrolyte abnormalities and an elevated blood urea nitrogen:creatinine ratio are characteristic in patients who are dehydrated (e.g., bowel obstruction or high-output fistula). An elevated **lactic acid** level reflects hypoperfusion of tissues and is often a late finding indicating tissue ischemia. Measurement of **albumin** and **prealbumin** levels allows for an assessment of nutritional status in patients with fistulae or Crohn's disease. In patients with suspected carcinoid tumors, obtaining a **5-HIAA** (a serotonin metabolite) level may help confirm the diagnosis.

> Carcinoids are neuroendocrine tumors that sometimes secrete serotonin. The small bowel is the second most common location for carcinoid tumors after the appendix.

II. **Abdominal Radiographs:** Abdominal radiographs are frequently obtained as part of an evaluation of abdominal symptoms. Dilation of the stomach and proximal bowel, air–fluid levels, and absent colonic gas suggest bowel obstruction. **Pneumoperitoneum,** typically seen as free air under the diaphragm, suggests perforation. An **obstruction series,** which consists of several radiographs obtained with the patient in different positions (typically, supine and upright abdominal and upright chest radiographs) may increase the sensitivity of the radiographic evaluation compared with a single image.

III. **CT Scan:** CT scans are valuable in determining the degree of bowel dilation, the presence of pneumoperitoneum, the viability of bowel, or the presence of a mass. When a CT scan is performed to evaluate a small bowel obstruction, failure of oral contrast to pass beyond a *transition point* between dilated and collapsed bowel suggests complete obstruction. The use of oral and intravenous contrast allows for more detailed images and should be administered, if possible.

> Pneumoperitoneum is best seen on an upright chest radiograph.

> INTRAVENOUS CONTRAST IS NEPHROTOXIC AND SHOULD BE AVOIDED IN PATIENTS WITH CHRONIC RENAL INSUFFICIENCY OR AN ACUTE INCREASE IN SERUM CREATININE LEVEL.

IV. **Miscellaneous Studies:** Several other studies may be useful in the evaluation of suspected small bowel pathology.

A. In an **upper GI series with small bowel follow-through,** the transit of oral contrast through the GI tract is observed under fluoroscopy. This study may help to localize points of obstruction, mucosal abnormalities, and fistulae.

B. A **fistulogram** involves the administration of contrast through an enterocutaneous fistula to delineate the anatomy of its tract.

C. A **Meckel's scan** involves intravenous administration of technetium-99, which is taken up by ectopic gastric mucosa and allows for visualization of the majority of Meckel's diverticula.

D. **CT angiography, magnetic resonance angiography,** and conventional **angiography** may be useful in the evaluation of acute mesenteric ischemia.

> Between 50% and 60% of Meckel's diverticuli contain ectopic gastric mucosa.

COMPONENTS OF THE PROCEDURE

Preoperative Considerations

I. Prophylactic **antibiotics** should be administered within 1 hour before skin incision.

II. Urinary catheterization is indicated to decompress the bladder and facilitate monitoring of intraoperative volume status.

III. An **NGT** is placed to decompress the stomach and proximal small bowel.

Patient Positioning and Preparation

The patient is placed in the supine position with the arms extended. The abdomen is prepped to the nipples superiorly, the pubic symphysis inferiorly, and the midaxillary lines laterally.

Incision and Exposure

I. Small bowel resection is typically performed through a midline incision large enough to allow for adequate exposure of the entire abdominal cavity.

II. After abdominal entry, the small bowel is inspected by *running the bowel.* This is accomplished using one of two techniques. In the first technique, the ligament of Treitz is identified and the small bowel is examined antegrade to the ileocecal valve (Fig. 11-2). The second technique involves identification of the cecum and retrograde inspection of the bowel to the ligament of Treitz.

Resection

I. Once the entire small bowel has been evaluated, attention is focused on the area of small bowel pathology. Selection of appropriate margins for resection is guided by the pathologic process. For example, small bowel tumors should be resected with wide margins. In contrast, resections for Crohn's disease should preserve as much bowel as possible.

II. An opening in the mesentery is created immediately adjacent to the bowel, at the proximal resection margin. Care must be taken to avoid injuring the vessels supplying the bowel margins, which will ultimately feed the anastomosis.

III. A surgical stapler is placed around the bowel, with the lower jaw inserted through the mesenteric opening. The stapler is fired, leaving two closed ends of transected bowel. The same technique is used to divide the bowel at the distal resection margin.

Figure 11-2
Identification of the ligament of Treitz. Visualization of the ligament of Treitz and the proximal jejunum requires cephalad retraction of the transverse colon. *(From Smith CE: Gastrointestinal surgery. In Rothrock JC, McEwen DR [eds]: Alexander's Care of the Patient in Surgery, 13th ed. St. Louis, Mosby, 2007, p 330.)*

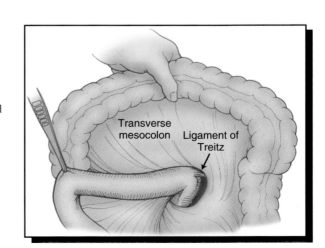

IV. The mesentery of the isolated bowel segment is ligated and divided, allowing for removal of the specimen from the abdomen.

Stapled Anastomosis

I. Corresponding corners of the proximal and distal staple lines are opened to expose the lumen of each bowel segment. A jaw of the surgical stapler is then inserted into each lumen, and the bowel segments are brought together side-to-side (i.e., lengthwise) by firing the stapler (Fig. 11-3).
II. The site of stapler insertion into the now common bowel lumen is closed.

> The stapler used to create small bowel anastomoses is called the *gastrointestinal anastomosis* (GIA). The GIA fires two staple lines and divides tissue between them.

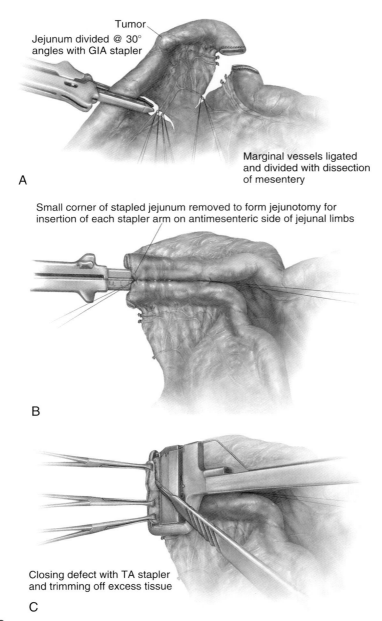

Tumor

Jejunum divided @ 30° angles with GIA stapler

Marginal vessels ligated and divided with dissection of mesentery

A

Small corner of stapled jejunum removed to form jejunotomy for insertion of each stapler arm on antimesenteric side of jejunal limbs

B

Closing defect with TA stapler and trimming off excess tissue

C

Figure 11-3

A, A gastrointestinal anastomosis (GIA) stapler is used to staple and cut proximal and distal small bowel resection margins. **B,** The jaws of the GIA stapler are placed into the openings made in each small bowel end. **C,** The remaining opening is closed with a thoracoabdominal (TA) stapler. *(From Martel G, Boushey RP: Stapled small bowel anastomoses. Operative Techniques in General Surgery 9:13–18, 2007.)*

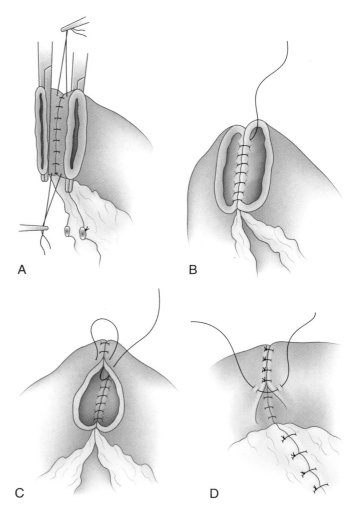

Figure 11-4 Hand-sewn two-layer small bowel anastomosis. **A,** Closure of the seromuscular layer of the posterior wall with interrupted sutures. **B,** Closure of the mucosa and inner layer of the posterior wall. **C,** Closure of the mucosa and inner layer of the anterior wall. **D,** Closure of the seromuscular layer of the anterior wall with interrupted stitches. *(From Liu KJM, Walker FW: Surgical procedures on the small intestines. In Zuidema GD [ed]: Shackelford's Surgery of the Alimentary Tract, 3rd ed. Philadelphia, Saunders, 1991, p 273.)*

Hand-Sewn Anastomosis

I. A small bowel anastomosis can be created without the use of surgical staplers. The small bowel is sharply divided with a scalpel, leaving two open ends that are brought together in two layers. An inner layer reapproximates the mucosa, and an outer layer reapproximates the seromuscular layers.

II. Typically, the posterior half of the seromuscular layer is sewn first. The inner layer is then sewn circumferentially. Finally, the anterior half of the seromuscular layer is completed (Fig. 11-4).

Irrigation and Closure of the Abdomen

The abdomen is irrigated with warm saline, and placement of the NGT within the stomach is verified before abdominal closure.

POSTOPERATIVE COURSE

The small bowel typically recovers function rapidly after surgery. Patients who undergo small bowel resection for bleeding or a tumor will often tolerate oral intake in the early postoperative period. In contrast, delayed return of bowel function is common after surgery for a bowel obstruction. This latter scenario often necessitates maintenance of an NGT, precluding feeding in the early postoperative period.

POTENTIAL COMPLICATIONS

I. In addition to technical complications, a number of factors increase the risk of **anastomotic dehiscence.** These factors include tension on the anastomosis, poor blood supply, infection, malnutrition, and immunosuppression. Anastomotic dehiscence may result in abscess or fistula formation. Patients with an anastomotic dehiscence may present with symptoms ranging from delayed bowel function to septic shock. Management is dependent on the timing and severity of symptoms. Stable patients are frequently managed with bowel rest, antibiotic therapy, and percutaneous drainage of intra-abdominal collections. Worsening clinical status and the presence of intra-abdominal collections that are not amenable to percutaneous drainage are indications for operative re-exploration.

> **TENSION MUST BE AVOIDED AND GOOD BLOOD SUPPLY ENSURED WHEN CREATING AN ANASTOMOSIS.**

II. A variety of devastating conditions (e.g., midgut volvulus, mesenteric vascular occlusion, and traumatic mesenteric vascular injuries) necessitate extensive bowel resections. **Short bowel syndrome** results when insufficient bowel remains to support a patient's nutritional needs. The syndrome is typically characterized by diarrhea, metabolic abnormalities, and nutritional deficiencies. Patients may require long-term nutritional support in the form of TPN delivered intravenously. However, long-term TPN is associated with a significant risk of infectious complications.

III. Resection of substantial segments of ileum may result in vitamin B_{12} malabsorption. Deficiencies of this vitamin cause megaloblastic **anemia and neuropathies.**

> Vitamin B_{12} and bile salts are absorbed in the ileum.

IV. Extensive loss of bile salts after ileal resection leads to **steatorrhea** and **fat-soluble vitamin deficiencies.**

SUGGESTED READINGS

Dayton MT: Small bowel obstruction. In Cameron JL (ed): Current Surgical Therapy, 8th ed. Philadelphia, Mosby, 2004, pp 105–110.

Evers BM: Small intestine. In Townsend CM, Beauchamp RD, Evers BM, Mattox KL (eds): Sabiston Textbook of Surgery: The Biological Basis of Modern Surgical Practice, 17th ed. Philadelphia, Saunders, 2004, pp 1323–1380.

Liu KJM, Walker FW: Surgical procedures on the small intestines. In Zuidema GD (ed): Shackelford's Surgery of the Alimentary Tract, 3rd ed. Philadelphia, Saunders, 1991, pp 264–285.

Smith CE: Gastrointestinal surgery. In Rothrock JC, McEwen DR (eds): Alexander's Care of the Patient in Surgery, 13th ed. St. Louis, Mosby, 2007, pp 297–355.

CHAPTER 12

Laparoscopic Cholecystectomy

E. Carter Paulson,   Robert E. Roses,   and   Jon B. Morris

Case Study

A 45-year-old female presents to the emergency department after several hours of persistent right upper abdominal pain, which became more severe after she ate dinner. She localizes the pain to the epigastrium and right upper quadrant and notes radiation to the right scapula. She recalls several less severe episodes of pain in a similar distribution over the previous year, typically after ingestion of fatty meals. These episodes usually resolved within 1 hour.

Her sclera are anicteric. Her abdomen is soft and nondistended. The right upper abdomen under the costal margin is exquisitely tender on palpation.

Laboratory evaluation is remarkable for mild leukocytosis. Other laboratory data, including liver function tests and pancreatic enzymes, are normal.

A right upper quadrant ultrasound is obtained, which shows gallstones and gallbladder wall thickening (Fig. 12-1). The common bile duct (CBD) is visualized and is of normal caliber.

BACKGROUND

The gallbladder is a pear-shaped organ located on the undersurface of the liver. The gallbladder functions as a concentrating reservoir for bile, which it delivers to the duodenum in response to meals. Gallbladder stones (cholelithiasis) and the complications associated with them are largely responsible for making cholecystectomy the most frequently performed gastrointestinal operation in the United States; approximately 700,000 cholecystectomies are performed annually.

The pathogenesis of cholesterol gallstones is multifactorial and involves excess cholesterol production by the liver as well as disordered gallbladder mucosal and motor function. **Biliary sludge,** a mixture of cholesterol crystals, calcium bilirubinate granules, and a

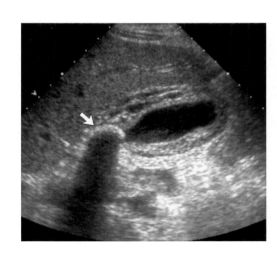

Figure 12-1
Gallbladder ultrasound demonstrating diffuse gallbladder wall thickening and shadowing from an impacted gallstone (*arrow*). *(From Goldman L, Ausiello DA: Cecil Medicine, 23rd ed. Philadelphia, Saunders, 2008.)*

mucin gel matrix, is observed frequently during prolonged fasting states. Mucin–bilirubin complexes are often found at the center of cholesterol stones, suggesting that sludge represents a precursor to stone formation.

Gallstones result from cholesterol supersaturation of bile. The primary components of bile (bile acids, phospholipids, and cholesterol) are normally maintained in solution in micelles. Cholesterol excess beyond a critical concentration may result in precipitation and stone formation. Although the majority of gallstones are composed of cholesterol (80%), a minority are composed of calcium bilirubinate and calcium palmitate, and are known as **pigment gallstones.** Pigment stones may be classified as **black,** usually associated with hemolytic conditions or cirrhosis, or **brown,** associated with disorders of biliary motility and bacterial infections.

Gallstones are common and are usually asymptomatic. Indeed, over a 20-year period, two thirds of individuals with gallstones remain asymptomatic. The remaining one third of individuals will either have pain (**biliary colic**) from transient obstruction of the cystic duct (the route of bile efflux from the gallbladder) or one of several complications of cholelithiasis. These complications include **acute cholecystitis, choledocholithiasis** with or without **cholangitis, gallstone pancreatitis,** and **gallstone ileus.** In general, cholecystectomy is not recommended for adults who have asymptomatic gallstones found on imaging or during surgery for another indication. Biliary colic and complicated gallstone disease, however, are indications for cholecystectomy and are discussed in more detail below.

INDICATIONS FOR CHOLECYSTECTOMY

I. **Biliary colic** (pain associated with transient obstruction of the cystic duct) is the most common indication for cholecystectomy. Episodes of biliary colic typically persist for 1 or more hours and may last as long as 24 hours. These episodes are characteristically precipitated by ingestion of fatty meals, although this is not always the case. Patients with symptomatic cholelithiasis are believed to be at higher risk for gallstone-related complications than are patients without symptoms. In addition to bringing about the resolution of symptoms, cholecystectomy in these patients serves to prevent the potential complications that comprise the other indications for this operation. Cholecystectomy is performed electively in patients with biliary colic, although severe or frequent symptoms may necessitate prompt intervention.

II. **Acute Calculous Cholecystitis:** More than 90% of cases of acute cholecystitis are related to gallstones. Persistent cystic duct obstruction leads to gallbladder distention and inflammation. Gallbladder ischemia and necrosis represent an endpoint of this process in severe cases. Patients typically present with persistent right upper quadrant pain, with or without nausea and vomiting. **Murphy's sign,** which is positive when a patient halts inspiration when the right upper quadrant of the abdomen is palpated, is characteristic. In rare instances, cholecystitis may present with systemic signs of sepsis. Cholecystectomy is the first-line treatment for acute cholecystitis and should be performed promptly after the diagnosis is confirmed. In selected cases, such as in the unstable or high-risk patient, **cholecystostomy** (drainage of the gallbladder) may be used as a temporizing measure. This procedure is commonly performed by interventional radiologists under fluoroscopic guidance, thus avoiding some of the risks associated with general anesthesia and conventional surgical management.

III. **Choledocholithiasis:** The preoperative evaluation of patients with calculous gallbladder disease should identify patients at risk for CBD stones. Signs and symptoms of choledocholithiasis may include jaundice, light-colored stools, dark-colored urine, elevated liver function test, and a dilated CBD on ultrasound (US) (>5 mm). Options for the evaluation and management of suspected choledocholithiasis include endoscopic retrograde cholangiopancreatography (ERCP), magnetic resonance cholangiopancreatography (MRCP), and intraoperative cholangiography at the time of cholecystectomy. Patients with choledocholithiasis may also present with **cholangitis,** a bacterial infection of the biliary ducts. The signs and symptoms of cholangitis include **Charcot's triad** (fever, jaundice, and abdominal pain) and **Reynold's pentad** (fever, jaundice, abdominal pain, hypotension, and mental status changes). The primary management of cholangitis is nonsurgical. Most cases resolve with antibiotics and supportive care. Gallstone-associated cholangitis that does not resolve after the initiation of medical management warrants endoscopic or percutaneous cholangiography, with biliary drainage and stone clearance, if possible. In rare circumstances, CBD exploration and T-tube (drain) placement may be lifesaving when other options are not feasible or have been unsuccessful.

IV. **Gallstone Pancreatitis:** Gallstones are responsible for the majority of cases of acute pancreatitis. Obstruction of the pancreatic duct by a CBD stone may resolve spontaneously after the passage of the stone into the duodenum. Worsening pancreatitis, however, sometimes reflects impaction of a common duct stone and persistent pancreatic duct obstruction. ERCP with stone extraction and sphincterotomy is the diagnostic and treatment modality of choice in patients with suspected gallstone pancreatitis, particularly when clinical indicators, including elevated levels of pancreatic enzymes, do not improve. Cholecystectomy should be performed after resolution of the symptoms of pancreatitis and normalization of pancreatic enzyme levels, but before hospital discharge. This recommendation is predicated on a high reported incidence of recurrent pancreatitis during the initial months after a first attack of gallstone pancreatitis.

V. **Biliary dyskinesia** resembles biliary colic in symptoms. The diagnosis is made when gallbladder imaging (US, CT scan) does not show gallstones. **Cholescintigraphy (HIDA)** demonstrating a decreased gallbladder ejection fraction confirms the diagnosis. Between 85% and 95% of patients with a low gallbladder ejection fraction and characteristic symptoms report improvement after cholecystectomy.

VI. **Acute acalculous cholecystitis** clinically resembles acute calculous cholecystitis. The pathogenesis of cholecystitis in the absence of stone disease is poorly understood, but acalculous cholecystitis most often afflicts the critically ill. Cholecystectomy is curative. **Cholecystotomy**, however, is frequently an appropriate management strategy in these patients, given their frequent high degree of acuity and the efficacy and potentially definitive nature of simple drainage of the gallbladder in the absence of gallstones.

VII. **Gallstone ileus** is a mechanical obstruction of the gastrointestinal tract. It is caused by the passage of a large-diameter gallstone through a spontaneous biliary–enteric fistula (most often between the gallbladder and the duodenum). Gallstone ileus most commonly affects elderly patients and mandates a laparotomy to relieve the bowel obstruction (usually with enterolithotomy). Cholecystectomy and biliary–enteric fistula take-down may be performed at the time of laparotomy or, if inflammation precludes safe dissection during the initial operation or the patient is unstable, at a subsequent time.

VIII. **Gallbladder cancer** is an aggressive malignancy that largely afflicts the elderly and is more common in women than in men. Unfortunately, most patients with gallbladder cancer have unresectable disease at the time of presentation, and the estimated 5-year survival rate among all patients with this malignancy is less than 15%. In the setting of suspected carcinoma of the gallbladder, open abdominal exploration should be undertaken. This approach facilitates an evaluation for metastatic disease and facilitates radical cholecystectomy (en bloc resection of the gallbladder and adjacent liver as well as regional lymphadenectomy), in the event that no metastases are identified. Importantly, suspicion of gallbladder cancer during laparoscopic cholecystectomy should prompt conversion to an open operation.

PREOPERATIVE EVALUATION

In addition to a review of standard preoperative studies, reassessment of all studies obtained in evaluating a patient with gallbladder pathology is essential because laboratory data and

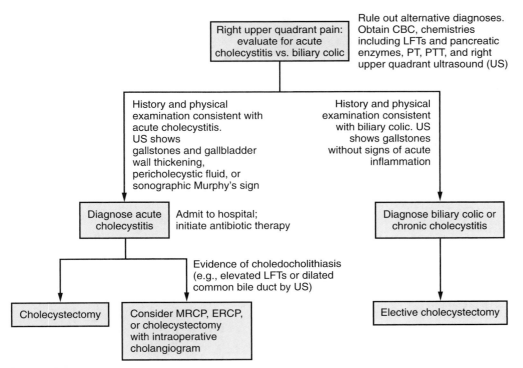

Figure 12-2
Algorithm for the evaluation of right upper quadrant pain suspicious for either biliary colic or acute cholecystitis, the two most common indications for cholecystectomy. CBC, complete blood count; ERCP, endoscopic retrograde cholangiopancreatography; LFT, liver function test; MRCP, magnetic resonance cholangiopancreatography; PT, prothrombin time; PTT, partial thromboplastin time.

study results significantly influence management (Fig. 12-2). Of particular importance are:

I. **Liver function tests** (LFTs), which include alanine aminotransferase, aspartate aminotransferase, bilirubin, alkaline phosphatase, and pancreatic enzymes (amylase and lipase), are essential to the evaluation of biliary pathology. Elevation of LFTs, particularly serum bilirubin, are predictive of CBD stones. Decisions to obtain a preoperative MRCP or ERCP or to perform an intraoperative cholangiogram at the time of cholecystectomy are sometimes predicated on these values. Elevated pancreatic enzymes are indicative of pancreatitis. These levels should be allowed to normalize before cholecystectomy, and interrogation of the CBD, whether by MRCP, ERCP, or intraoperative cholangiogram, is performed in conjunction with cholecystectomy after gallstone pancreatitis.

> Should your patient undergo preoperative ERCP or additional imaging to evaluate the common bile duct?

II. **Abdominal Ultrasound:** In addition to documenting the presence of gallstones, notable findings on preoperative US include pericholecystic fluid, gallbladder wall thickening, and a sonographic Murphy's sign, all of which are consistent with cholecystitis. A dilated CBD is suggestive of the presence of, or recent passage of, a CBD stone.

III. **Cholescintigraphy (HIDA):** This noninvasive modality can provide important diagnostic information and is most frequently obtained when acute cholecystitis is suspected, but US findings are equivocal. Technetium-labeled analogues of iminodiacetic acid are administered intravenously. These compounds are rapidly excreted into the biliary tract. Enhancement of the liver, gallbladder, CBD, and duodenum within 1 hour is anticipated under normal circumstances. Nonvisualization of the gallbladder, with filling of the CBD and duodenum, suggests cystic duct obstruction and is consistent with acute cholecystitis.

IV. **CT scan** is frequently obtained in the evaluation of nonspecific abdominal pain. Although it is not sensitive for the detection of gallstones, it is sensitive for the diagnosis of acute cholecystitis.

COMPONENTS OF THE PREOCEDURE AND APPLIED ANATOMY

Patient Positioning and Preparation

I. The patient is placed in the supine position with the arms extended.
II. The abdomen is prepared to the xiphoid superiorly, to the pubic bone inferiorly, and to the midaxillary lines laterally.

Preoperative Considerations

I. Prophylactic **antibiotics** for elective laparoscopic cholecystectomy are advocated by some surgeons. Antibiotics are routinely administered to patients with acute cholecystitis at the time of admission and should be continued throughout the perioperative period.
II. **Urinary catheter** placement before cholecystectomy is often unnecessary. If conversion to an open cholecystectomy is likely or if there is reason to believe that the procedure will take longer than usual, urinary catheter placement should be considered.

Port Placement

In general, laparoscopic cholecystectomy is performed through four operative ports (Fig. 12-3).

I. **Placement of the Umbilical Port**
A. Access to the abdomen may be obtained with a "blind" percutaneous technique using a Veress needle or an open technique. Although each approach has its proponents, the open technique is more commonly used. It is important to note that the open technique is mandatory for patients who are pregnant or have had previous abdominal surgery.
B. Open technique umbilical port placement
1. A horizontal incision is made above the umbilicus.
2. Subcutaneous soft tissue is bluntly dissected to expose the anterior rectus muscle fascia.
3. The fascia and underlying peritoneum are divided at the midline under direct vision.

> Has your patient had previous abdominal surgery?

Figure 12-3
Port placement for laparoscopic cholecystectomy. *(From Cameron J: Atlas of Surgery, vol 2. Philadelphia, Decker, 1994.)*

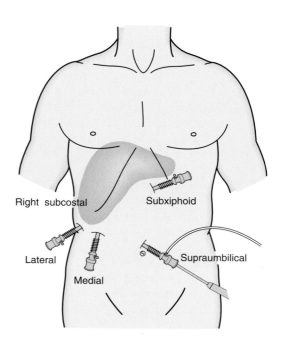

4. Fascial sutures are placed to secure the port and minimize CO_2 leakage and loss of pneumoperitoneum.
5. The port is inserted through the incision with a blunt-tipped trocar.
6. CO_2 is insufflated through the port. The abdomen should distend symmetrically and become uniformly tympanic. If this does not happen, extraperitoneal port placement should be suspected.
7. The laparoscope is inserted through the umbilical port, and the peritoneal cavity is surveyed.

II. **Placement of the Remaining Ports**
   A. After the laparoscope is inserted, the remaining three ports are inserted under direct intra-abdominal visualization. A cutting (sharp) introducer is used to penetrate the fascia and enter the peritoneal cavity.
   B. Epigastric port placement
      1. An epigastric port serves as the main operating port for the case.
      2. The port is usually placed at the midline at the approximate level of the gallbladder on the abdominal wall and angled to the right of the falciform ligament on insertion into the peritoneal cavity.
   C. First (medial) accessory port placement
      1. This port is used for retraction of the gallbladder fundus.
      2. The port is generally placed at the midclavicular line, just beneath the costal margin.
   D. Second (lateral) accessory port placement
      1. The second port is used for retraction of the gallbladder infundibulum.
      2. The port is generally placed at the anterior axillary line, halfway between the costal margin and the anterior superior iliac spine.

Exposure

I. Clear visualization of the gallbladder is sometimes obscured by adhesions involving the gallbladder, liver edge, omentum, duodenum, and colon. When possible, these adhesions should be gently dissected away from the gallbladder without the use of electrocautery to avoid injury to adjacent organs.
II. The fundus of the gallbladder is grasped, and the gallbladder is retracted cephalad toward the patient's left shoulder.
III. With a second instrument, the gallbladder is grasped near the infundibulum, and lateral and inferior traction is applied. This maneuver allows for exposure of the triangle of Calot and increases the angle between the cystic duct and the CBD, allowing for safer dissection (Fig. 12-4).
IV. Exposure is further facilitated by elevating the head of the bed (reverse Trendelenburg positioning), with the left side of the table down.

> The triangle of Calot is the space bounded by the liver edge, the cystic duct, and the common hepatic duct.

Dissection

I. With a curved dissector, the peritoneum is stripped from the base of the gallbladder, beginning at the infundibulum and continuing medially toward the junction of the gallbladder and the cystic duct.
II. Surrounding tissue is bluntly dissected away from the cystic duct. The cystic artery, which is most often cephalad and posterior to the cystic duct, is exposed in similar fashion (Fig. 12-5).

Division of the Cystic Duct and Cystic Artery

I. Three surgical clips, two placed proximally and one placed distally, are applied to the exposed cystic duct.
II. The duct is divided sharply between the proximal and distal clips.
III. The same technique is used to divide the cystic artery.

> THE CYSTIC DUCT AND ARTERY MUST BE CLEARLY DEFINED BEFORE THE APPLICATION OF SURGICAL CLIPS TO AVOID INADVERTENT COMMON BILE DUCT INJURIES.

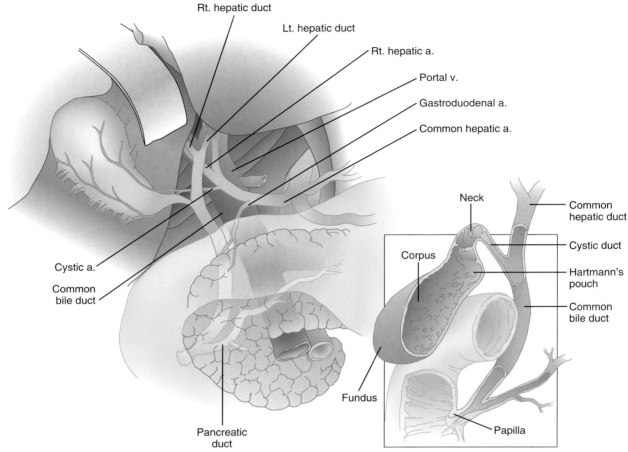

Figure 12-4

The gallbladder sits on the undersurface of the liver within the gallbladder fossa. It is partially covered by the peritoneum. The gallbladder may be divided into the fundus, body (corpus), infundibulum, and neck. The gallbladder empties into the cystic duct, which joins the common hepatic duct to form the common bile duct. The cystic artery, which supplies the gallbladder, is most often a branch of the right hepatic artery and runs medial and parallel to the cystic duct. The artery courses through the triangle of Calot, the space bounded by the liver edge, the cystic duct, and the common hepatic duct. *(From Townsend CM, Beauchamp RD, Evers BM, Mattox KL [eds]: Sabiston Textbook of Surgery: The Biological Basis of Modern Surgical Practice, 17th ed. Philadelphia, Saunders, 2004.)*

Removal of the Gallbladder from the Liver Bed

INSPECT THE GALLBLADDER FOSSA FOR ACTIVE BLEEDING BEFORE DIVISION OF THE FINAL ATTACHMENTS BETWEEN THE GALLBLADDER AND LIVER.

I. The gallbladder is retracted downward and to the right to expose the plane between it and the gallbladder fossa.
II. Electrocautery is used to dissect the gallbladder free from the liver.
III. Toward the conclusion of the dissection, retraction of the gallbladder over the top of the liver to expose the plane of dissection between the posterior wall of the gallbladder and the liver is often helpful.
IV. Before division of the final attachments between the liver and the gallbladder, the liver bed is irrigated and inspected for ongoing bleeding (Fig. 12-6).

Extraction of the Gallbladder

I. The camera is inserted through the epigastric port.
II. If the gallbladder is small and intact, it can be removed directly through the umbilical port. Alternatively, it may be removed in a sterile bag, which is introduced through the umbilical port, closed around the gallbladder, and withdrawn (Fig. 12-7).

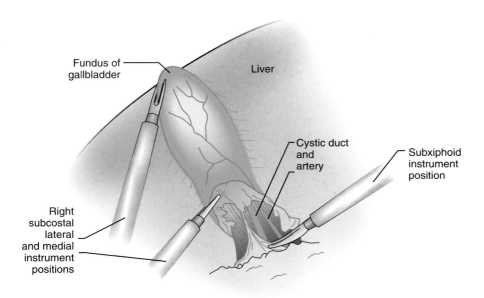

Figure 12-5
Dissection. *(From Cameron J: Atlas of Surgery, vol 2. Philadelphia, Decker, 1994.)*

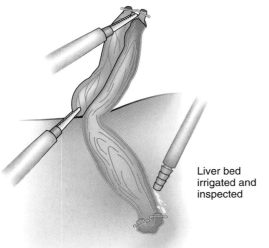

Figure 12-6
Removal of the gallbladder from the liver bed. *(From Cameron J: Atlas of Surgery, vol 2. Philadelphia, Decker, 1994.)*

Removal of the Ports and Closure of the Port Sites

I. The trocars are then removed sequentially under direct vision to evaluate for bleeding.

II. The fascia is reapproximated at the umbilical port site.

III. The four incisions are closed.

ADDITIONAL OPERATIVE CONSIDERATIONS

I. Routine or selective **drainage** of the gallbladder bed is advocated by some surgeons. The presence of a drain in the initial postoperative period may facilitate the early diagnosis of a bile leak or postoperative bleeding. When a drain is placed, the absence of bilious bloody drainage on the first postoperative day is frequently an indication for drain removal.

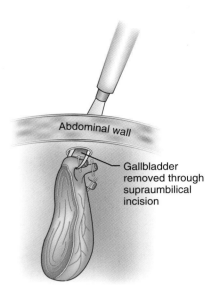

Figure 12-7
Extraction of the gallbladder. *(From Cameron J: Atlas of Surgery, vol 2. Philadelphia, Decker, 1994.)*

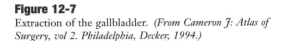

Should your patient undergo an intraoperative cholangiogram?

II. Although routine **intraoperative cholangiography** has its proponents, most surgeons apply this technique selectively. Most often, intraoperative cholangiogram is performed when a patient undergoing cholecystectomy has a history, signs, or symptoms consistent with choledocholithiasis (e.g., history of pancreatitis, elevated serum bilirubin level, dilated CBD by US), but has not undergone MRCP or ERCP preoperatively. In these instances, a cholangiogram consistent with CBD stones prompts either CBD exploration or, more often, postoperative ERCP.

III. The rate of **conversion to open cholecystectomy** during an elective laparoscopic cholecystectomy is 5%. This rate is significantly higher (30%) in the setting of acute cholecystitis, where inflammation can make the identification of normal anatomy and tissue planes, and the dissection, more challenging. Conversion to an open approach, usually performed through a right subcostal incision, may facilitate the identification of anatomic landmarks and allow for safer dissection and better hemostasis. Patients should be counseled about the possibility of conversion to open surgery in advance. Conversion to an open procedure should not be viewed as a complication, but as an important surgical option.

POSTOPERATIVE COURSE

I. After an uncomplicated laparoscopic cholecystectomy for biliary colic and gallstones, patients frequently feel well with limited analgesia and can tolerate a regular diet. Laparoscopic cholecystectomy for this indication is increasingly being performed as an outpatient procedure.

II. After laparoscopic cholecystectomy for acute cholecystitis, patients should be observed overnight. These patients can often tolerate a liquid diet, if not a regular diet, in the immediate postoperative period. If a drain is left in place and the drainage is nonbilious and nonbloody on the morning of the first postoperative day, it may be removed. Postoperative laboratory work is usually unnecessary in the absence of concerning postoperative symptoms.

Complications

A number of intraoperative and long-term complications are associated with laparoscopic cholecystectomy. In addition to the always present risks of surgical site infection and bleeding, these include:

I. **Bowel Injuries:** Bowel injuries can occur during port placement or during dissection of adhesions. Thermal injuries from the electrocautery device can occur at sites distant from the operative field due to arcing of the electrical current in the abdomen. Bowel injuries recognized at the time of surgery are repaired immediately. Those injuries that are discovered postoperatively usually mandate operative re-exploration.

II. **CBD Injuries:** CBD injuries are rare (<1%), but serious complications of laparoscopic cholecystectomy. CBD transection may result from misidentification of anatomic landmarks because of anomalous anatomy, inadequate exposure, or overaggressive retraction that brings the CBD and cystic duct into alignment. These injuries may or may not be evident at the time of surgery. They are frequently associated with significant short- and long-term morbidity and often mandate complex biliary reconstructive procedures.

III. **Bile Leaks:** Bile leaks most commonly emanate from the ducts of Luschka (cholecystohepatic ducts). These ducts form a communication between the gallbladder and the right lobe of the liver, and they can be transected when the gallbladder is dissected from the liver bed. The cystic duct stump may leak bile as a result of inadequate placement of surgical clips, because of clip failure or displacement, or from a traction injury. Patients may present with bilious output from a surgical drain or some combination of abdominal discomfort, leukocytosis, elevated LFTs, and fever. Depending on the patient's clinical presentation, a suspected bile leak may be evaluated with US, cholescintigraphy, ERCP, laparoscopy, laparotomy, or some combination of these.

> PROLONGED OR SEVERE ABDOMINAL PAIN AFTER CHOLECYSTECTOMY SHOULD RAISE SUSPICION FOR A BILE LEAK OR BILIARY OBSTRUCTION.

IV. **Retained Gallstones:** Retained gallstones are stones left in the cystic duct stump or biliary system after a laparoscopic cholecystectomy. Patients may present with signs or symptoms of choledocholithiasis as long as 2 years after cholecystectomy. A number of modalities allow for the diagnosis of retained stones, including cholescintigraphy, MRCP, and ERCP, which may also be therapeutic in this setting.

Postoperative Evaluation for Suspected Complications

Patients with postoperative symptoms, such as severe abdominal pain, a prolonged ileus, a persistent fever, or jaundice, should be carefully evaluated for a surgical complication. In addition to a thorough physical examination and basic laboratory work, the evaluation of these patients may include the following tests:

I. **LFTs** are frequently elevated in the setting of a bile leak, biloma (intraperitoneal bile collection), or choledocholithiasis.

II. **Abdominal US** frequently allows for identification of postoperative fluid collection, sometimes indicating a bile leak or postoperative abscess.

III. **Cholescintigraphy** frequently identifies bile leaks and obstruction from stones or aberrantly placed clips.

IV. In addition to diagnosing bile leaks and biliary duct obstruction with great sensitivity, **ERCP** is potentially therapeutic. Endoscopists can frequently retrieve retained CBD stones or stent the CBD to decrease pressure in the biliary tree, facilitating cystic duct stump leak closure.

SUGGESTED READINGS

Ahrendt SA, Pitt HA: Biliary tract. In Townsend CM, Beauchamp RD, Evers BM, Mattox KL (eds): Sabiston Textbook of Surgery: The Biological Basis of Modern Surgical Practice, 17th ed. Philadelphia, Saunders, 2004, pp 1597–1622.

Collins C, Maguire D, Ireland A, et al: A prospective study of common bile duct calculi in patients undergoing laparoscopic cholecystectomy: natural history of choledocholithiasis revisited. Ann Surg 239:28–33, 2004.

CHAPTER 13

Hepatectomy

Paige M. Porrett   and   Kim M. Olthoff

Case Study

A 52-year-old male is found to have a mass in his sigmoid colon during a screening colonoscopy. Pathologic evaluation of the biopsy specimens confirms the diagnosis of adenocarcinoma. An elective sigmoidectomy is planned; however, a preoperative computed tomography (CT) scan of his abdomen to evaluate for metastatic disease shows a 3-cm hypodense solitary mass within the right lobe of the liver. Results of liver function tests (LFTs), complete blood count, chemistry panel, and coagulation studies (prothrombin time [PT], partial thromboplastin time [PTT], and international normalized ratio [INR]) are all within normal limits. He is otherwise healthy, without any known medical comorbidities, and the rest of the metastatic workup is normal.

BACKGROUND

Although once associated with significant morbidity and high mortality rates, improvements in surgical technique, anesthetic management, and postoperative care have made liver resection a viable treatment option for a variety of benign and malignant processes. At centers specializing in hepatobiliary surgery, overall mortality and morbidity rates are now estimated at 1% to 5% and 30% to 40%, respectively.

After resection, a residual liver volume of 25% to 40% is usually sufficient. Fatty infiltration of the liver (steatosis), advanced age, fibrosis, and cirrhosis limit the extent of resection that can be performed safely.

A variety of liver resections are commonly performed, including limited resections (e.g., tumor *enucleation* or *wedge resection*) and anatomic resections (i.e., removal of a segment or lobe of the liver). The extent of hepatic resection undertaken is, in part, dictated by the type of pathology and its anatomic location. Additionally, the choice of operation depends on the patient's hepatic reserve. Up to 80% of the liver parenchyma can be removed from a normal liver because the remaining segment will hypertrophy and hepatic function will be restored within days to weeks. In the presence of underlying liver disease, however, significantly less liver parenchyma can be safely removed. The Child's classification and its modifications are commonly used to assess a patient's hepatic functional reserve (Table 13-1). In patients classified as Child's class C, hepatic resection should not be attempted because of the very high risk of postoperative liver failure. Even in patients with well-compensated cirrhosis who are classified as Child's class A, only limited hepatic resection should be performed.

Does your patient have normal underlying liver function?

INDICATIONS FOR HEPATECTOMY

There are three primary indications for partial hepatectomy in adults: neoplasm, infection, and to provide a liver lobe for transplantation.

I. **Neoplasm:** The majority of liver resections in the United States are performed for malignant disease, most commonly for metastatic cancer. Additionally, the increasing burden of hepatocellular carcinoma (HCC) in the United States because

TABLE 13-1 Child-Pugh Criteria for Hepatic Functional Reserve

Criterion	Score		
	1	**2**	**3**
Encephalopathy (grade)	None	1 or 2	3 or 4
Ascites	None	Mild	Moderate
Bilirubin (mg/dL)	≤2	2.1–3	≥3.1
Albumin (g/dL)	≥3.5	2.8–3.4	≤2.7
Prothrombin time	1–4	4.1–6	≥6.1
Class	**Total Points**		
A	5–6		
B	7–9		
C	10–15		

Data from Blumgart LH (ed): Surgery of the Liver, Biliary Tract, and Pancreas, 4th ed. Philadelphia, Saunders, 2007.

of chronic hepatitis C virus infection and cirrhosis has made liver resection and transplantation for HCC more common. In contrast, hepatic resection for cholangiocarcinoma remains relatively uncommon because the majority of patients with this malignancy present with advanced, unresectable disease.

A. **Malignant Neoplasms**
1. **Metastatic cancer:** The liver is the first site of metastases in most patients with advanced **colorectal cancer.** The 5-year survival rate is improved by hepatic resection in appropriately selected patients with colorectal metastases. Generally, patients with three or fewer lesions confined to one lobe of the liver are considered candidates for resection, as are patients with more than three lesions that shrink in response to chemotherapy. Hepatic resection of metastases is rarely beneficial unless it renders the patient free of disease. Contraindications to partial hepatectomy include: (1) involvement of more than six of the eight anatomic liver segments with tumor, (2) involvement of more than 70% of the liver, and (3) involvement of all three hepatic veins. Although optimal margins for resection have not been clearly defined, some studies suggest that patients who undergo anatomic resection (i.e., resection of a lobe or segment of the liver) have superior outcomes compared with those who receive wedge resection. Combinations of resection with local ablative techniques (e.g., radiofrequency ablation) have also been explored for the treatment of patients with multiple metastases.

   > Partial hepatectomy may be considered for the treatment of metastatic breast cancer and melanoma, in addition to metastatic colon cancer.

2. **Hepatocellular carcinoma:** The surgical management of HCC is frequently complicated by the presence of cirrhosis. Patients who have limited disease and undergo expeditious liver transplantation have superior disease-free survival compared with those who undergo hepatic resection. The United Network for Organ Sharing (UNOS) prioritizes patients who have HCC for transplantation on the basis of the *Milan criteria*; these include solitary tumors smaller than 5 cm or three or fewer masses, each less than 3 cm in size. Currently, most patients who receive priority listing receive transplants within 90 to 120 days. In contrast, limited resection should be considered in patients with well-compensated cirrhosis (i.e., Child's class A or no portal hypertension). In the absence of cirrhosis, anatomic hepatic resection is the treatment of choice for HCC (Fig. 13-1).

3. **Cholangiocarcinoma:** Cholangiocarcinomas are malignancies of the biliary epithelia. These tumors may be classified as intrahepatic, perihilar, or distal extrahepatic. Surgical resection of the bile duct and associated hepatic parenchyma affords the only chance for cure. However, because of their

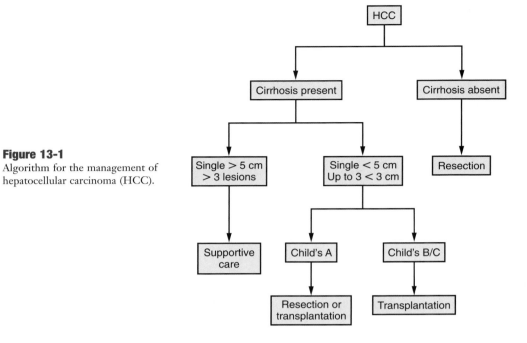

Figure 13-1
Algorithm for the management of
hepatocellular carcinoma (HCC).

aggressive nature, a minority (<10%) of these tumors are resectable. Partial
hepatectomy is indicated in patients with intrahepatic or perihilar disease,
whereas pancreaticoduodenectomy (i.e., Whipple procedure) is performed
in patients with resectable distal disease.

B. **Benign neoplasms:** The majority of liver masses are benign. Most are discovered incidentally and do not require resection in the absence of symptoms. The
most common benign tumors are **hemangiomas**, **focal nodular hyperplasia**,
and adenomas. Hepatic **adenomas** are associated with a risk of spontaneous
intra-abdominal hemorrhage and malignant degeneration and sometimes
require resection. Adenomas have been linked to the use of oral contraceptives
(OCPs), and discontinuation of these agents constitutes first-line therapy.
Indications for resection of adenomas include size greater than 2 cm in the
absence of OCP use and subcapsular location. Enucleation or wedge resection
is usually adequate therapy.

II. **Infection:** Infection is a rare indication for hepatic resection. Percutaneous drainage of liver abscesses has supplanted hepatic resection and open surgical drainage
in the majority of cases of bacterial or fungal infection. However, hepatic resection
still plays an important role in the management of parasitic cystic diseases of the
liver. Some cysts are treated with drainage and obliteration of the cyst cavity or
total cyst excision (pericystectomy). These more conservative surgical procedures
are not appropriate for the treatment of large intrahepatic **echinococcal cysts**
(hydatid cysts). Although patients with hydatid cysts are generally treated with
albendazole, in many patients, medical treatment is unsuccessful and surgery is
required. Such cysts are best treated with partial hepatectomy to avoid spillage of
the cyst contents into the peritoneal cavity, which is associated with disseminated
cystic disease and a risk of anaphylaxis.

III. **Living-Related Liver Transplantation:** Living-related liver transplantation has
evolved in response to the severe shortage of organ donors. The donation of liver
lobes from adults into pediatric recipients has been widely practiced since the
1980s. These operations typically involve resection and transplantation of a small
left lateral segment. Living-related transplantation is more challenging in adults

**INTRAPERITONEAL SPILLAGE
OF THE CONTENTS OF A
HYDATID CYST CAN RESULT IN
DISSEMINATED DISEASE AND
ANAPHYLAXIS.**

because of the requirement for greater hepatic mass. Right hepatic lobectomy is usually necessary to provide sufficient liver volume.

PREOPERATIVE EVALUATION

The preoperative evaluation for partial hepatectomy focuses on determining: (1) the amount and location of hepatic parenchyma that should be resected and (2) whether the remaining liver will be sufficient to sustain the patient physiologically.

I. **Radiographic Evaluation:** Contrast-enhanced CT scan and magnetic resonance imaging (MRI) are the imaging modalities of choice during the planning of a partial hepatectomy. The extent of involvement of venous, arterial, and biliary structures in the potential resection specimen must be delineated. Cross-sectional imaging techniques, such as magnetic resonance angiography and magnetic resonance cholangiography, can also be extremely useful for preoperative planning, particularly for living-related donor hepatectomy. Additionally, *volumetric CT and MRI* allow measurement of hepatic volume and can assist in estimating postoperative remnant volume before planned partial hepatectomy.

> Cross-sectional imaging can also identify evidence of portal hypertension, such as splenomegaly or the presence of venous collaterals.

II. **Laboratory Evaluation:** Liver function may be estimated by serologic tests, including LFTs (serum aspartate aminotransferase [AST], alanine aminotransferase [ALT], total bilirubin, and alkaline phosphatase) and coagulation parameters (PT, PTT, INR). Albumin may be used as a marker of long-term protein production, and thrombocytopenia may reflect hypersplenism and portal hypertension. Serum α-fetoprotein levels can be useful in confirming the diagnosis of HCC and can be followed after resection to detect recurrence.

III. **Tests of Metabolic Capacity:** A variety of tests can be performed to more accurately assess physiologic hepatic function. Tests that measure protein synthesis, microsomal and cytosolic function, hepatic perfusion, and functional hepatocyte mass are available at some centers. *Clearance of indocyanine green* from the bloodstream can be used to assess hepatic function and has been shown to predict hospital mortality and survival rates after hepatic resection in patients with cirrhosis. Other tests that measure quantitative hepatic metabolic capacity include erythromycin breath tests, galactose elimination capacity, and salivary caffeine clearance.

IV. **Liver Biopsy:** Biopsy of the liver can provide important information about the presence or absence of normal hepatic architecture, fibrosis, cirrhosis, and fatty infiltration. Liver histology can be helpful preoperatively in determining how much liver can be resected (Fig. 13-2).

COMPONENTS OF THE PROCEDURE AND APPLIED ANATOMY

Resection Nomenclature

Cantlie's line divides the liver into the right hemiliver (segments V–VIII) and the left hemiliver (segments II–IV), which are the segments that are commonly resected during right and left **hepatectomy,** respectively. Resection of the hepatic parenchyma to the left of the falciform ligament (segments II and III) is called **left lateral segmentectomy.** Resection of the hepatic parenchyma to the right of the falciform ligament (segments IV–VIII) has multiple names, including **extended right hepatectomy, right trisegmentectomy,** and **right lobectomy,** depending on which nomenclature system is used (Fig. 13-3 and Box 13-1). Other limited *anatomic resections,* including specific segmental resections that follow the segmental anatomy of the liver, can be performed as well. During nonanatomic *wedge resections,* the parenchyma and vessels are divided without consideration of the internal hepatic anatomy. Wedge resections are most commonly used for small peripheral tumors in patients with benign disease or in patients with malignant disease who cannot tolerate a formal lobectomy.

> What operation does your patient require?

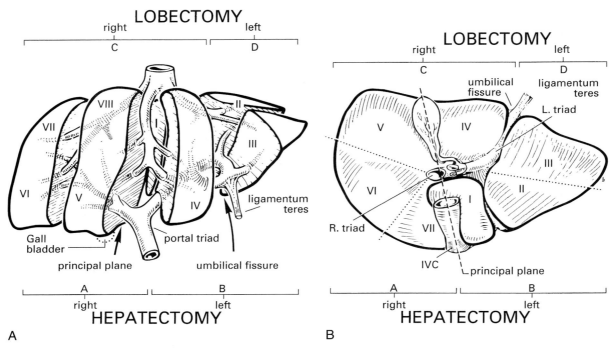

LOBECTOMY
right   left
C   D

VIII
VII   I
VI   V   II
III
IV
Gall
bladder
principal plane
portal triad
umbilical fissure
ligamentum
teres
A
right   left
A   B
HEPATECTOMY

A

LOBECTOMY
right   left
C   D

umbilical
fissure
ligamentum
teres
V   IV
L. triad
VI   I   III
R. triad   II
VII
IVC   principal plane
A
right   left
A   B
HEPATECTOMY

B

Figure 13-2
The internal segmental anatomy of the liver. **A,** Exploded anterior view. The liver is divided into the right and left *hemiliver* by *Cantlie's line,* which connects the gallbladder bed and the inferior vena cava. Each hemiliver is additionally divided into *sectors* (separated by the hepatic veins that run through the vertically oriented scissurae) and eight *segments* supplied by individual portal pedicles. Each pedicle consists of a portal venous branch, an arterial branch, and a branch of the common hepatic duct. All segments are drained by the three main hepatic veins that empty posteriorly into the retrohepatic inferior vena cava (IVC). Although the liver is externally divided by the falciform ligament, this division does not correspond to the internal segmental anatomy. **B,** Inferior view of the liver. Cantlie's line from the gallbladder bed to the IVC is shown. *(Adapted from Blumgart LH [ed]: Surgery of the Liver, Biliary Tract, and Pancreas, 4th ed. Philadelphia, Saunders, 2007.)*

Figure 13-3
Commonly performed hepatic resections. Shading indicates the portion of liver removed during the procedures. **A,** Right hepatectomy. **B,** Left hepatectomy. **C,** Right trisegmentectomy. **D,** Left lateral segmentectomy. **E,** Left trisegmentectomy. *(Adapted from Blumgart LH [ed]: Surgery of the Liver, Biliary Tract, and Pancreas, 4th ed. Philadelphia, Saunders, 2007.)*

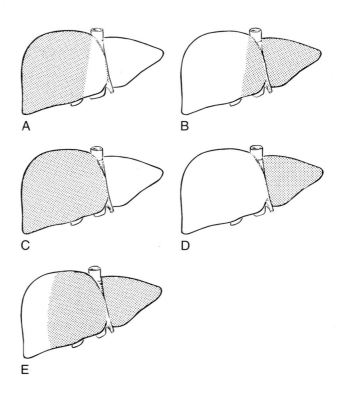

BOX 13-1 Nomenclature of Hepatic Resections

Couinaud (1957)

Right hepatectomy (segments V, VI, VII, VIII)

Left hepatectomy (segments II, III, IV)

Right lobectomy* (segments IV, V, VI, VII, VIII)

Left lobectomy (segments II, III)

Extended left hepatectomy† (segments II, III, IV, V, VIII) [see Fig. 13-3B]

Goldsmith and Woodburne (1957)

Right hepatic lobectomy

Left hepatic lobectomy

Extended right hepatic lobectomy*

Left lateral segmentectomy

Extended left lobectomy†

*Also referred to as a right trisegmentectomy (Starzl, 1975, 1980).
†Also referred to as a left trisegmentectomy (Starzl, 1982).
Data from Blumgart LH [ed]: Surgery of the Liver, Biliary Tract, and Pancreas, 4th ed. Philadelphia, Saunders, 2007.

Preoperative Considerations

I. Preoperative **antibiotics** that cover gram-positive and gram-negative organisms are given within 1 hour before incision.

II. **Urinary catheterization** is indicated to decompress the bladder and monitor intraoperative and postoperative volume status.

III. Placement of a **nasogastric tube** is indicated to decompress the stomach and enhance exposure.

IV. Liver resections may be associated with substantial blood loss, large fluid requirements, and wide fluctuations in blood pressure. **Arterial lines** are commonly indicated to allow for continuous blood pressure monitoring. **Central venous catheters** are often inserted to provide durable venous access and allow for the assessment of volume status.

Patient Positioning and Preparation

I. The patient is placed in the supine position.

II. The sterile preparation should extend to the nipples superiorly, to the pubis inferiorly, and to the posterior axillary lines laterally.

Incision and Exposure

I. Although most hepatic resections can be performed through a right subcostal incision, additional exposure sometimes requires midline or left subcostal extension. Very rarely, a median sternotomy is required to access the intrapericardial inferior vena cava (IVC) (Fig. 13-4).

II. The abdominal cavity is entered, and the abdomen is explored. The liver is evaluated by inspection and bimanual palpation.

III. In many circumstances, especially in patients with malignant disease, an intraoperative ultrasound is useful in confirming the findings of preoperative studies and determining the relationship of the tumor to major vascular structures within the hepatic parenchyma. Enlarged lymph nodes may be sent for frozen section examination to rule out extrahepatic metastases.

IV. The liver is mobilized by selectively dividing its peritoneal attachments. For most resections, the liver is mobilized from the anterior abdominal wall by dividing the falciform ligament (Fig. 13-5).

V. The liver's attachments to the diaphragm, including the right and left triangular ligaments, are selectively divided, depending on the portion of the liver to be

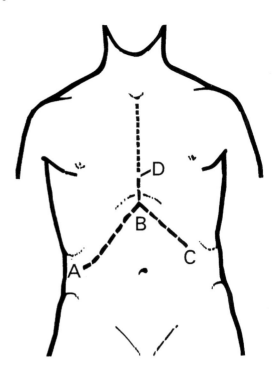

Figure 13-4
Incisions for partial hepatectomy. Liver resection is most often performed via a right subcostal incision with midline extension (ABD). Alternatively, a right subcostal incision with left subcostal extension (ABC) may be used. (*Adapted from Blumgart LH [ed]: Surgery of the Liver, Biliary Tract, and Pancreas, 4th ed. Philadelphia, Saunders, 2007.*)

removed (Figs. 13-6 and 13-7). If an anterior wedge resection is to be performed, these ligaments do not have to be divided.

Inflow and Outflow Control

I. Vascular inflow (i.e., hepatic artery and portal vein) and outflow (i.e., hepatic veins and IVC) control are obtained to minimize bleeding during parenchymal transection.

II. If a total lobectomy is to be performed, the hepatic artery and portal vein to that lobe can be dissected and divided. This can be achieved either through dissection of the extrahepatic right or left hepatic arteries or through transection of these pedicles within the liver substance after an opening is created in the liver parenchyma (i.e., hepatotomy) near the liver hilum. More selective inflow control can be obtained by dissecting branches of the hepatic artery or portal vein to specific segments.

III. Outflow control is achieved by dissecting and encircling the specific hepatic vein to the lobe or segment to be removed. Often, these veins are not divided until some portion of the parenchymal dissection has been performed, to allow for decompression of the lobe (Figs. 13-8 and 13-9).

IV. Total hepatic vascular exclusion is an alternative method by which vascular control is obtained. This technique is performed by clamping the IVC above and below the liver. The hepatic artery and the portal vein are controlled via Pringle's maneuver (Fig. 13-10). Total vascular exclusion of the liver can be associated with significant hemodynamic changes. Therefore, this procedure is used only in select patients in whom more selective methods of inflow and outflow control are inadequate (e.g., patients with large tumors in close proximity to the major hepatic veins or IVC).

Parenchymal Transection

I. The hepatic parenchyma can be divided with a fracture technique, crushing the liver with clamps (Fig. 13-11). Newer devices, such as the ultrasonic dissector or

BEFORE MAJOR HEPATIC RESECTION, PATIENTS SHOULD BE CROSSMATCHED FOR BLOOD.

Pringle's maneuver is performed by transiently occluding the portal triad and can be used to limit bleeding during hepatic transection. Five-minute periods of portal triad occlusion followed by 1-minute periods of reperfusion are generally well tolerated by patients with normal underlying liver function.

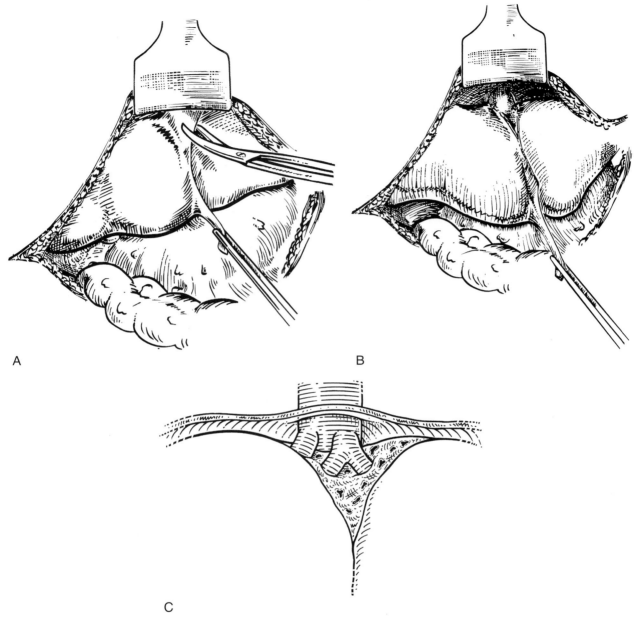

A

B

C

Figure 13-5
Mobilization of the liver from the anterior abdominal wall via division of the falciform ligament. **A** and **B**, The falciform ligament is divided.
C, The hepatic venous outflow and vena cava are exposed. *(Adapted from Blumgart LH [ed]: Surgery of the Liver, Biliary Tract, and Pancreas, 4th ed. Philadelphia, Saunders, 2007.)*

water-jet dissector, are effective and may offer an additional degree of safety because they help to expose blood vessels before division.

II. Bleeding from the cut hepatic surface is controlled with electrocautery, an argon beam coagulator, or suture ligation. Pringle's maneuver may be helpful in limiting bleeding from the hepatic remnant during hepatic transection.

ADDITIONAL OPERATIVE CONSIDERATIONS

I. **Laparoscopic liver resections** are being performed with increasing frequency as surgeons become more comfortable with this technique. Laparoscopic resection is typically limited to wedge resection of small peripheral lesions. Although major

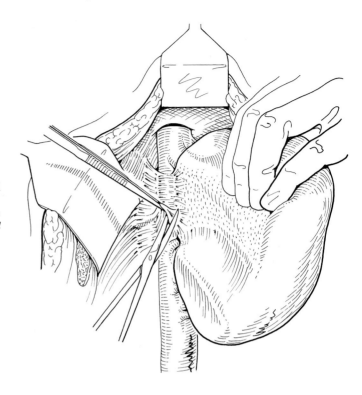

Figure 13-6
Mobilization of the right hemiliver. The right triangular ligament between the liver and the diaphragm is divided. This maneuver exposes the right lateral margin of the inferior vena cava and allows for additional exposure of the right hepatic vein. *(Adapted from Blumgart LH [ed]: Surgery of the Liver, Biliary Tract, and Pancreas, 4th ed. Philadelphia, Saunders, 2007.)*

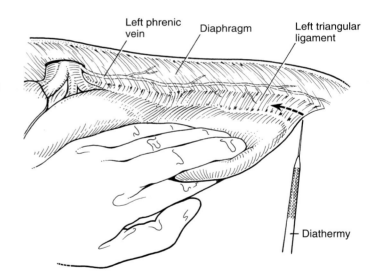

Figure 13-7
Mobilization of the left hepatic lobe. The left hepatic lobe is suspended from the diaphragm by the left triangular ligament. Division of this ligament is required for left hepatectomy and left lobectomy. *(Adapted from Blumgart LH [ed]: Surgery of the Liver, Biliary Tract, and Pancreas, 4th ed. Philadelphia, Saunders, 2007.)*

anatomic hepatectomy has been performed laparoscopically, this approach has not been widely adopted. In patients who undergo laparoscopic resection, decreased length of stay has been reported.

II. Placement of a closed suction **drain** near the transected liver edge may facilitate monitoring for bleeding and bile leakage in the immediate postoperative period.

POSTOPERATIVE COURSE

I. Most patients who undergo uncomplicated major anatomic hepatectomy will be discharged from the hospital within 5 to 10 days. Intravenous or epidural analgesia is often necessary in the early postoperative period.

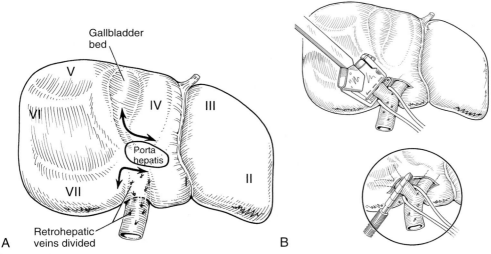

Figure 13-8

Selective approach to the right portal pedicle. **A,** *Curved arrows* indicate where the hepatotomy will be performed to access the right portal pedicle. **B,** After the hepatic parenchyma overlying the right portal pedicle is divided, it is encircled with a vessel loop. A stapler can then be used to divide the pedicle. *(Adapted from Blumgart LH [ed]: Surgery of the Liver, Biliary Tract, and Pancreas, 4th ed. Philadelphia, Saunders, 2007.)*

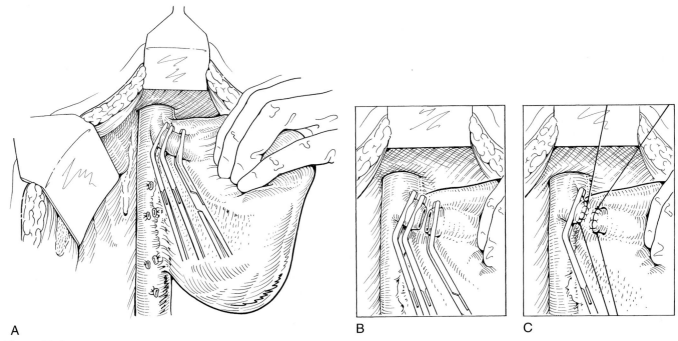

Figure 13-9

Selective approach to the right hepatic vein. **A,** After mobilization of the right hepatic lobe, the right hepatic vein is exposed. Clamps are placed on the vein before division. **B,** The vein is divided between two clamps. **C,** The venous stumps are oversewn. *(Adapted from Blumgart LH [ed]: Surgery of the Liver, Biliary Tract, and Pancreas, 4th ed. Philadelphia, Saunders, 2007.)*

II. Complications

A. A **bile leak** from the cut surface of the liver, and development of a biloma (bile collection), can complicate postoperative recovery. This complication presents within days of surgery and may be heralded by the appearance of bile in the surgical drain, abdominal pain, or an elevated white blood cell count. Infection of a biloma can result in abscess formation.

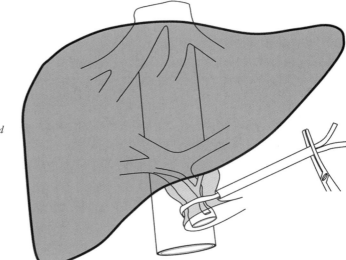

Figure 13-10
Pringle's maneuver. Hepatic pedicle clamping occludes hepatic arterial and portal inflow. *(Adapted from Blumgart LH [ed]: Surgery of the Liver, Biliary Tract, and Pancreas, 4th ed. Philadelphia, Saunders, 2007.)*

> What is the character of the drain output (e.g., bilious or bloody)?

B. **Postoperative bleeding** from the cut surface of the liver is a relatively rare complication of liver resection. Hemoglobin levels and hemodynamic parameters are monitored closely postoperatively.

C. **Biliary stricture or obstruction** is typically a later complication and presents with jaundice, elevations in total bilirubin, persistent pain in the right upper quadrant, and anorexia.

D. Hepatic function is also closely monitored in the postoperative period, because **hepatic insufficiency** can occur. This is most commonly observed in patients with compromised liver function who undergo major anatomic resection. In patients with a normal liver, serum ALT and AST levels peak 6 hours after surgery and remain elevated for approximately 3 days. After partial hepatectomy, levels of serum AST and ALT (transaminases) do not usually increase more than 10- to 15-fold; this increase is due to injury of hepatocytes during the procedure. In contrast to this expected mild *transaminitis*, elevation of coagulation parameters (e.g., INR) several days after hepatectomy is suggestive

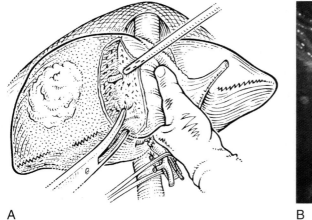

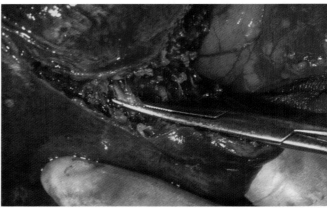

A   B

Figure 13-11
Parenchymal transection during right hepatectomy. Individual intrahepatic vessels are exposed and ligated as parenchymal transection progresses. Transection proceeds along a line of demarcation that develops after division of the right portal triad. **A,** Schematic. **B,** Intraoperative photograph. An intrahepatic vessel is encountered and clamped during parenchymal transection. *(Adapted from Blumgart LH [ed]: Surgery of the Liver, Biliary Tract, and Pancreas, 4th ed. Philadelphia, Saunders, 2007.)*

of hepatic insufficiency. Unfortunately, if severe hepatic insufficiency persists, no curative therapy is available other than liver transplantation.

SUGGESTED READINGS

Are C, Gonen M, Zazzali K, et al: The impact of margins on outcome after hepatic resection for colorectal metastasis. Ann Surg 246:295–300, 2007.

Baccarani U, Benzoni E, Adani GL, et al: Superiority of liver transplantation versus resection for the treatment of small hepatocellular carcinoma. Transplant Proc 39:1898–1900, 2007.

Blumgart LH (ed): Surgery of the Liver, Biliary Tract, and Pancreas, 4th ed. Philadelphia, Saunders, 2007.

Mazzaferro V, Regalia E, Doci R, et al: Liver transplantation for the treatment of small hepatocellular carcinomas in patients with cirrhosis. N Engl J Med 334:693–699, 1996.

Olthoff KM, Merion RM, Ghobrial RM, et al: Outcomes of 385 adult-to-adult living donor liver transplant recipients: a report from the A2ALL Consortium. Ann Surg 242:314–323, 2005.

Pawlik TM, Choti MA: Surgical therapy for colorectal metastases to the liver. J Gastrointest Surg 11:1057–1077, 2007.

CHAPTER 14

Pancreatic Resection

Paul J. Foley   and   Jeffrey A. Drebin

Case Study

A 65-year-old male is referred to a surgeon for evaluation of a pancreatic mass. He reports a 2-month history of progressive jaundice, anorexia, and loss of 15 pounds. Additionally, he notes intermittent dull upper abdominal pain, light-colored stools, and tea-colored urine. He was recently seen by a gastroenterologist and underwent endoscopic retrograde cholangiopancreatography (ERCP), which showed narrowing of the distal common bile duct and pancreatic duct; a biliary stent was placed during the procedure. A subsequent computed tomography (CT) scan of the abdomen and pelvis showed a mass in the head of the pancreas without evidence of metastases or vascular encasement or invasion (Fig. 14-1).

On physical examination, his sclerae are icteric. His abdomen is soft and nontender. No mass or lymphadenopathy is appreciated. Results of laboratory testing are remarkable for a conjugated hyperbilirubinemia and an elevated CA 19-9 level. Liver enzymes, amylase, and lipase levels are within normal limits.

BACKGROUND

The pancreas is a retroperitoneal structure located behind the stomach and lesser omentum; it is composed of four anatomic regions: head, neck, body, and tail. The head lies medial to the C-loop of the duodenum. The neck lies anterior to the mesenteric vessels and portal vein. The body and tail extend obliquely toward the hilum of the spleen. The uncinate process, an extension of the pancreatic head, wraps posteriorly around the superior mesenteric vessels.

The majority of pancreatic resections are performed for neoplasia. Generally, pancreaticoduodenectomy (Whipple procedure) is performed for lesions near the head of the pancreas and ampulla of Vater. Distal pancreatectomy is reserved for lesions of

Figure 14-1
Computed tomography scan. There is a mass in the head of the pancreas (*black arrowhead*) adjacent to the duodenum (*white arrowhead*). A stent is seen in the intrapancreatic segment of the common bile duct (*asterisk*). The superior mesenteric artery (*black arrow*) and the superior mesenteric vein (*white arrow*) are not involved.

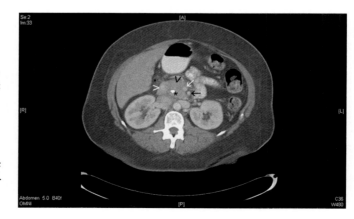

the body and tail. Total pancreatectomy, an infrequently performed procedure, is indicated for rare pancreatic malignancies that involve the entire gland. This chapter focuses on indications for and technical aspects of pancreaticoduodenectomy and distal pancreatectomy.

INDICATIONS FOR PANCREATIC RESECTION

Malignancies of the periampullary region are the most common indication for pancreaticoduodenectomy. These include primary pancreatic head and neck malignancies, distal common bile duct lesions, cancer of the ampulla of Vater, and periampullary duodenal cancers. Lesions localized to the body and tail of the pancreas (to the left of the mesenteric vessels) can be treated with distal pancreatectomy.

I. **Pancreatic Adenocarcinoma:** Surgical resection remains the only potentially curative therapy for adenocarcinoma of the pancreas. Pancreaticoduodenectomy is indicated for tumors of the pancreatic head, whereas body and tail lesions are treated with distal pancreatectomy and splenectomy. Because of the aggressive nature of most pancreatic tumors, most are diagnosed at an advanced stage and only 20% of lesions are resectable at the time of diagnosis. Locally advanced cancers are deemed unresectable if they extend beyond the pancreatic parenchyma and invade or encase adjacent vascular structures (e.g., the mesenteric vessels or portal vein). Patients with locally advanced tumors may be candidates for neoadjuvant therapy consisting of chemotherapy and radiation. Resection in this patient population is sometimes possible after treatment if tumor characteristics are favorable on repeat imaging studies. Patients with metastatic disease receive no survival benefit from pancreaticoduodenectomy, but may be offered palliative therapies. Nonsurgical palliative interventions include biliary stenting, chemotherapy, radiation, and chemical neurolysis of the celiac plexus. Surgical palliation, including Roux-en-Y hepaticojejunostomy or choledocojejunostomy to relieve biliary obstruction and gastrojejunostomy to relieve duodenal obstruction, are often performed simultaneously (i.e., *double bypass*) when metastatic disease is discovered at the time of surgical exploration. In patients with pancreatic cancer, the median survival time after resection with curative intent is 16 to 24 months. Patients with metastatic disease fare much worse, with a median survival of less than 6 months.

Pancreatic cancer is the fourth leading cause of cancer-related death in the United States.

II. **Pancreatic Cystic Neoplasms:** Cystic neoplasms of the pancreas include serous cystic neoplasms, mucinous cystic neoplasms, and intraductal papillary mucinous neoplasms (IPMNs). Combined, these represent fewer than 10% of all pancreatic neoplasms. Distinguishing cystic neoplasms from inflammatory pseudocysts, which are much more common, often poses a considerable diagnostic challenge. Smaller mucinous cystic neoplasms (<3 cm) with favorable imaging criteria and serous cystic neoplasms, which are almost always benign, may be monitored with serial imaging. In contrast, IPMNs are more likely to harbor invasive carcinoma and should generally be resected.

III. **Pancreatic Neuroendocrine Tumors:** Neuroendocrine tumors of the pancreas are a rare and heterogeneous group of lesions that includes insulinomas, glucagonomas, gastrinomas, somatostatinomas, and VIPomas. These tumors can arise sporadically or as a part of the multiple endocrine neoplasia (MEN) I syndrome. Symptoms result from overproduction of biologically active hormones. Gastrinomas are associated with the Zollinger-Ellison syndrome, which is characterized by gastric acid hypersecretion and intractable peptic ulcer disease. Gastrinomas and somatostatinomas are frequently malignant and should be resected with appropriate margins. Insulinomas are most often benign and can be enucleated. Insulinomas and glucagonomas are most often found in the body and tail of the pancreas. In contrast, somatostatinomas and gastrinomas are more often found in the pancreatic head.

MEN I is a hereditary syndrome characterized by parathyroid hyperplasia and tumors of the pancreatic islet cells and pituitary gland.

IV. **Ampulla of Vater Neoplasms:** Ampullary adenomas may be sporadic or associated with familial cancer syndromes, such as familial adenomatous polyposis (FAP).

These adenomas are associated with a risk of malignant degeneration and are therefore treated with resection.

V. **Periampullary Duodenal Neoplasms:** Like ampullary adenomas, duodenal adenomas may be sporadic or may be associated with familial cancer syndromes, such as FAP or Peutz-Jeghers syndrome. Duodenal adenomas can progress to adenocarcinoma and should be removed when discovered. Inability to achieve complete excision, either endoscopically or via a transduodenal surgical approach, is an indication for pancreaticoduodenectomy. Duodenal adenocarcinoma is likewise treated with pancreaticoduodenectomy.

VI. **Distal Common Bile Duct Strictures:** Obstructive jaundice may result from benign or malignant biliary strictures. The most common cause of a benign stricture is iatrogenic injury (e.g., during cholecystectomy). Other causes include recurrent or chronic pancreatitis and choledocholithiasis. Malignant etiologies include primary bile duct cancers (cholangiocarcinoma) and pancreatic neoplasms. Pancreaticoduodenectomy is indicated if a malignant stricture is diagnosed or suspected.

VII. **Sequelae of Chronic Pancreatitis:** Inflammation of the pancreas can lead to scarring and stenosis of the pancreatic duct and common bile duct. Inflammatory masses in the setting of chronic pancreatitis and ductal strictures are often difficult to distinguish from pancreatic neoplasia. If the diagnosis of neoplasia cannot be excluded, such masses should be resected. Pancreatic resections may also be indicated for the management of intractable pain in the setting of chronic pancreatitis, although other operative procedures may be preferable.

VIII. **Trauma:** Injury to the pancreas may result from blunt or penetrating trauma. The management of pancreatic trauma is largely dependent on the severity and location of injury. Penetrating injuries to the head of the pancreas are typically associated with concomitant injuries to surrounding structures, including the duodenum, bile duct, or liver. Severe devitalizing injuries to the pancreatic head, duodenum, and distal common bile duct may require pancreaticoduodenectomy. The mortality rate associated with a Whipple procedure performed in this setting approaches 60%. Injuries localized to the body and tail are best treated with a distal resection, with or without splenectomy.

PREOPERATIVE EVALUATION

I. **History and Physical Examination:** In the patient with a pancreatic mass, a history of abdominal pain, back pain, loss of appetite, vomiting, weight loss, and jaundice, should be elicited. Back pain may indicate invasion of a tumor into the retroperitoneum. Vomiting suggests a gastric outlet obstruction. In the presence of metastatic disease, physical examination may reveal an umbilical nodule (Sister Mary Joseph's node) or left supraclavicular lymphadenopathy (Virchow's node). Digital rectal examination may reveal peritoneal implants in the pelvis (Blumer's shelf).

II. **Computed Tomography and Magnetic Resonance Imaging:** An enhanced CT scan of the abdomen and pelvis with fine cuts through the pancreas is useful for localizing a mass, delineating its relationship to the superior mesenteric vessels and portal vein, and detecting metastatic disease. Magnetic resonance imaging may be helpful if CT scan findings are equivocal and is of particular utility in the evaluation of suspected liver metastases.

III. **Endoscopy:** Esophagogastroduodenoscopy and ERCP allow for the evaluation of the stomach, duodenum, common bile duct, and pancreatic duct. Biliary stenting can be performed in conjunction with ERCP for the treatment of obstructive jaundice. Endoscopic ultrasound and ultrasound-guided fine-needle aspiration (FNA) may be used to evaluate the pancreas and peripancreatic lymph nodes for the presence of disease, to determine the relationship of a tumor to adjacent vascular structures, and to obtain a tissue diagnosis. Although preoperative FNA of pancreatic masses is commonly performed, preoperative tissue diagnosis is not essential before proceeding with a pancreatic resection if pancreatic cancer is strongly suspected.

IV. **Laboratory Testing:** Preoperative laboratory testing should include a complete blood count and electrolyte panel, including blood urea nitrogen and creatinine levels. Serum albumin, liver-associated enzyme, bilirubin, prothrombin time, and partial thromboplastin time should be measured because many patients with pancreatic disease are malnourished and have impaired liver synthetic function and some degree of biliary obstruction. The level of CA 19-9, a serum tumor marker, is often elevated in patients with pancreatic cancer and should be measured preoperatively. In cases of suspected pancreatic endocrine neoplasia, laboratory confirmation of hormone hypersecretion should be sought. A type and screen with crossmatch should be obtained for all patients before pancreatic resection.

V. **Diagnostic Laparoscopy:** In some series, up to 30% of patients with pancreatic carcinoma that is determined to be resectable by preoperative imaging are found to have metastatic disease to the liver or peritoneal surfaces at the time of exploration. Laparoscopy can be used to explore the abdomen before commiting to an unnecessary laparotomy (Fig. 14-2). Some surgeons use laparoscopic ultrasonography to allow for a more sensitive examination of the liver. The indications for diagnostic laparoscopy in pancreatic cancer are evolving.

> Is the lesion resectable?

COMPONENTS OF PANCREATIC RESECTION AND APPLIED ANATOMY

See Figure 14-3.

Preoperative Considerations

I. Preoperative antibiotics covering bowel and biliary flora are administered within 1 hour before skin incision.

II. A Foley catheter is placed to decompress the bladder and facilitate intraoperative assessment of volume status.

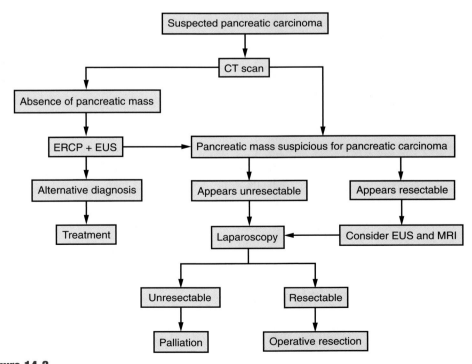

Figure 14-2
The evaluation of a suspected pancreatic carcinoma. CT, computed tomography; ERCP, endoscopic retrograde cholangiopancreatography; EUS, endoscopic ultrasound; MRI, magnetic resonance imaging.
(Modified from Cameron JL [ed]: Current Surgical Therapy, 8th ed. Philadelphia, Mosby, 2004.)

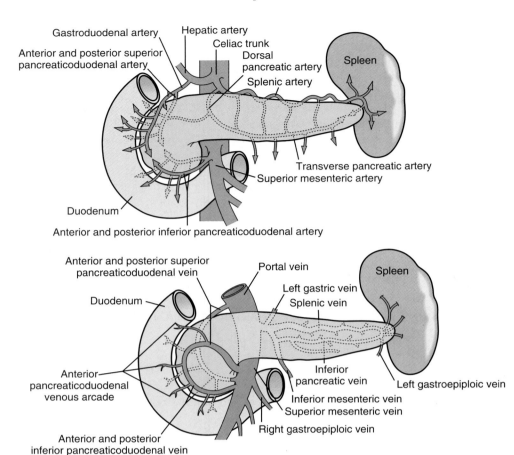

Figure 14-3
Arterial supply (*top*) and venous drainage (*bottom*) of the pancreas and duodenum. *(From Skandalakis JE, Gray SW, Rowe JS Jr, et al: Anatomical complications of pancreatic surgery. Contemp Surg 15:17–50, 1979. Reprinted with permission.)*

   III. A central venous catheter is often inserted to facilitate hemodynamic monitoring
        and intraoperative resuscitation.

Patient Positioning and Preparation

   I. The patient is placed in the supine position.
   II. The sterile preparation should extend to the nipples superiorly, the inguinal
        regions inferiorly, and the midaxillary lines laterally.

Whipple Procedure

The classic pancreaticoduodenectomy includes a gastric antrectomy. Most surgeons today
perform a pylorus-preserving operation, which is associated with a shorter operative time
and less blood loss. The pylorus-preserving operation is described.

   I. **Incision and Exploration**
      A. Pancreaticoduodenectomy may be performed through either a vertical midline
         or a bilateral subcostal incision.
      B. On entering the peritoneal cavity, a thorough exploration of all peritoneal
         surfaces, the liver, and omentum is undertaken. Suspicious lesions are identi-
         fied, and biopsy specimens are obtained and sent for frozen section examina-
         tion. If metastases are discovered, the planned resection is aborted and a
         palliative bypass procedure may be performed.

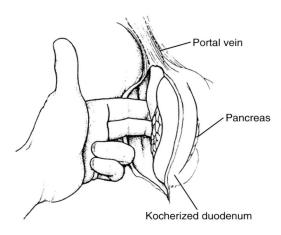

Portal vein

Pancreas

Kocherized duodenum

Figure 14-4
Kocher maneuver. The peritoneum lateral to the duodenum is incised, and the duodenum and pancreatic head are rotated to the patient's left. *(From Cameron JL [ed]: Current Surgical Therapy, 8th ed. Philadelphia, Mosby, 2004.)*

II. Right Colon Mobilization and Kocher Maneuver
A. The right colon and hepatic flexure are mobilized by dividing the peritoneal attachments along the white line of Toldt, exposing the duodenum.
B. Peritoneal attachments lateral to the duodenum are incised (Kocher maneuver) to allow for medial rotation of the duodenum and pancreatic head (Fig. 14-4).
C. Mobilization of the third portion of the duodenum allows for assessment of the relationship between the tumor and the superior mesenteric artery (SMA) and vein (SMV) as they pass posterior to the pancreatic neck.

III. Cholecystectomy and Periportal Dissection
A. The gallbladder is dissected off the liver bed with electrocautery, beginning at the fundus and continuing toward the neck. The cystic artery and duct are ligated and divided separately.
B. After removal of the gallbladder, dissection of the porta hepatis is performed and the portal vein, hepatic artery, and common bile duct and common hepatic duct are identified. The common hepatic duct is dissected free from adjacent vascular structures and transected above the cystic duct stump. Regional lymph nodes are dissected down toward the resection specimen.
C. The gastroduodenal artery (GDA) is identified as it arises from the common hepatic artery and is divided. The remaining stump is doubly ligated to minimize the risk of rebleeding. Division of the GDA allows for clear exposure of the portal vein as dissection continues behind the pancreatic neck.
D. The dissection is continued inferiorly along the avascular plane between the anterior surface of the portal vein and the neck of the pancreas.
E. The plane behind the pancreatic neck is then developed from an inferior approach. The gastrocolic omentum is divided between clamps to allow for access to the lesser sac. The stomach is retracted superiorly and the transverse colon is retracted inferiorly to expose the pancreas. The SMA and SMV are identified by following the middle colic vessels down to their origin. The pancreas is then dissected off the anterior surface of the SMV until the pancreatic neck is free.

IV. Division of the Pancreas, Duodenum, and Proximal Jejunum (Removal of the Specimen)
A. The postpyloric duodenum is divided with a surgical stapler.
B. The pancreatic neck is sharply divided. Bleeding from the distal cut edge of the pancreas confirms adequate perfusion to support healing of the pancreaticojejunostomy. If the cut edge does not bleed, the distal pancreas may be cut back further.
C. The uncinate process is dissected away from the SMA and SMV. Vascular branches in this region are divided between ties.

D. The small bowel is divided with a stapler at a point approximately 10 to 20 cm distal to the ligament of Treitz. The mesenteric branches supplying the isolated segment of jejunum and distal duodenum are divided. The ligament of Treitz is fully mobilized, and the distal duodenum and jejunum are passed beneath the SMA and SMV. As the specimen is reflected back toward the patient's right, any remaining duodenal attachments or vascular branches between the superior mesenteric vessels and the pancreas are divided.

E. The specimen is oriented for the pathologist with sutures placed on the pancreatic neck, uncinate process, and common hepatic duct.

V. **Reconstruction (Pancreaticojejunostomy, Hepaticojejunostomy, and Duodenojejunostomy)** (Fig. 14-5)

A. An opening is created in the transverse mesocolon to the right of the middle colic vessels through which the distal end of the divided jejunum is delivered. A pancreatic duct–to–small bowel mucosa anastomosis is performed in an end-to-side fashion (i.e., end of pancreatic duct to side of jejunum). If the pancreatic duct is small, the anastomosis can be performed over a stent (typically, a small-caliber feeding tube) to maintain the patency of the duct during healing. Reinforcing sutures are placed between the pancreatic capsule and the seromuscular layer of the jejunum.

B. An end-to-side hepaticojejunostomy is created distal to the pancreaticojejunostomy.

C. A mobile segment of the jejunum distal to the hepaticojejunostomy is brought up to the duodenum in an antecolic fashion (in front of and over the top of the transverse colon). The duodenal staple line is opened, and an end-to-side anastomosis (end of duodenum to side of jejunum) is performed. After completion of the duodenojejunostomy, the nasogastric tube can be advanced past the anastomosis.

D. The abdomen is irrigated, inspected to confirm hemostasis, and then closed.

Distal Pancreatectomy

I. **Incision and Exploration**

A. Distal pancreatectomy may be performed through either a vertical midline or a left subcostal incision.

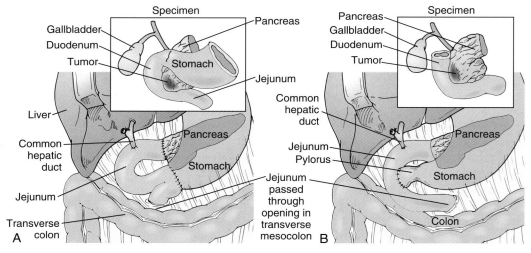

Figure 14-5
Reconstructed anatomy after a classic (**A**) and pylorus-preserving (**B**) Whipple procedure. *(From Cameron JL: Current status of the Whipple operation for periampullary carcinoma. Surg Rounds 77–87, 1988.)*

B. On entering the peritoneal cavity, a thorough exploration of all peritoneal surfaces, the liver, and the omentum is undertaken. If suspicious lesions are found, biopsy specimens are obtained and sent for frozen section examination. If metastases are discovered at this point, the planned resection is aborted.

II. **Exposure and Mobilization of the Spleen and Pancreatic Body and Tail**

A. The lesser sac is entered by dividing the gastrocolic omentum. The stomach is retracted superiorly and the colon is retracted inferiorly to allow for exposure of the pancreatic body and tail.

B. The peritoneum overlying the inferior border of the pancreas is incised, and the body and tail of the pancreas are mobilized bluntly along the avascular plane posterior to the splenic vessels.

C. The splenocolic ligament is divided, and the spleen is gently rotated medially to free the lateral peritoneal attachments. The splenorenal ligament is then divided, allowing for complete mobilization of the spleen and pancreatic tail.

III. **Resection of the Distal Pancreas and Spleen**

A. The splenic artery and vein are dissected away from surrounding tissues, ligated, and divided.

B. The pancreas is divided with a stapling device, and the specimen is removed. Bleeding sites on the proximal pancreas are oversewn. Some surgeons seal the distal staple line with fibrin glue before irrigating the abdomen.

Additional Operative Considerations

I. **Drains:** A nasogastric tube is maintained after both pancreaticoduodenectomy and distal pancreatectomy. Placement of closed-suction drains posterior to the hepaticojejunostomy and the pancreaticojejunostomy at the conclusion of pancreaticoduodenectomy sometimes facilitates postoperative management and is advocated by some surgeons. A drain may be placed adjacent to the pancreatic staple line after distal pancreatectomy.

II. **Gastrostomy and Feeding Tubes:** Gastrostomy tubes and feeding jejunostomy tubes are sometimes placed after pancreaticoduodenectomy. Gastrostomy tubes are particularly helpful in cases of postoperative delayed gastric emptying; however, it is difficult to reliably predict which patients will encounter this complication.

III. **Laparoscopy:** Laparoscopic distal pancreatectomy is performed routinely at some centers. Although the positioning and approach are somewhat different than with the open procedure, the basic concepts of exposure and resection are similar. Laparoscopic pancreaticoduodenectomy has been reported in the literature, but is infrequently performed.

POSTOPERATIVE COURSE

After pancreaticoduodenectomy, patients are routinely followed in the intensive care unit for 24 to 48 hours. Patients who undergo distal pancreatectomy are likewise closely monitored in the early postoperative period, although recovery is generally quicker and admission to the intensive care unit is often unnecessary. Nasogastric tubes are typically removed on the second postoperative day. Patients are subsequently allowed clear liquids and advanced to a regular diet as tolerated. Surgical drains are monitored closely for the quantity and character of output and are typically maintained until a regular diet is tolerated.

COMPLICATIONS

I. **Bleeding** after pancreatic resection is relatively common because patients with pancreatic neoplasms may be malnourished and have impaired liver synthetic function. Coagulopathy should be aggressively corrected in the postoperative period. Rarely, re-exploration for surgical bleeding is necessary.

II. **Pancreatic leak** (pancreatic fistula) is the most common complication of pancreatic resection. Such leaks are often heralded by high-volume, amylase-rich output from the surgical drain. After a Whipple procedure, many surgeons routinely measure amylase levels in the drainage fluid several days after surgery or after patients resume a regular diet, regardless of the rate of drainage. CT scanning is sometimes useful in identifying undrained intra-abdominal fluid collections, which generally mandate percutaneous drainage. Low-output leaks can typically be managed with maintenance of drainage alone. High-output leaks require a more aggressive approach, including bowel rest and total parenteral nutrition.

III. **Bile leaks** after pancreaticoduodenectomy are rare. When they do occur, they are most often managed with closed-suction drainage. Persistent leaks may require percutaneous transhepatic drainage to divert bile flow from the hepaticojejunostomy.

IV. **Delayed gastric emptying** is one of the most common complications after a Whipple procedure, occurring in 20% to 70% of patients. The etiology of delayed gastric emptying is poorly understood, and in most cases, symptoms improve with time. An upper gastrointestinal study should be obtained to rule out a mechanical obstruction if delayed gastric emptying continues beyond the first postoperative week. Promotility agents, such as metoclopramide and erythromycin, are sometimes helpful.

SUGGESTED READINGS

Brugge WR, Lauwers GY, Sahani D, et al: Cystic neoplasms of the pancreas. N Engl J Med 351:1218–1226, 2004.

Steer ML: Exocrine pancreas. In Townsend CM, Beauchamp RD, Evers BM, Mattox KL (eds): Sabiston Textbook of Surgery: The Biological Basis of Modern Surgical Practice, 17th ed. Philadelphia, Saunders, 2004, pp 1667–1674.

Thayer SP, Warshaw AL: Periampullary cancer. In Cameron JL (ed): Current Surgical Therapy, 8th ed. Philadelphia, Elsevier Mosby, 2004, pp 494–504.

Appendectomy

Joseph Anthony P. Rodriguez, Robert E. Roses, and Benjamin Braslow

Case Study

A 19-year-old male presents to the emergency room complaining of severe right-sided lower abdominal pain, nausea, and anorexia, which began 24 hours earlier. On physical examination, he has a fever of 100.5°F. His abdomen is focally tender on palpation of the right lower quadrant. His white blood cell count is within the normal range. A computed tomography (CT) scan of the abdomen and pelvis shows a thickened appendix and peri-appendiceal inflammation (Fig. 15-1).

BACKGROUND

The **appendix** is a blind-ended tubular structure arising from the cecum approximately 2 cm below the ileocecal valve (Fig. 15-2). Obstruction of the lumen of the appendix by fecal material (i.e., **fecalith**), a tumor, or **lymphoid hyperplasia** may result in elevated intraluminal pressures, vascular congestion, stasis, bacterial overgrowth, and inflammation. Without intervention, the resulting **appendicitis** may progress to wall necrosis and appendiceal perforation. Prompt diagnosis and management are critical to the successful treatment of appendicitis. Despite the high incidence of appendicitis, however, its diagnosis is not always straightforward. The differential diagnosis of appendicitis is broad and may include gastroenteritis, Meckel's diverticulitis, colonic diverticulitis, inflammatory bowel disease, urinary tract infection, epididymitis, and gastrointestinal and reproductive tract malignancies. Women of childbearing age who present with abdominal pain pose a particular diagnostic challenge because pelvic inflammatory disease, ovarian cysts, and ovarian torsion can also mimic appendicitis.

This chapter focuses on the perioperative and operative management of diseases of the appendix. Both laparoscopic and open approaches to appendectomy are frequently in use and are discussed.

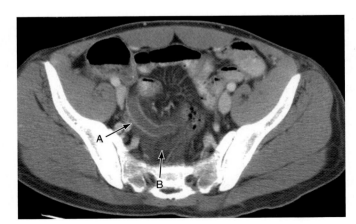

Figure 15-1

Computed tomography scan showing a thickened appendix (**A**) and adjacent inflammation (**B**). *(From Rakel RE [ed]: Textbook of Family Medicine, 7th ed. Philadelphia, Saunders, 2007, courtesy of Dr. Perry Pernicano, Department of Radiology, University of Michigan Medical School, Ann Arbor, MI.)*

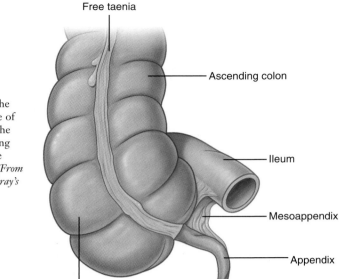

Figure 15-2
The appendix and mesoappendix. The appendix is located at the confluence of the three taenia coli, at the base of the cecum. The mesoappendix, containing the appendiceal vessels, suspends the appendix from the terminal ileum. *(From Drake RL, Vogl W, Mitchell AWM: Gray's Anatomy for Students. Philadelphia, Churchill Livingstone, 2005.)*

INDICATIONS FOR SURGERY

I. **Appendicitis:** Appendectomy is indicated in all cases of suspected nonperforated appendicitis. Laparoscopic and open approaches are largely equivalent; however, each approach has advantages in selected situations. The open technique is generally less costly and is associated with shorter operative times. Laparoscopy allows for superior visualization of the peritoneal cavity and exclusion of other pathology when the diagnosis of appendicitis is equivocal. For this reason, laparoscopic appendectomy is often the preferred operation in women of childbearing age in whom the differential diagnosis for appendicitis is especially broad. Obese patients particularly benefit from the superior visualization and smaller incisions afforded by the laparoscopic approach as well.

II. In cases of **perforated appendicitis,** a role for nonoperative management, coupled with percutaneous drainage of periappendiceal collections, has emerged. Such an approach is supported by the relatively high complication rates and long recovery times associated with immediate operative management. Clinically stable patients with well-circumscribed abscesses at the time of presentation are typical candidates for such an approach. Most surgeons will perform an interval appendectomy, usually 6 to 8 weeks later. However, some have advocated forgoing this in light of the relatively low frequency and typically mild course of recurrent appendicitis in patients managed nonoperatively.

III. **Neoplasm:** Tumors of the appendix are present in approximately 5% of specimens after appendectomy for appendicitis, but are rarely diagnosed preoperatively. Carcinoid tumors are the most common malignancy of the appendix; most of these are small (<1 cm) and are adequately treated with simple appendectomy. Carcinoid tumors larger than 2 cm are associated with higher rates of metastases and should be treated with right hemicolectomy, as should tumors of any size located at the base of the appendix. Adenocarcinomas of the appendix are extremely rare and are generally treated with right hemicolectomy.

PREOPERATIVE EVALUATION

I. **History**

A. Patients with acute appendicitis typically provide a history of initial vague periumbilical or epigastric pain, reflecting distention of the appendix and stimulation of the visceral fibers of the autonomic nervous system. The pain subsequently becomes more severe and localizes to the right lower quadrant of the abdomen as the appendix becomes progressively more inflamed and irritates the adjacent peritoneum. Appendicitis is usually associated with anorexia. Nausea, emesis, and low-grade fever may also be present and typically follow the onset of pain.

B. Appendiceal perforation may be heralded by high fever, tachycardia, and more diffuse pain. Alternatively, some patients experience an interval of decreased pain and nausea immediately after perforation as a result of decompression of the distended appendix. Very young or elderly patients are more likely to present atypically and to be diagnosed after appendiceal perforation.

II. **Physical Examination**

A. Patients with appendicitis typically have a low-grade fever. High fevers (>101°F) are more common in the setting of appendiceal perforation. Focal tenderness in the right lower quadrant is usually present. **McBurney's point,** located two thirds of the distance between the umbilicus and the anterior superior iliac crest, typically overlies the appendix and is, therefore, the point of maximal tenderness. Importantly, tenderness may be remote from McBurney's point, reflecting the variable position of the appendix (Fig. 15-3).

B. Other signs associated with appendicitis include Rovsing's sign, the psoas sign, and the obturator sign.

1. **Rovsing's sign** is positive when right lower quadrant abdominal pain is exacerbated by palpating the left lower quadrant, reflecting the site of local peritoneal irritation.

2. The **psoas sign** is present when pain is elicited by extending the right hip with the patient lying on the left side. The presence of a psoas sign suggests a retrocecal appendix.

3. The **obturator sign** is present when pain is elicited by flexing and internally rotating the rig, and suggests a pelvic appendix.

III. **Laboratory Tests**

A. **Leukocytosis** may accompany appendicitis. A white blood cell count of greater than 18,000 cells/mm^3 is unusual in the absence of perforation or an abscess.

> Is your patient hungry?

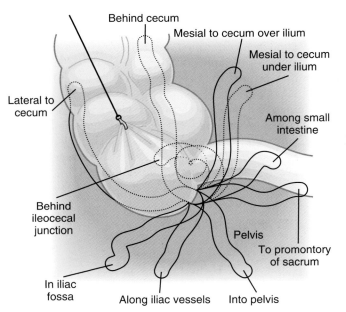

Figure 15-3
Variable position of the appendix. *(From Kelly HA, Hurdon E: The Vermiform Appendix and Its Diseases. Philadelphia, WB Saunders, 1905.)*

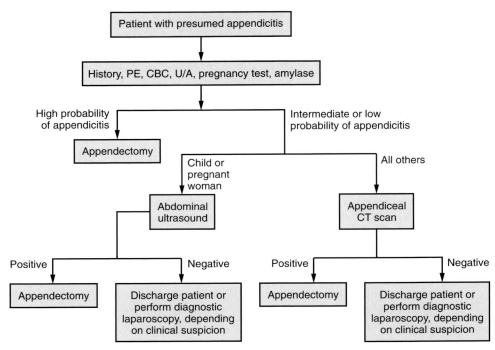

Figure 15-4

Evaluation for suspected appendicitis. CBC, complete blood count; CT, computed tomography; PE, physical examination; U/A, urinalysis. *(Adapted from Feldman M, Friedman LS, Brandt LJ [eds]: Sleisenger and Fordtran's Gastrointestinal and Liver Disease, 8th ed. Philadelphia, Saunders, 2006.)*

Does your patient exhibit signs or symptoms consistent with appendiceal perforation?

B. Urinalysis is helpful in excluding alternative diagnoses; however, red and white blood cells are sometimes detected in the urine during appendicitis when the inflamed appendix abuts the right ureter or bladder.

IV. **Radiographic Studies**

    A. **Abdominal radiographs** are frequently obtained but are rarely helpful in the diagnosis of appendicitis. They may, however, point to alternative diagnoses (e.g., renal or ureteral calculi). Rarely, a radio-opaque fecalith in the right lower quadrant or free intraperitoneal air from an appendiceal perforation is visible.

    B. **Ultrasonography** is both sensitive and specific for the diagnosis of appendicitis but is highly operator dependent. Ultrasonographic findings suggestive of appendicitis include a noncompressible appendix, an appendix with an antero-posterior diameter of 7 mm or greater, the presence of a fecalith, and periappendiceal fluid.

    C. **CT scanning** of the abdomen and pelvis with intravenous and oral contrast has a sensitivity and specificity of greater than 95% for the diagnosis of appendicitis. Periappendiceal inflammation and appendiceal wall thickening are diagnostic of appendicitis (Fig. 15-4). CT scanning is also of utility in identifying abscesses or phlegmons associated with perforated appendicitis.

COMPONENTS OF THE PROCEDURE AND APPLIED ANATOMY

Preoperative Considerations

    I. Once the diagnosis of acute appendicitis is established, broad-spectrum antibiotic therapy should be initiated.

    II. Before laparoscopy, an orogastric tube and a urinary catheter should be placed for decompression of the stomach and urinary bladder, respectively.

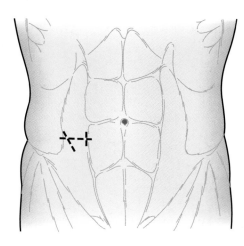

Figure 15-5
Common incisions for open appendectomy (*dashed lines*). (*From Ortega JM, Ricardo AE: Surgery of the appendix and colon. In Moody FG [ed]: Atlas of Ambulatory Surgery. Philadelphia, WB Saunders, 1999.*)

Open Appendectomy

I. **Incision and Exposure**
   A. Open appendectomy is most often performed through either a transverse (*Rocky-Davis*) or an oblique (*McBurney*) incision (Fig. 15-5). If greater exposure is required, the transverse incision can more readily be extended past the lateral edge of the rectus sheath than can the oblique incision. Therefore a transverse incision is generally preferred.
   B. Regardless of whether a transverse or an oblique incision is chosen, a muscle-splitting (sparing) technique is used. Subcutaneous fat is bluntly dissected away to expose the external oblique aponeurosis. The external and internal oblique aponeuroses are sharply divided. The transversus abdominis muscle fibers are retracted to expose the underlying transversalis fascia, which, along with the underlying peritoneum, is sharply incised.
   C. If murky or purulent fluid is encountered on entry into the peritoneal cavity, it is sampled and sent for Gram stain and culture to aid in postoperative antibiotic selection if postoperative antibiotic therapy is indicated.
   D. The appendix is delivered into the wound with a gentle finger sweep from lateral to medial in the right paracolic gutter. Alternatively, the teniae of the right colon are followed to their convergence to identify the base of the appendix.

II. **Appendectomy**
   A. The mesoappendix, which contains the appendiceal artery, is divided between ties (Fig. 15-6). The base of the appendix is then divided between clamps. The base is ligated, and the appendix is removed.
   B. The mucosa of the appendiceal stump is cauterized to prevent mucocele formation.
   C. The appendiceal stump can be inverted by placement of a *Z-stitch* (Fig. 15-7) or a purse-string suture.

III. **Irrigation and Closure**
   A. The right lower quadrant is irrigated, and the transversalis fascia and peritoneum, internal oblique aponeurosis, and external oblique aponeurosis are closed in three layers.
   B. If the appendix was nonperforated, the skin is typically closed. If the appendix was perforated, the skin is either left open, left to close secondarily, or loosely closed with staples.

> Inversion of the appendiceal stump is controversial because the resulting bulge in the cecal wall can be mistaken for a polypoid lesion on subsequent colonoscopy.

Laparoscopic Appendectomy

I. **Port Placement**
   A. Laparoscopic appendectomy is generally performed through three operative ports: a port for the camera (most often through or below the umbilicus), a

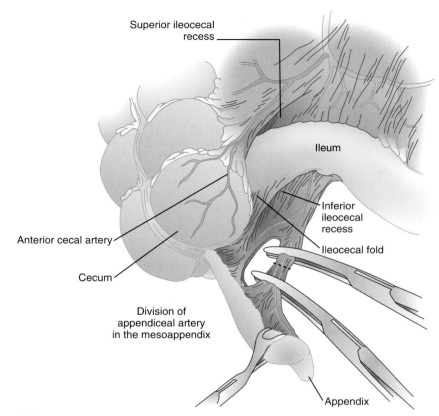

Figure 15-6

Division of the mesoappendix. *(From Ortega JM, Ricardo AE: Surgery of the appendix and colon. In Moody FG [ed]: Atlas of Ambulatory Surgery. Philadelphia, WB Saunders, 1999.)*

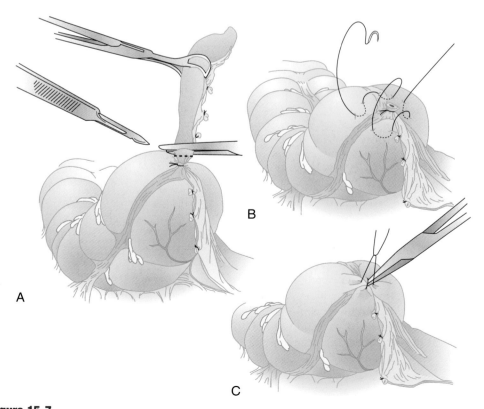

Figure 15-7

Division of the appendix. **A,** The appendix is divided after ligation. **B,** A Z- or purse-string stitch is placed in the cecum. **C,** The appendiceal stump is inverted. *(From Ortega JM, Ricardo AE: Surgery of the appendix and colon. In Moody FG [ed]: Atlas of Ambulatory Surgery. Philadelphia, WB Saunders, 1999.)*

12-mm port through which a surgical stapler can be passed, and an additional port to aid in retraction and dissection. The location of the latter two ports is highly variable.

B. Access to the abdomen is obtained with a Veress needle using a "blind" percutaneous technique or an open technique. The open technique is more commonly used.

C. **Open technique for placement of the first port**
1. A horizontal incision is made below the umbilicus.
2. Subcutaneous soft tissue is bluntly dissected to expose the linea alba. The fascia and underlying peritoneum are divided at the midline under direct vision.
3. Fascial sutures are placed to secure the port and minimize CO_2 leakage and loss of pneumoperitoneum. The port is inserted through the incision with a blunt-tipped trocar.
4. CO_2 is insufflated through the port. The abdomen should distend symmetrically and become uniformly tympanic.
5. The laparoscope is inserted through the umbilical port, and the peritoneal cavity is surveyed.

D. **Placement of the remaining ports:** The remaining two ports are inserted under direct intra-abdominal visualization. Cutting (sharp) introducers are used to penetrate the fascia and enter the peritoneal cavity.

II. Exposure and Appendectomy

A. The abdominal cavity is surveyed before identification of the appendix in the right lower quadrant.

B. The tip of the appendix is retracted anteriorly to expose the mesoappendix. A dissector is used to bluntly create an opening in the mesoappendix adjacent to the base of the appendix.

C. The bottom jaw of a surgical stapler is passed through the opening in the mesoappendix, and the stapler is fired across the base of the appendix. The stapler is then used to divide the mesoappendix separately (Fig. 15-8).

III. Irrigation and Closure

A. The right lower quadrant is irrigated with normal saline and inspected for hemostasis. The umbilical fascia is closed.

B. All skin incisions are closed with absorbable suture.

> **THE VERESS NEEDLE APPROACH SHOULD NOT BE USED IN PATIENTS WHO HAVE HAD PREVIOUS ABDOMINAL SURGERY.**

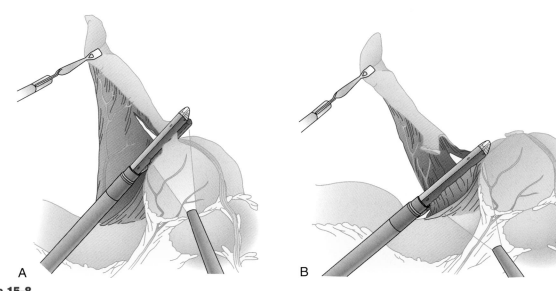

Figure 15-8
A, Division of the appendix using an endostapler. **B,** Division of the mesoappendix with an endostapler. *(From Ortega JM, Ricardo AE: Surgery of the appendix and colon. In Moody FG [ed]: Atlas of Ambulatory Surgery. Philadelphia, WB Saunders, 1999.)*

Additional Considerations

I. **Appendicitis in Pregnancy**
   A. Appendicitis is the most common indication for surgery in pregnant patients. The diagnosis of appendicitis is particularly challenging in this setting because early signs and symptoms of appendicitis, including nausea, emesis, and leukocytosis, are also attributable to pregnancy. Additionally, the gravid uterus may push the appendix away from its normal location, resulting in an atypical distribution of pain. As a result, diagnosis is frequently delayed until symptoms become relatively severe.
   B. Prompt diagnosis and treatment are particularly important because perforated appendicitis is associated with fetal mortality rates of as high as 35%. Ultrasound poses no risk to the fetus and is frequently used to aid in diagnosis. In contrast, CT scanning should be used judiciously to minimize unnecessary radiation exposure. Magnetic resonance imaging is emerging as a reliable, and likely safe, alternative to CT scanning when the diagnosis of appendicitis is equivocal. Open appendectomy remains the most common approach to appendectomy in the setting of pregnancy, although the laparoscopic approach is increasingly being used as well.

II. **The Normal Appendix:** When a noninflamed appendix is encountered during open exploration through a right lower quadrant incision, generally, the appendix should still be removed to avoid future diagnostic confusion. It is less clear whether a noninflamed appendix should be removed during laparoscopic exploration.

III. **Inflammatory Bowel Disease:** Crohn's disease may mimic appendicitis. Indeed, the diagnosis of inflammatory bowel disease after surgical exploration for appendicitis is not uncommon. When evidence of Crohn's disease rather than appendicitis is encountered during operative exploration, generally, the appendix should still be removed to avoid future diagnostic confusion. Inflammation involving the cecum and the base of the appendix sometimes precludes safe appendectomy.

POSTOPERATIVE COURSE

> **FORMAL PATHOLOGIC EVALUATION OF THE SURGICAL SPECIMEN SHOULD BE REVIEWED TO EXCLUDE A MISSED NEOPLASM.**

Patients typically have little postoperative pain after appendectomy. Urinary catheters should be removed before emergence from anesthesia. A clinically significant postoperative ileus is uncommon, and patients can be fed shortly after recovery from anesthesia. Postoperative antibiotic therapy is unnecessary. Most patients are discharged within 48 hours of surgery.

Perforated appendicitis is associated with a more protracted postoperative recovery. Ileus is common, and diet should be advanced gradually. Postoperative antibiotic therapy is indicated, at least until the patient is afebrile for more than 24 hours and the white blood cell count normalizes.

COMPLICATIONS

I. Surgical site **infections** and intra-abdominal abscess formation are particularly common after appendectomy for perforated appendicitis. By leaving the skin open and allowing for closure by secondary intention, the risk of superficial infection is minimized. Intra-abdominal abscesses are usually amenable to percutaneous drainage and rarely require reoperation.

II. Although it is uncommon, significant intraoperative or postoperative **bleeding** may result from inadequate ligation of the mesoappendix and appendiceal artery.

SUGGESTED READINGS

Lally KP, Cox CS, Andrassy RJ: Appendix. In Townsend CM, Beauchamp RD, Evers BM, Mattox KL (eds): Sabiston Textbook of Surgery: The Biological Basis of Modern Surgical Practice, 17th ed. Philadelphia, Saunders, 2004.

Paulson EK, Kalady MF, Pappas TN: Clinical practice: suspected appendicitis. N Engl J Med 348:236–242, 2003.

CHAPTER 16

Colectomy

E. Carter Paulson   and   Najjia N. Mahmoud

Case Study

A 65-year-old female is found to be anemic on routine laboratory testing. A subsequent colonoscopy shows multiple diverticula in her sigmoid colon and a 5-cm sessile mass in her right colon. A biopsy reveals moderately differentiated adenocarcinoma.

BACKGROUND

The colon is a tubular digestive organ that is mainly responsible for water absorption and storage. It is 4 to 6 feet in length and extends from the ileocecal valve to the anus. The wall of the colon consists of five distinct layers: mucosa, submucosa, inner circular muscle, outer longitudinal muscle, and serosa. The outer longitudinal muscle forms three distinct muscular bands (*teniae coli*), which converge proximally at the appendix and distally at the rectum, where the outer longitudinal muscle layer is circumferential. The cecum, the first portion of the colon, connects to the terminal ileum via the ileocecal valve and is the portion of the colon with the largest diameter. It is fixed in the right lower quadrant by attachments to the lateral abdominal wall. The ascending colon, which is retroperitoneal, extends from the cecum to the hepatic flexure in the right upper quadrant. The hepatic flexure marks the transition to the transverse colon, which is a mobile, intraperitoneal structure. The colon becomes retroperitoneal again at the splenic flexure, which marks the transition to the more fixed descending colon. In the left lower quadrant, the descending colon becomes the sigmoid colon, which is the most narrow, muscular part of the large intestine and is extremely mobile. The rectum begins at the approximate level of the sacral promontory and terminates at the anus.

There are many indications for both partial and total colectomy. These include malignant, benign, ischemic, inflammatory, and infectious processes. The most common indications for colon and rectal resection are addressed individually later in the chapter. Common terms used to describe the types of colon and rectal operations are described in Table 16-1.

INDICATIONS FOR COLORECTAL RESECTION

I. **Sporadic Cancer and Inherited Polyposis Syndromes**
   A. **Colon adenocarcinoma** is the third most frequently diagnosed cancer and the second most common cause of cancer death in the United States. Surgical resection is the initial treatment of choice for most colon cancers, although postoperative (adjuvant) chemotherapy plays an important role in the management of patients with nodal metastases. Surgery is aimed at removing the primary cancer with tumor-free margins, as well as the associated bowel mesentery and regional lymph nodes. In practice, the extent of resection is dictated by the location of the lesion and the colonic blood supply. For example, cecal tumors are treated with right hemicolectomy, an operation that involves ligation of the ileocolic, right colic, and right branch of the middle colic vessels, and resection of the segment of colon fed by these vessels. When curative

TABLE 16-1 Common Colon Procedures

Type of Resection	Description
Segmental colectomy	Removal of a portion of the colon (e.g., right, transverse, left, or sigmoid).
Total abdominal colectomy	Removal of the entire abdominal colon, leaving the rectum and creation of an end ileostomy or ileorectal anastomosis.
End stoma	Intestinal diversion involving division and exteriorization of the colon (colostomy) or terminal ileum (ileostomy) through the skin. The distal colon is then either brought out as a mucous fistula or left in the abdomen as a Hartmann's pouch.
Loop stoma	A loop of either colon or ileum is exteriorized and opened, but not divided.
Hartmann's pouch	An end stoma is created from proximal bowel; distal bowel is closed and remains in the pelvis.
Ileal pouch–anal anastomosis (Park's pouch, J-pouch)	After total proctocolectomy, the terminal ileum is used to create a reservoir that is connected to the anus as a "neorectum."
Total mesorectal excision	En bloc removal of the mesorectum along with the rectum for rectal cancers of the mid and distal rectum. This is carried out by dissection in the plane between the fascia propria of the rectum and the presacral fascia.
Low anterior resection	Resection of the upper rectum; an anastomosis is formed between the colon and distal rectum.
Abdominoperineal resection	Total mesorectal excision of the rectum, surrounding tissues, and lymph nodes via abdominal and perineal approaches; creation of an end stoma.
Total proctocolectomy	Removal of the entire colon and rectum. Ileoanal pouch reconstruction or end ileostomy is required.

resection is not possible, resection of the primary tumor is often still indicated to prevent complications associated with large tumors (e.g., obstruction and bleeding).

B. **Rectal Adenocarcinoma:** Because of the extraperitoneal position of the rectum within the pelvis (which allows for the administration of radiation therapy) and its proximity to parasympathetic and sympathetic nerves, rectal cancers are treated differently than are cancers of the colon. In the absence of nodal metastases, smaller lesions are typically treated with surgical resection and regional lymphadenectomy or with transanal *local* excision. The treatment of more advanced rectal cancers includes radiation and chemotherapy given before surgical excision of the tumor (i.e., neoadjuvant therapy). Large tumors may shrink significantly after chemoradiation, allowing for resection of most rectal cancers, with preservation of the anal sphincters (i.e., low anterior resection). In contrast, the distal location of some rectal cancers precludes sphincter preservation, despite neoadjuvant therapy, and mandates abdominoperineal resection (APR).

C. **Adenomatous Polyps:** Most colorectal carcinomas are believed to develop from adenomatous polyps. Polyps are generally classified by gross appearance as either pedunculated (i.e., with a stalk) or sessile (i.e., flat). Histologically, polyps are classified as tubular, tubulovillous, or villous. Tubular adenomas are the most common subtype, constituting 75% or more of colorectal adenomas, and have the least malignant potential of the three subtypes. Villous polyps constitute approximately 10% of colorectal adenomas, are most often found in the rectum, and have the greatest malignant potential. Polyps identified at colonoscopy should be excised completely. If complete endoscopic excision is not possible, segmental colectomy is indicated. If invasive carcinoma is found in the head of a pedunculated polyp, endoscopic resection is adequate treatment. Poorly differentiated histology, lymphovascular invasion, and the presence of invasive tumor within 1 mm of the resection margin mandate segmental colectomy.

D. **Familial adenomatous polyposis (FAP)** is an autosomal dominant genetic syndrome most often associated with mutations of the APC gene. Patients with FAP have in excess of 100 precancerous polyps throughout the colon as early as their teens. If untreated, nearly all of these patients have colon cancer by age 40 years. Attenuated FAP is a phenotypic variant of the classic syndrome that is characterized by later onset of polyps, fewer polyps, and rectal sparing. The treatment of FAP is prophylactic surgical resection, usually performed after the onset of puberty. Surgical options include total proctocolectomy with permanent end ileostomy, total proctocolectomy with ileal pouch–anal anastomosis (IPAA) and total abdominal colectomy with ileorectal anastomosis. The latter option should be offered only to carefully selected patients because it leaves the rectum in place, necessitating close subsequent surveillance. Patients with the attenuated FAP phenotype are sometimes offered a rectal sparing procedure, whereas patients with classic FAP are generally offered total proctocolectomy.

E. **Hereditary nonpolyposis colon cancer (HNPCC)** accounts for 5% to 7% of all colon cancer diagnoses. HNPCC is inherited in an autosomal dominant pattern and has been linked to mutations in DNA mismatch repair genes. The Amsterdam criteria are used to identify patients at high risk for HNPCC. In such patients, screening colonoscopy is recommended beginning at age 20 to 25 years. Total abdominal colectomy with ileorectal anastomosis is recommended if an adenomatous polyp or a colon carcinoma is identified. Patients with HNPCC are at an increased risk for rectal cancer, and annual proctoscopy is mandatory after colectomy.

II. **Inflammatory Bowel Disease**

A. **Ulcerative colitis (UC)** is a chronic inflammatory disease of the large intestine. The disease is marked by inflammation and ulceration of the bowel mucosa beginning at the rectum and extending proximally. UC is associated with a significantly elevated risk of colorectal cancer, and patients require frequent colonoscopic surveillance. There is no medical cure for UC, and current medical treatment is aimed at suppressing the inflammatory process. Although many patients remain symptom-free for prolonged periods, up to one third of patients ultimately require surgery.

1. Indications for surgery include intractable symptomatic disease despite medical therapy and the presence of dysplasia or cancer. Total proctocolectomy with ileostomy and total proctocolectomy with IPAA are curative and eliminate the risk of colon or rectal cancer.

2. Emergent indications for surgery in patients with UC include massive bleeding and toxic megacolon. Toxic megacolon occurs in approximately 10% of patients with UC and is characterized by acute dilation of the colon, accompanied by diarrhea, abdominal pain, fever, tachycardia, and leukocytosis. Initial treatment involves aggressive intravenous hydration, antibiotics, steroids, and cessation of narcotic pain medications. A worsening clinical appearance mandates surgical intervention, typically, total abdominal colectomy and creation of an end ileostomy.

B. **Crohn's disease** is an inflammatory disease that may affect any segment of the gastrointestinal (GI) tract. Disease limited exclusively to the colon occurs in approximately 15% of patients. As with UC, the initial treatment for Crohn's colitis is medical. Surgical indications include failure of medical management, intestinal obstruction, fistula, fulminant colitis, toxic megacolon, massive bleeding, cancer, and malnutrition. Because more than half of all patients with Crohn's disease experience a recurrence within 10 years of surgery, conservation of bowel length is an important surgical principle. The amount of colon resected depends on the extent and location of disease.

Malignancy is present in approximately 5%, 20%, and 40% of tubular, tubulovillous, and villous adenomas, respectively.

Amsterdam criteria:

Three affected relatives with colon cancer
One affected person is a first-degree relative of the other two affected persons
Two successive generations affected
At least one case diagnosed before age 50 years
Familial adenomatous polyposis excluded

Crohn's disease may spare the rectum and is frequently accompanied by anal disease, whereas ulcerative colitis always involves the rectum and never involves the anus.

III. Benign Conditions

A. **Diverticulitis** results from microperforation of colonic diverticula. In **uncomplicated diverticulitis,** this perforation is contained and manifests as colonic and pericolonic inflammation. Diverticulitis may be complicated by abscess formation, fistulization between the colon and adjacent structures, free perforation, or obstruction. Initial episodes of uncomplicated diverticulitis are treated medically with antibiotics and dietary restriction until symptoms resolve. Recurrent uncomplicated diverticulitis and complicated diverticulitis are indications for surgical resection. In the stable patient with **recurrent or complicated diverticulitis,** medical treatment should be instituted to treat symptoms and reduce inflammation. After symptoms have subsided for at least 3 weeks, a colonoscopy should be performed to confirm the presence of diverticula, document the extent of disease, and exclude the presence of a neoplasm. Segmental resection of the involved colon, most commonly the sigmoid colon, with primary anastomosis can then be performed. Patients with complicated diverticulitis and evidence of free colonic perforation or sepsis should be operated on emergently and resection of the involved colon undertaken. Creation of a temporary colostomy, rather than an anastomosis, is often the preferred approach in such settings.

> A perforated colon cancer may mimic diverticulitis.

B. **Sigmoid volvulus** results from the torsion of the colon on its mesenteric axis. Volvulus may result in partial or complete obstruction of the bowel lumen, vascular compromise, bowel wall ischemia, and perforation. More than 80% of colonic volvuli involve the sigmoid colon. Patients are typically elderly, chronically debilitated, immobile, and institutionalized and present with abdominal distention, pain, and obstipation. Evidence of perforation and clinical deterioration are indications for emergent operative intervention, including sigmoid resection. In patients who are stable, reduction of the volvulus may be accomplished initially via colonoscopy or proctoscopy. Recurrence rates after endoscopic decompression are as high as 80% to 90%, and elective sigmoid resection should subsequently be undertaken.

C. **Cecal volvulus,** which is less common than sigmoid volvulus, is most commonly caused by congenital incomplete peritoneal fixation of the cecum in the right lower quadrant. Presenting symptoms are similar to those associated with sigmoid volvulus. Plain radiographs of the abdomen show a dilated cecum, often displaced to the left side of the abdomen. Endoscopic decompression is rarely successful. Treatment of suspected cecal volvulus, therefore, should include prompt right hemicolectomy, even in stable patients. In patients who cannot tolerate a lengthy procedure, surgical decompression and cecopexy (i.e., detorsion of the colon and fixation of the cecum in the right lower quadrant) is an acceptable alternative procedure, albeit one associated with a significant rate of recurrence.

D. **Lower GI bleeding** is most often caused by diverticulosis (50%) or arteriovenous malformations (30%). The initial treatment of lower GI bleeding includes resuscitation, correction of coagulopathy if present, and localization of the bleeding site. In 80% of patients with a diverticular bleed, bleeding stops spontaneously. In other patients, colonoscopic approaches or angioembolization can be used to control bleeding. Patients who continue to bleed require surgical intervention. Optimally, the site of bleeding is localized preoperatively with angiography, Technetium-99m–tagged red blood cell nuclear medicine scan, or colonoscopy, allowing for segmental resection of the involved colon. When preoperative localization is not possible, total abdominal colectomy is the procedure of choice.

E. **Infectious colitis** is most often treated with antibiotics, but occasionally necessitates colectomy. **Pseudomembranous colitis** is caused by the toxin-secreting bacterium *Clostridium difficile.* Most prevalent in hospitals and nursing home settings, pseudomembranous colitis is almost always associated with the previous use of antibiotics. Patients typically present with watery diarrhea and crampy abdominal pain. Generally, a course of oral metronidazole or vancomycin is adequate treatment for uncomplicated pseudomembranous colitis. Rarely, severe infection can lead to progressive colonic dilation, ischemia, and even perforation. In such fulminant cases, total abdominal colectomy with temporary ileostomy is required. The rectum is spared and an ileorectal anastomosis can be performed months later, when the patient is stable and well nourished.

F. **Ischemic colitis** occurs when there is insufficient blood flow to a portion of the colon. Risk factors for ischemic colitis include aortic aneurysms and transient hypotension. Most often, ischemia is confined to the mucosa and is transient. Occasionally, full-thickness ischemia may progress to perforation and sepsis, requiring emergency segmental colectomy. Evidence of perforation, massive bleeding, or clinical deterioration mandates operative exploration. Revascularization of the colon is rarely successful; thus, the procedure of choice is segmental colectomy with an end stoma, which may be reversed 3 to 4 months later.

PREOPERATIVE EVALUATION

I. **Colonoscopy:** In general, patients should undergo colonoscopy before any elective colon resection to localize and determine the extent of disease and identify other pathology that could influence the surgical approach. Active inflammatory conditions (e.g., acute diverticulitis) may predispose to perforation and are, therefore, relative contraindications to colonoscopy.

> Has your patient undergone a preoperative colonoscopy?

II. **Proctoscopy:** Every patient diagnosed with rectal cancer should undergo preoperative rigid proctoscopy to determine the distance of the tumor from the anal verge, because this distance influences recommendations for preoperative chemotherapy and radiation as well as the surgical approach. Proctoscopic evaluation is also important for ruling out bleeding hemorrhoids or rectal varices as sources for lower GI bleeding and in establishing the presence of inflammation in patients with inflammatory bowel disease.

III. **Endorectal Ultrasound (ERUS):** ERUS allows for an assessment of mesorectal lymph nodes and the depth of invasion of rectal cancers and is critical to preoperative staging.

IV. **Barium Enema:** A barium enema allows for the detection of polyps, cancers, diverticula, strictures, and fistulas, and is particularly useful when colonoscopy cannot be completed before surgery because of difficult anatomy or structural features (e.g., strictures) that prevent passage of the scope.

V. **Computed Tomography (CT):** A CT scan of the abdomen and pelvis is generally obtained on all patients with colon or rectal cancer to evaluate for adenopathy, tumor invasion of adjacent structures, and distant metastatic disease. In patients with abdominal pain and tenderness, CT scan can show evidence of bowel perforation (e.g., pneumoperitoneum) and provide information about the extent and location of inflammation, ischemia, or obstruction.

VI. **Magnetic Resonance Imaging (MRI):** MRI provides similar information to CT. Advantages of MRI compared with CT include more accurate delineation of the depth of rectal cancer invasion and identification of liver metastases. MRI may serve as an alternative to ERUS in the preoperative evaluation of patients with rectal cancers. Generally, MRI provides a more accurate assessment of nodal status, whereas ERUS provides a more accurate assessment of the depth of tumor invasion.

VII. **Laboratory Tests**

A. **Carcinoembryonic antigen (CEA)** is a serum glycoprotein that may be elevated in patients with primary or metastatic colon cancer. A serum CEA level is obtained before resection to establish a baseline level. Serial CEA levels are also followed after resection to screen patients for evidence of cancer recurrence.

B. **Liver function tests,** including alkaline phosphatase, aspartate aminotransfer-ase, and alanine aminotransferase, should be obtained before surgery in patients with colon cancer. Elevation of these enzymes in the presence of a diagnosis of colon cancer should raise suspicion for liver metastases.

VIII. **Additional Preoperative Considerations**

A. Until recently, it was widely accepted that all patients should undergo **bowel preparation** prior to elective colon resection to purge the colon of fecal contents and reduce colonic bacterial counts. Recently, studies of elective colorectal resections with primary anastomoses, with or without bowel prep-aration, have shown similar rates of anastomotic leak and wound infection. Despite these findings, most surgeons still prescribe bowel preparations to their patients before surgery. Bowel preparations are contraindicated in patients who require emergent intervention, have an obstruction, or have toxic colitis.

B. In the setting of severe pericolonic inflammation (e.g., in patients with UC, Crohn's disease, or diverticulitis) or scarring (e.g., after pelvic radiation or previous abdominal surgery), the ureters may be difficult to identify intraop-eratively and are vulnerable to iatrogenic injury. In such cases, preoperative placement of **ureteral stents** is recommended.

> Should your patient have preoperative ureteral stents placed?

COMPONENTS OF THE PROCEDURE AND APPLIED ANATOMY

The next section provides a detailed description of an open right colectomy. The pre-operative considerations and many of the operative principles described also apply to other colon resections, whether open or laparoscopic.

Preoperative Considerations

I. One dose of **antibiotics,** typically a second- or third-generation cephalosporin, should be administered 30 to 60 minutes before incision. If the procedure lasts longer than 4 hours, a second dose can be given.

II. A **urinary catheter** is inserted before colon resections to decompress the bladder and facilitate assessment of fluid status.

III. An **oro-** or **nasogastric tube** is placed to decompress the stomach.

IV. If **stoma** placement is anticipated, a site should be marked preoperatively. Opti-mally, the patient is evaluated in both sitting and standing positions. Stomas are generally created through the rectus abdominis muscle, avoiding skin creases and beltlines.

Open Right Hemicolectomy

See Figure 16-1.

I. **Patient Positioning and Preparation**

A. The patient is placed in the supine position with the arms extended at 90 degrees.

B. The sterile preparation should extend from the nipples superiorly, to the groin inferiorly, and to the midaxillary lines laterally.

II. **Incision and Exploration**

A. Right hemicolectomy may be performed through a variety of incisions, includ-ing vertical midline, transverse supraumbilical, and right paramedian. A vertical midline incision provides good exposure and is used most commonly.

B. Often, a self-retaining retractor (e.g., Bookwalter or Balfour) is used to main-tain exposure.

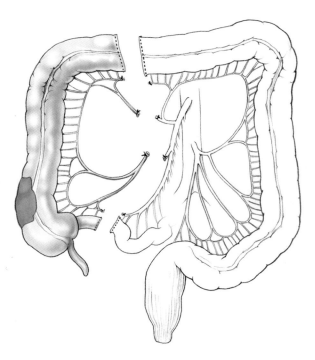

Figure 16-1
Right hemicolectomy. *(From Cameron JL [ed]: Current Surgical Therapy, 7th ed. Philadelphia, Mosby, 2001.)*

    C. Full abdominal exploration is undertaken. This is particularly important during operations for malignancy to exclude peritoneal and liver metastases.

  III. **Mobilization of the Right Colon**
    A. The small bowel is reflected to the patient's left and packed out of the operative field.
    B. The colon is then reflected medially by dividing the white line of Toldt (the lateral reflection of the peritoneum over the mesentery of the ascending colon).
    C. Care is taken to identify and remain anterior to the retroperitoneal right ureter and gonadal vessels.
    D. As dissection is continued around the hepatic flexure, the duodenum is identified.
    E. Once the ascending colon and hepatic flexure have been mobilized, the lesser sac is entered by dissecting the greater omentum away from the transverse colon as far as is necessary to allow for division of the colon with an adequate resection margin.

  IV. **Division of the Bowel**
    A. Proximal and distal sites for division of the colon are identified. When a right hemicolectomy is performed in a patient who has cancer, the ileocolic, right colic, and right branch of the middle colic vessels are ligated. The bowel is typically divided at the terminal ileum proximally and the transverse colon to the right of the main trunk of the middle colic vessels distally; this ensures adequate vascular supply to the bowel that will be used to form an anastomosis.
    B. At the sites chosen for bowel division, the bowel is cleared of mesenteric fat and small windows are bluntly created in the mesentery directly adjacent to the bowel wall to allow for passage of clamps or a surgical stapler.
    C. The bowel is divided proximally and distally with a stapling device.

  V. **Mesenteric Resection and Vessel Ligation**
    A. The mesentery of the right and proximal transverse colon is then divided in small segments to ensure vascular control.
    B. Mesenteric fat and small vessels may be divided using electrocautery.

> **IDENTIFY AND AVOID THE RETROPERITONEAL URETER AND DUODENUM DURING MOBILIZATION OF THE RIGHT COLON AND HEPATIC FLEXURE.**

C. The ileocolic, right, and middle colic vessels are identified by visual inspection and palpation of the colonic mesentery.

D. The large mesenteric vessels are divided between clamps. Each end of the cut vessels is ligated.

E. After division of the mesentery, the specimen is removed.

VI. **Bowel Anastomosis:** The anastomosis between the ileum and transverse colon can be hand sewn or stapled in an end-to-end, end-to-side, or side-to-side configuration. The stapled side-to-side approach is most often used and is discussed in detail. The hand-sewn end-to-side approach is also discussed.

A. **Stapled Anastomosis**

1. The distal ileum and transverse colon are aligned along their antimesenteric borders.

2. The divided ends of bowel are opened to permit the insertion of one jaw of a gastrointestinal anastomosis (GIA) stapler into each lumen.

3. The anastomosis is created by firing the stapler.

4. The remaining open end of bowel through which the GIA stapler was inserted is closed using a thoracoabdominal (TA) stapling device.

B. **Hand-Sewn Anastomosis**

1. The end of the ileum is cleaned of mesenteric fat and positioned along the side of the transverse colon. The staple line is resected, opening the bowel lumen.

2. A colotomy (i.e., an opening in the colon), comparable in diameter to the small bowel opening, is created.

3. A two-layer anastomosis is created between the open end of the small bowel and the colotomy, with an inner layer of running, absorbable suture followed by an outer layer of interrupted, nonabsorbable sutures.

VII. **Closing the Mesenteric Defect:** Closure of the defect between the ileal and transverse colon mesenteries is performed using interrupted or running sutures. Although some surgeons do not close the mesenteric defect, proponents argue that closure reduces the incidence of postoperative internal hernia formation.

> The gastrointestinal anastomosis stapler fires two parallel rows of staples and divides the intervening tissue.

Other Operative Procedures

I. An **ileocolic resection** is a limited resection of the terminal ileum, cecum, and appendix. Indications include ileocecal Crohn's disease, benign lesions, and incurable cancers arising in the terminal ileum, cecum, and, occasionally, the appendix. The ileocolic vessels are ligated and divided, and a primary anastomosis is created between the distal small bowel and the ascending colon.

II. Lesions at the hepatic flexure or proximal transverse colon may require an **extended right colectomy.** This procedure involves the ligation and division of the middle colic vessels at their origins and resection of the majority of the transverse colon, in addition to standard right colectomy (Fig. 16-2). A primary anastomosis is created between the ileum and the distal transverse colon. After division of the middle colic vessels, the anastomosis is supplied by the marginal artery of Drummond.

III. **Transverse colectomy,** which involves ligation of the middle colic vessel and a right colon–left colon anastomosis, is rarely performed. In general, lesions in the transverse colon are amenable to an extended right colectomy with anastomosis of the ileum to the descending colon.

IV. **Left colectomy** is performed for pathology of the distal transverse colon, splenic flexure, and descending colon. The left branches of the middle colic vessel, the left colic vessel, and the first branches of the sigmoid vessels are ligated; the distal transverse and descending colon are resected; and a colocolonic anastomosis is created (Fig. 16-3).

A. The splenic flexure of the colon is attached to the inferior pole of the spleen via the splenocolic ligaments. Traction on the flexure can tear the splenic capsule at the site of the colonic attachments and should be avoided to the degree possible during dissection.

> The marginal artery of Drummond is a source of collateral flow between the middle colic artery and the left colic artery (a branch of the inferior mesenteric artery).

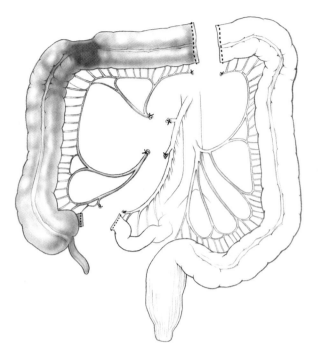

Figure 16-2
Extended right hemicolectomy. *(From Cameron JL [ed]: Current Surgical Therapy, 7th ed. Philadelphia, Mosby, 2001.)*

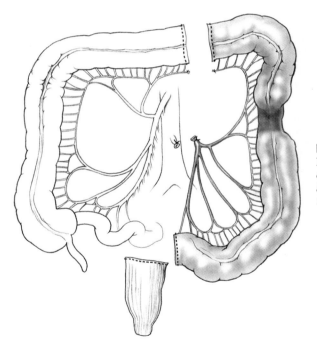

Figure 16-3
Left hemicolectomy for descending colon cancer. *(From Cameron JL [ed]: Current Surgical Therapy, 7th ed. Philadelphia, Mosby, 2001.)*

    B. The tail of the pancreas, left ureter, and left gonadal vessels should also be identified and protected during mobilization of the left colon.

V. **Sigmoid colectomy** is frequently performed for recurrent complicated sigmoid diverticulitis, and occasionally for sigmoid adenocarcinoma. Sigmoid colectomy involves ligation and division of the sigmoid branches of the inferior mesenteric artery, resection of the entire sigmoid colon, and creation of an anastomosis between the descending colon and the upper rectum (Fig. 16-4). Full mobilization of the splenic flexure is often required to create a tension-free anastomosis.

VI. Curiously, the terms "subtotal" and "total" **abdominal colectomy** are often used interchangeably; both describe the removal of the colon and preservation of the rectum. The ileocolic, right colic, middle colic, and inferior mesenteric vessels are

TRACTION ON THE SPLENIC FLEXURE CAN TEAR THE SPLENIC CAPSULE.

IDENTIFY AND AVOID THE HYPOGASTRIC NERVE PLEXUS NEAR THE TAKE-OFF OF THE INFERIOR MESENTERIC ARTERY.

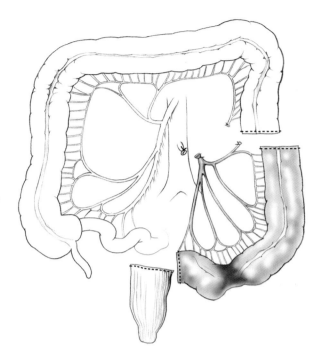

Figure 16-4
Sigmoid colectomy for sigmoid colon
cancer. *(From Cameron JL [ed]: Current
Surgical Therapy, 7th ed. Philadelphia, Mosby,
2001.)*

ligated and divided. After colon resection, an anastomosis is created between the
ileum and the upper rectum (Fig. 16-5). If an anastomosis is contraindicated, an
ileostomy is created and the remaining rectum is left in place as a **Hartmann's
pouch.**

VII. All of these procedures can be performed using laparoscopic or laparoscopically
assisted approaches. The indications for **laparoscopic colon resections** are essen-
tially the same as those for the corresponding open procedures. Generally, laparoscopic approaches are associated with longer operative times, and emergent
procedures should be performed using an open approach. The laparoscopic
approach to right colectomy is described.

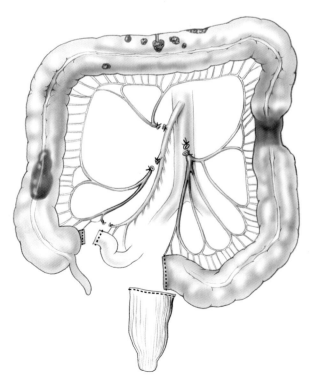

Figure 16-5
Total colectomy for synchronous colon
cancers. *(From Cameron JL [ed]: Current
Surgical Therapy, 7th ed. Philadelphia, Mosby,
2001.)*

VIII. **Laparoscopic Right Colectomy**
  A. Positioning
     1. The patient is placed in the supine position with the arms extended at 90 degrees.
     2. The sterile preparation should extend from the nipples superiorly, to the groin inferiorly, and to the midaxillary lines laterally.
  B. Port placement
     1. The first port is placed just above or below the umbilicus using either a "blind" percutaneous (Veress needle) or an open technique. The open technique is mandatory in pregnant patients and those who have had previous abdominal surgery.
     2. After the laparoscope is inserted through the umbilical port, two additional ports are placed under laparoscopic visualization. The second port is placed in the left or right upper quadrant, 2 cm below the costal margin and lateral to the epigastric vessels. The third post is placed in the midline just above the pubis.
  C. Mobilization of the colon terminal ileum, cecum, and ascending colon: Mobilization of the right colon is carried out as described for open colectomy.
  D. Exteriorization, mesenteric division, and anastomosis: Division of the bowel, ligation of the mesenteric vessels, and creation of the anastomosis during a laparoscopic colectomy may be performed extracorporeally (i.e., outside of the body) or intracorporally, using endoscopic stapling devices. The extracorporeal approach is described.
     1. The supraumbilical port site incision is extended transversely to the right of the umbilicus by 4 to 6 cm. Alternatively, a small midline incision may be made.
     2. The cecum is delivered through this incision, and the freely mobile right colon and hepatic flexure are exteriorized.
     3. Division of the bowel, resection of the mesentery, and bowel anastomosis proceed as in a standard open right colectomy.
     4. Once the anastomosis is complete, the bowel is returned into the abdomen. The anastomosis is inspected with the laparoscope.

> **CHECK TO ENSURE THAT THE ILEAL AND COLONIC MESENTERIES ARE NOT TWISTED BEFORE CREATION OF THE ANASTOMOSIS.**

IX. **Low anterior resection** is indicated for rectal lesions that are high enough to allow for adequate oncologic resection and preservation of the anal sphincters. Resection of cancers involving the lower half of the rectum should include excision of the entire mesorectum (which contains the lymph channels draining the tumor bed) in continuity with the rectum. This **total mesorectal excision** results in lower rates of local recurrence, impotence, and bladder dysfunction.
  A. Patient positioning and preparation
     1. The patient is placed in the lithotomy position.
     2. The sterile preparation should extend from the nipples superiorly, to the mid-thighs inferiorly, and to the midaxillary lines laterally, and should include the groin and perineum.
  B. Incision
     1. A midline incision is made, extending from 2 cm above the umbilicus to the pubic symphysis, and the peritoneum is opened.
     2. A self-retaining retractor is inserted into the abdomen, and the small bowel is packed into the right upper quadrant.
  C. Mobilization and division of the bowel
     1. The sigmoid colon and rectum are mobilized along the white line of Toldt from the peritoneal reflection anteriorly to the splenic flexure.
     2. The ureters are identified as they course in the retroperitoneum over the internal iliac vessels.
     3. The inferior mesenteric artery (IMA) is identified at the base of the mesentery, and the adjacent peritoneum is incised.
     4. The IMA is divided between two clamps. Each end is ligated.
     5. The mid or proximal sigmoid colon is divided with a stapler.

6. The proximal bowel is packed into the left upper quadrant.
7. Total mesorectal excision is performed by dissecting between the presacral fascia and the fascia propria of the rectum. The thin, avascular fibers encountered in the presacral space are often referred to as **Waldeyer's fascia.**
8. The hypogastric nerves are identified at the sacral promontory. These nerves descend into the presacral space and must be preserved to maintain postoperative sexual function.
9. Dissection proceeds down to the pelvic floor circumferentially. Anteriorly, the seminal vesicles and prostate in males and the vagina in females are protected.
10. The distal rectum is divided with a thoracoabdominal stapler, and the specimen is removed.

D. Creating the anastomosis
1. The proximal staple line is resected, and the "anvil" of the end-to-end anastomosis stapling device is inserted and secured in place.
2. The stapler is inserted through the anus. A trocar, attached to the stapler, is advanced through the rectal stump. The trocar is then removed, and the tip of the anvil is advanced into the end of the stapling device. The stapler is fired to create the anastomosis.
3. A proctoscopic examination with insufflation is performed to test for anastomotic leaks.
4. The abdomen is irrigated, and the fascia and skin are closed.

| Is the anastomosis well vascularized and tension-free? |

X. **Abdominoperineal resection** is required for the management of tumors that involve the anal sphincters and sphincter preservation or are too close to the sphincters to allow for resection with adequate margins. Patients with an unfavorable body habitus or poor preoperative sphincter control may require APR as well. The abdominal portion of APR, including rectal mobilization and nerve preservation, is identical to a low anterior resection. The perineal portion of the operation involves excision of the anus, the anal sphincters, and the distal rectum through an elliptical incision that extends around the anus from the perineal body anteriorly to the coccyx posteriorly. A permanent end colostomy is brought out through the left lower aspect of the anterior abdominal wall.

XI. **Total proctocolectomy with IPAA** allows for resection of the colon and rectum with restoration of GI continuity. Disadvantages of IPAA include frequent, loose bowel movements and relatively high complication rates. Notwithstanding, IPAA has become the treatment of choice in properly selected patients with UC requiring colon resection and FAP.

A. Controversy exists as to whether this operation should be performed in one stage (without ileostomy) or two (with ileostomy). The one-stage approach eliminates the need for a second operation and precludes complications that may accompany an ileostomy. Disadvantages include an increased risk of pelvic sepsis and symptomatic leaks of the pouch or ileoanal suture line. Most surgeons favor the two-stage operation, particularly in patients with UC, many of whom are immunosuppressed.

B. Ileal pouch–anal anastomosis involves mobilization of the ileal mesentery from the retroperitoneum (sometimes with division of the ileocolic artery to provide for adequate mesenteric length), rectal transection at the level of the levator muscles, and creation of an ileal pouch from the distal 20 cm of ileum (Fig. 16-6). A stapled anastomosis is constructed between the apex of the ileal pouch and the anus using an end-to-end anastomosis stapler.

POSTOPERATIVE COURSE

I. Postoperative care varies greatly, depending on the type of resection performed and the indication for surgery. Most patients are maintained on either intravenous narcotics or epidural analgesia. Oral pain medication is not initiated until the

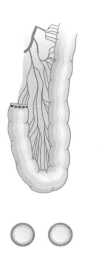
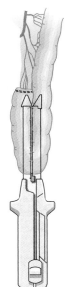
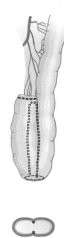

Figure 16-6
Creation of an ileal J-pouch. A reservoir is created from the distal ileum. A stapler is used to connect two limbs of intestine. *(From Townsend CM, Beauchamp RD, Evers BM, Mattox KL [eds]: Sabiston Textbook of Surgery: The Biological Basis of Modern Surgical Practice, 17th ed. Philadelphia, Saunders, 2004.)*

patient is tolerating oral intake. In patients without epidural analgesia, the urinary catheter can often be removed on the first postoperative day. Patients who undergo sigmoid or rectal resections are at relatively high risk for postoperative urinary retention as a result of dissection near the pelvic nerves, and may require more prolonged catheterization.

II. Twenty percent of patients who undergo elective colon resection will develop a postoperative ileus requiring the use of a nasogastric tube. Many surgeons remove the tube immediately after surgery and replace it if necessary; others advocate nasogastric decompression until the return of bowel function. Typically, a clear liquid diet is initiated with the return of bowel function and is advanced as is tolerated by the patient. Alternatively, oral intake may be initiated in the early postoperative period; however, the development of nausea and vomiting with oral intake should prompt a period of bowel rest. Antiemetics should be avoided because they may mask clinically important symptoms.

III. After low anterior resection or total proctocolectomy with ileoanal anastomosis, no medications should be administered per rectum. Digital rectal examinations and endoscopy should be used judiciously, if at all, to avoid anastomotic disruption.

COMPLICATIONS

I. **Anastomotic leak** most often develops between the third and seventh days after surgery. Patients may present with vague abdominal pain, fever, or leukocytosis.

A. Most often, leaks result in contained pelvic collections in the region of the anastomosis. Rarely, significant anastomotic disruption leads to diffuse peritoneal contamination. Lastly, an enterocutaneous fistula may result when a tract develops from the site of the leak to the skin. Fistulas are sometimes associated with concomitant fluid collections.

B. The management of a leak depends on the patient's clinical presentation. Stable patients are generally managed with bowel rest, antibiotic therapy, and percutaneous drainage of intra-abdominal collections. Reoperation with intestinal diversion is an acceptable initial strategy as well. Peritonitis and clinical deterioration are indications for urgent operative intervention, which usually involves abdominal washout, drainage, and creation of a diverting ostomy. Reoperation is also necessary when fistulas do not resolve after conservative management.

II. **Ureteral injury** is a serious complication of colectomy and is more common when significant inflammation is present (e.g., in complicated diverticulitis). If recognized intraoperatively, the ureter should be repaired immediately. Postoperatively, patients with a ureteral injury may present with abdominal pain or fever. CT may show an intra-abdominal fluid collection. Intravenous pyelogram can be obtained to confirm the diagnosis and will show urine extravasation from the disrupted ureter. Often, a percutaneous nephrostomy tube is required for urinary diversion, followed by a delayed ureteral repair.

III. **Anastomotic strictures** and associated bowel obstruction can complicate colon resection. Strictures are most common after low anastomoses involving the rectum or anus. When strictures present early in the postoperative course, they are usually caused by edema at the site of anastomosis and leak. More often, strictures present weeks to months after surgery as a result of scar formation related to low-grade ischemia of the anastomosis. Symptoms may include nausea, distention, small-caliber stools, and tenesmus. Digital rectal examination (for low strictures) and sigmoidoscopy or colonoscopy may aid in the diagnosis. Endoscopic dilation of the narrowed segment of bowel is sometimes an effective treatment. Strictures that are not amenable to endoscopic dilation may require operative revision of the anastomosis.

SUGGESTED READING

Mahmoud N, Rombeau J, Ross HM, Fry RD: Colon and rectum. In Townsend CM, Beauchamp RD, Evers BM, Mattox KL (eds): Sabiston Textbook of Surgery: The Biological Basis of Modern Surgical Practice, 17th ed. Philadelphia, Saunders, 2004, pp 1401–1481.

CHAPTER 17

Procedures for Benign Anorectal Disease

Hooman Noorchashm   and   David J. Maron

HEMORRHOIDS

Case Study

A 45-year-old multiparous female presents to a general surgeon's office complaining of intermittent painless bright red blood per rectum during bowel movements. She also notes anal discharge and perianal pruritis. She reports a long-standing history of constipation. Anoscopy is performed and shows redundant anorectal mucosa in the right anterolateral and right posterolateral positions.

BACKGROUND

Hemorrhoids are cushions of fibromuscular tissue that line the anal canal. Three main bundles of hemorrhoidal tissue are located at the right anterolateral, right posterolateral, and left lateral positions and play a role in anal continence. As it is used clinically, the term *hemorrhoid* connotes the pathologic engorgement of a cushion of hemorrhoidal tissue. Constipation, prolonged straining, and pregnancy may contribute to hemorrhoid development.

Hemorrhoids are broadly categorized as external or internal. **External hemorrhoids** develop distal to the dentate line and are associated with pain when they thrombose. **Internal hemorrhoids** develop proximal to the dentate line and are typically painless. Common presentations of internal hemorrhoids include bleeding and prolapse with defecation. The following classification system is used to describe internal hemorrhoids: (1) *first-degree* hemorrhoids are nonprolapsed, (2) *second-degree* hemorrhoids prolapse and spontaneously reduce, (3) *third-degree* hemorrhoids prolapse and must be digitally reduced, and (4) *fourth-degree* hemorrhoids are irreducible.

> The dentate line is the junction between the columnar epithelium of the upper anal canal and the squamous epithelium of the lower anal canal, also known as the anoderm.

INDICATIONS FOR SURGERY

I. **Failure of Medical Therapy:** Hemorrhoids often improve with Sitz baths, avoidance of excessive straining, stool softeners, and fiber supplementation. Patients with symptomatic hemorrhoids that do not improve with conservative management are candidates for more aggressive treatment. First-, second-, and third-degree hemorrhoids refractory to medical treatment are often treated with rubber band ligation, which can be performed in the office. Extensive third- and fourth-degree hemorrhoids are rarely amenable to conservative management or rubber band ligation and are typically treated with hemorrhoidectomy.

II. **Thrombosed External Hemorrhoids:** Acute thrombosis of an external hemorrhoid may be associated with severe pain. Patients who present early after thrombosis (<72 hours) may benefit from incision and clot enucleation.

PREOPERATIVE EVALUATION

I. **History:** Internal hemorrhoids are typically painless and may cause bright red bleeding or prolapse with defecation. Patients with external hemorrhoids may

COLORECTAL CANCER MUST ALWAYS BE EXCLUDED AS A SOURCE OF BLEEDING PER RECTUM.

Has your patient undergone colonoscopy?

complain of swelling and discomfort. In the absence of thrombosis, pain should not be attributed to hemorrhoids and alternative diagnoses should be sought.

II. **Physical Examination:** Physical examination of patients with hemorrhoids should include a digital rectal examination and anoscopy. In the absence of prolapse, anoscopic evaluation of internal hemorrhoids may show redundant anorectal mucosa. In patients who present with bleeding, endoscopic evaluation must be undertaken to exclude colorectal cancer.

COMPONENTS OF THE PROCEDURE AND APPLIED ANATOMY

Rubber band ligation can be performed in the office setting and is frequently used for the treatment of first-, second-, and some third-degree hemorrhoids. Traditional **open** and **closed** hemorrhoidectomy procedures are technically similar and lead to comparable outcomes. As its name implies, the closed technique involves closure of the defect created by hemorrhoid excision and is the approach most frequently used in the United States. Stapled hemorrhoidopexy is an increasingly popular alternative that may be associated with less postoperative pain than traditional hemorrhoidectomy.

I. **Preoperative Considerations**
A. Bowel preparation is administered preoperatively.
B. Antibiotics to cover gram-negative and anaerobic bacteria are administered preoperatively.
C. Rubber band ligation is often performed without anesthesia in the office setting. Hemorrhoidectomy and stapled hemorrhoidopexy may be performed under general or spinal anesthesia.

II. **Patient Positioning and Preparation:** The patient is placed in the **prone jack-knife position** (supine and flexed at the hips). The perianal region is prepared and draped.

III. **Surgical Approach**
A. Rubber band ligation:
1. A speculum is inserted into the anal canal and the hemorrhoidal bundles are identified.
2. With a band applicator, two rubber bands are applied to each hemorrhoidal cluster above the dentate line (Fig. 17-1).

APPLICATION OF RUBBER BANDS BELOW THE DENTATE LINE IS ASSOCIATED WITH SEVERE PAIN BECAUSE THE ANODERM DISTAL TO THE DENTATE LINE IS INNERVATED BY SOMATIC PAIN FIBERS.

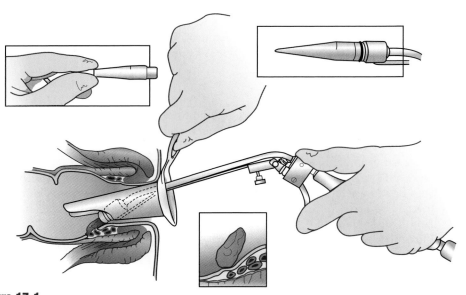

Figure 17-1
Rubber band ligation of hemorrhoids. Rubber bands are loaded onto the applicator, which is introduced into the anal canal. The hemorrhoidal bundles are suctioned into the applicator and bands are applied. *(From Townsend CM, Beauchamp RD, Evers BM, Mattox KL [eds]: Sabiston Textbook of Surgery: The Biological Basis of Modern Surgical Practice, 17th ed. Philadelphia, Saunders, 2004.)*

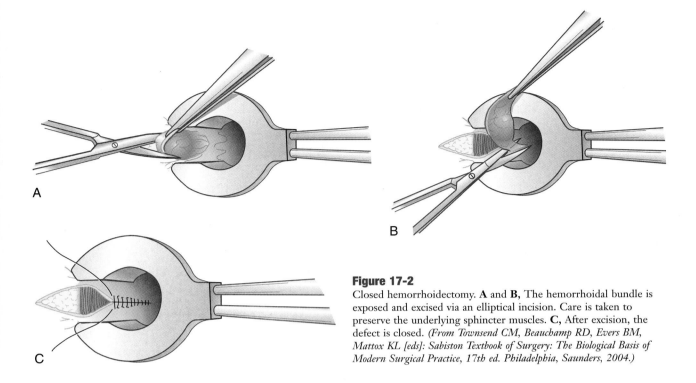

Figure 17-2

Closed hemorrhoidectomy. **A** and **B**, The hemorrhoidal bundle is exposed and excised via an elliptical incision. Care is taken to preserve the underlying sphincter muscles. **C,** After excision, the defect is closed. *(From Townsend CM, Beauchamp RD, Evers BM, Mattox KL [eds]: Sabiston Textbook of Surgery: The Biological Basis of Modern Surgical Practice, 17th ed. Philadelphia, Saunders, 2004.)*

B. **Closed hemorrhoidectomy:**
   1. A retractor is inserted into the anal canal, and the hemorrhoidal bundles are identified.
   2. Enlarged hemorrhoidal tissues are excised with an elliptical incision. Care is taken to preserve the underlying muscle fibers of the anal sphincters.
   3. When multiple bundles are excised, intervening bridges of anoderm are preserved to avoid subsequent stenosis.
   4. After excision, defects are closed with absorbable suture (Fig. 17-2).
C. **Stapled hemorrhoidopexy:** A circular anal dilator/stapler is inserted into the anal canal. A purse-string suture is placed through the mucosa and submucosa of the anal canal, 3 to 4 cm above the dentate line, to draw the hemorrhoidal tissue into the stapling device. The stapler is fired to excise a 4-cm ring of rectal mucosa (Fig. 17-3).

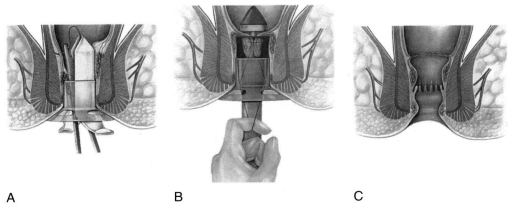

Figure 17-3

Stapled hemorrhoidopexy. A suture is placed through the mucosa and submucosa (**A**), which are drawn into the stapling device (**B**). The stapler is fired to excise a ring of hemorrhoidal tissue (**C**). *(From Cameron J: Current Surgical Therapy, 8th ed. Philadelphia, Mosby, 2004.)*

POSTOPERATIVE COURSE

Hemorrhoidectomy is typically performed as an outpatient procedure. Patients may experience substantial postoperative pain and should be prescribed analgesic agents and stool softeners. Use of a doughnut cushion may improve comfort when sitting.

COMPLICATIONS

I. **Perineal sepsis** is a well-described complication of hemorrhoidectomy. Severe postprocedure pain, inability to void, and fever may herald the onset of sepsis and should prompt emergent evaluation.

II. **Bleeding** is common after hemorrhoidectomy. Bleeding is usually self-limited, but occasionally requires operative intervention.

III. **Urinary retention** is common after hemorrhoidectomy. Although it is typically self-limited, temporary placement of a urinary catheter is sometimes necessary.

IV. **Stricture formation** after hemorrhoidectomy has been associated with circumferential excision of anoderm. Preservation of intervening islands of anoderm between excised bundles may lessen the risk of stricture formation.

ANORECTAL ABSCESS

Case Study

A 35-year-old male presents to a surgeon's office complaining of perianal pain and purulent discharge for the last 2 days. His symptoms preclude him from sitting or walking comfortably. One month earlier, the patient underwent incision and drainage of a perirectal abscess and began a course of oral antibiotics.

BACKGROUND

The majority of anorectal abscesses result from infection originating in the anal crypts located at the dentate line. Abscesses are classified as **perianal** (60%), **ischiorectal** (20%), **intersphincteric** (10%), or **supralevator** (9%), depending on their location (Fig. 17-4). **Deep postanal space abscesses** represent a particular challenge. The deep postanal space is protected from view by the sacrum, and abscesses originating in this cavity may track circumferentially into the ischiorectal, intersphincteric, or supralevator space before they are diagnosed (Fig. 17-5). This pattern of spread results in what is known as a *horseshoe abscess*.

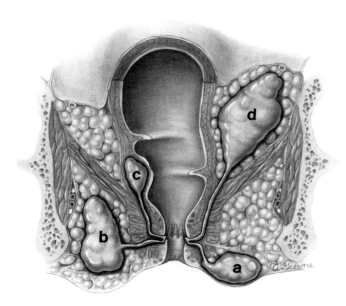

Figure 17-4
Common anatomic locations of anorectal abscesses: perianal (a), ischiorectal (b), intersphincteric (c), and supralevator (d). *(From Noble J [ed]: Textbook of Primary Care Medicine, 3rd ed. Philadelphia, Mosby, 2001.)*

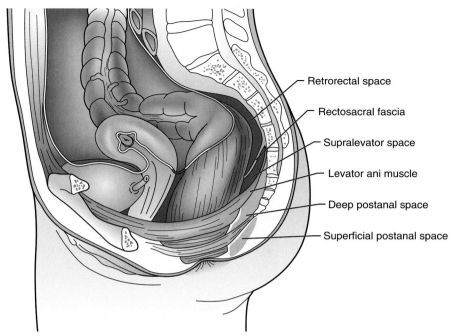

Figure 17-5
Lateral view of the deep postanal space. *(From Cameron J: Current Surgical Therapy, 8th ed. Philadelphia, Mosby, 2004.)*

Anorectal abscesses are often caused by normal intestinal tract flora (e.g., *Escherichia coli* and *Bacteroides splanchnicus*). Alternatively, infections of the perianal skin caused by gram-positive organisms may evolve into perianal abscesses.

INDICATIONS FOR SURGERY

Anorectal abscesses should be treated with prompt surgical drainage. Septic and immunosuppressed patients should be taken to the operating room emergently. Although some abscesses may be drained at the bedside, drainage in the operating room allows for better patient positioning, exposure, and anesthesia.

PREOPERATIVE EVALUATION

I. **History:** Patients with anorectal abscesses may complain of pain, fevers, chills, and purulent discharge. A history of recurrent abscesses and immunosuppression (e.g., HIV/AIDS and diabetes) should be elicited.

II. **Physical Examination:** Although digital rectal examination should be performed when tolerated by the patient, examination under anesthesia (EUA) is required to define the anatomy of the anorectal abcess. An EUA is typically combined with drainage of the abcess.

   A. Superficial abscesses (i.e., perianal and ischiorectal abscesses) typically present with tenderness, fluctuance, and erythema.

   B. Perianal abscesses are found adjacent to the anal verge.

   C. Ischiorectal abscesses are typically larger and present with a buttock mass.

   D. Intersphincteric and supralevator abscesses may present with tenderness and fullness within the anal canal.

III. **Laboratory Studies:** Leukocytosis is frequently noted on complete blood count.

IV. **Imaging Studies:** Computed tomography (CT) scanning or magnetic resonance imaging (MRI) of the pelvis may be helpful in delineating the anatomy of an abscess, particularly when examination findings are equivocal.

COMPONENTS OF THE PROCEDURE AND APPLIED ANATOMY

I. **Preoperative Considerations**
   A. Broad-spectrum antibiotics are administered preoperatively, when the diagnosis of abscess is made.
   B. In the case of superficial abscesses, local anesthetics are used to infiltrate the surrounding area. Drainage of complex abscesses may be performed under conscious sedation or general, epidural, or spinal anesthesia.

II. **Patient Positioning and Preparation:** The patient is placed in the **prone jack-knife position.** The perianal region is prepared and draped.

III. **Surgical Approach**
   A. Perianal and ischiorectal abscesses
      1. Perianal and ischiorectal abscesses are superficial and readily drained by incising the skin overlying the abscess cavity. Both are typically associated with appreciable fluctuance and are therefore readily localized by external examination.
      2. An elliptical or cruciate incision is made over the area of maximal fluctuance. A finger or instrument is inserted into the abscess cavity to break any loculations. The abscess cavity is then irrigated with sterile saline. The skin edges are trimmed to prevent rapid closure of the incision and ensure ongoing drainage.
      3. When draining an ischiorectal abscess, care must be taken not to violate the levator muscle (which lies superior to the ischiorectal fossa) because this can result in the development of a supralevator abscess.
   B. Intersphincteric abscesses
      1. Intersphincteric abscesses are generally located posteriorly. Unlike perianal and ischiorectal abscesses, they are not usually evident on external examination. However, a tender mass is sometimes appreciable on digital rectal examination.
      2. To access the intersphincteric space, a posterior transverse incision is made in the anoderm. The plane between the internal and external sphincters is developed bluntly, and the abscess cavity is opened and irrigated with sterile saline.
      3. A mushroom catheter is placed in the cavity and sutured in place.
   C. Supralevator abscesses: Supralevator abscesses may develop from upward extension of intersphincteric or ischiorectal abscesses. Abscesses that develop from extension of infections of the intersphincteric space are drained directly through the rectal mucosa, whereas abscesses that communicate with ischiorectal abscesses are drained through the ischiorectal fossa (as described under "Perianal and Ischiorectal Abscesses").
   D. Deep postanal space abscesses: To access the deep postanal space, a posterior transverse incision is made in the anoderm. The plane between the internal and external sphincters is developed bluntly. Dissection is continued superiorly through the puborectalis muscle to enter the deep postanal space. A drainage catheter placed in the abscess cavity and sutured in place.

THE LEVATOR MUSCLE SHOULD NOT BE VIOLATED DURING DRAINAGE OF AN ISCHIORECTAL ABSCESS.

Failure to leave a drainage catheter in the intersphincteric space after abscess drainage results in a high rate of recurrence.

POSTOPERATIVE COURSE

After drainage of anorectal abscesses, patients are prescribed analgesia, local anesthetics, stool softeners, and mild laxatives. Antibiotic therapy should be continued during the postoperative period, particularly in immunosuppressed patients (e.g., those with HIV/AIDS or diabetes).

COMPLICATIONS

I. **Recurrence** rates after abscess drainage may be as high as 30%. Incomplete drainage of a deep postanal space abscess is one example of a technical error, which can result in recurrent ischiorectal abscesses.

II. Rates of **fistula formation** after drainage of anorectal abscesses are also high (40%), and careful postoperative follow-up is essential.

ANORECTAL FISTULAE

Case Study

A 32-year-old male presents to a surgeon's office complaining of intermittent purulent anal discharge. His medical history is significant for inflammatory bowel disease and recurrent anorectal abscesses. He is afebrile and has a normal white blood cell count. On examination, several draining perianal sinuses are noted anteriorly.

BACKGROUND

A fistula is defined as the abnormal communication between two epithelial-lined surfaces. Most anorectal fistulae begin as abscesses of the anal crypts. The offending organisms are almost always enteric bacteria. A communication between the epithelial surface of the perianal region and the infected anal crypt may form spontaneously or iatrogenically after surgical drainage. Anorectal fistulae are classified by the anatomic relationship of the tract to the anal sphincters as intersphincteric, trans-sphincteric, suprasphincteric, or extrasphincteric (Fig. 17-6).

> Spontaneous anorectal fistulae are caused by inflammatory bowel disease, congenital desmoids, chronic pelvic sepsis, tuberculosis, and actinomycosis.

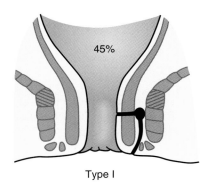

Type I

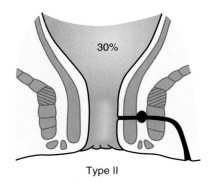

Type II

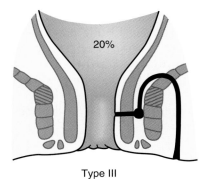

Type III

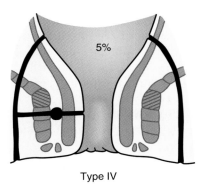

Type IV

Figure 17-6

Anatomic classification of anorectal fistulae. Intersphincteric fistulae (type I) are confined to the intersphincteric plane. Trans-sphincteric fistulae (type II) traverse the external sphincter. Suprasphincteric fistulae (type III) traverse the levator muscle above the sphincter. Extrasphincteric fistulae (type IV) form a communication between the rectum and perianal skin, external to the sphincters. The puborectalis muscle is identified by *cross-hatching* and forms the superior boundary of the external sphincter. *(From Parks AG, Gordon PH, Hardcastle JD: A classification of fistula-in-ano. Br J Surg 63:5, 1976. Copyright British Journal of Surgery Society Ltd. Reproduced with permission. Permission is granted by John Wiley & Sons Ltd. on behalf of the BJSS Ltd.)*

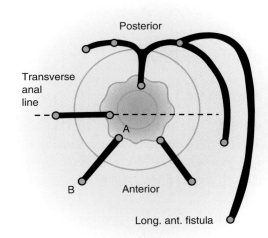

Figure 17-7
Goodsall's rule. Posterior external openings communicate with the anal canal at the posterior midline through a curved tract (**A**). Anterior external openings directly communicate with the closest anal crypt along a straight path (**B**). The long anterior fistula is an exception to the rule and may also communicate with the anal canal through an internal opening at the posterior midline. *(From Schrock TR: Benign and malignant disease of the anorectum. In Fromm O [ed]: Gastrointestinal Surgery. New York, Churchill Livingstone, 1985, p 612.)*

The path of fistulae generally follows *Goodsall's rule* (Fig. 17-7), which states that posterior external openings communicate with the anal canal at the posterior midline through a curved tract, whereas anterior external openings communicate directly with the closest anal crypt along a straight path. Multiple anterior external openings typically have separate internal openings. Multiple posterior external openings usually have a common posterior midline internal opening.

INDICATIONS FOR SURGERY

Failure of Medical Management: Persistent anorectal fistulae require operative management. Surgical treatment of anorectal fistulae in the setting of inflammatory bowel disease is optimally undertaken when the inflammatory process is relatively quiescent.

PREOPERATIVE EVALUATION

I. **History:** Patients typically report a history of anorectal abscesses. A history of a predisposing medical condition (e.g., inflammatory bowel disease) should also be elicited.
II. **Physical Examination:** Proctoscopy and sigmoidoscopy are useful in identifying the location of the internal fistula openings and evaluating for the presence of underlying pathology, respectively. These evaluations are usually undertaken at the time of surgery. Additionally, **methylene blue or hydrogen peroxide** can be injected into the external opening to identify the internal fistula opening when it is not readily apparent.
III. **Imaging Studies:** Magnetic resonance imaging is sometimes useful for delineating the anatomy of complex fistulae.

COMPONENTS OF THE PROCEDURE AND APPLIED ANATOMY

I. **Preoperative Considerations**
   A. Bowel preparation is administered preoperatively.
   B. Broad-spectrum antibiotics are often administered in the perioperative setting.
   C. Fistulae may be approached under general, epidural, or spinal anesthesia.
II. **Patient Positioning and Preparation:** The patient is placed in the prone jack-knife position. The perianal region is prepared and draped.

III. **Surgical Approach**
   A. The surgical approach to a fistula tract depends on whether it traverses the anal sphincters or the puborectalis muscle. Fistulae that do not traverse these muscles are typically treated with a simple fistulotomy. Those involving the sphincter muscle are treated with seton fistulotomy, fibrin glue, an anal fistula plug, or a mucosal advancement flap to preserve anal continence.
   B. Fistulotomy
      1. A malleable probe is gently inserted into the fistula tract.
      2. The skin and epithelium overlying the tract are divided with cautery. If more than a few muscle fibers are encountered in the course of this dissection, the procedure is converted to a seton fistulotomy.
   C. Seton fistulotomy (cutting seton)
      1. Soft rubber tubing or heavy silk suture (i.e., a seton) is threaded through a malleable probe and passed through the fistula tract.
      2. The perianal skin and only the most superficial fibers of the internal sphincter overlying the fistula tract are typically divided.
      3. The seton is held in place while the probe is removed from the tract. The ends of the seton are tied together to create a loop through the tract.
      4. The seton may be intermittently tightened in the office setting to allow for gradual division and healing of the sphincter (i.e., *a cutting seton*).
   D. **Fibrin Glue and Anal Fistula Plug:** The fistula tract is irrigated and injected with either fibrin glue or a decellularized porcine collagen plug. Both are intended to occlude the fistula tract. The collagen plug also serves as a "bioscaffold" on which scar tissue may form.
   E. Mucosal advancement flap
      1. The fistula tract is excised from the external opening to the sphincter muscles.
      2. The internal opening is visualized with the aid of a retractor.
      3. A mucosal flap incorporating the internal fistula opening is raised off the underlying internal sphincter muscle. The opening of the fistula is sharply excised from the flap.
      4. The flap is pulled down and sutured in place over the exposed muscle.

POSTOPERATIVE COURSE

Adequate analgesia, antibiotic coverage, and local hygiene are critical to a successful outcome. After seton fistulotomy, patients should be examined at regular intervals. The seton may be tightened biweekly to gradually divide the involved portion of sphincter muscle. By the second or third postoperative visit, the seton has usually divided through the sphincter muscle and may have fallen out spontaneously.

COMPLICATIONS

   I. **Recurrence** is common after surgery, particularly in the setting of an under-lying inflammatory process. Careful postoperative follow-up in the office is required.
   II. **Incontinence** may result from dissection of the anal sphincter muscles. This complication is more common in the setting of complex fistulae.

FISSURE IN ANO

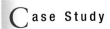

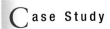ase Study

A 30-year-old female presents to a surgeon's office 3 months postpartum from an uneventful vaginal delivery. She complains of intense anal pain during defecation, accompanied by mild bleeding on the toilet paper. On physical examination, a small, shallow anal ulcer is seen at the anterior midline of the anal margin.

BACKGROUND

Anal fissures are caused by a split in the highly sensitive squamous epithelium of the anal canal below the dentate line. **Primary fissures** are typically associated with constipation and local trauma. Ninety percent of primary fissures occur in the posterior midline. However, postpartum fissures sometimes occur in the anterior aspect of the anal canal during childbirth. **Secondary fissures** are complications of AIDS, anal tuberculosis, or Crohn's disease. These fissures may occur away from the midline.

INDICATIONS FOR SURGERY

Failure of Medical Therapy: Anal fissures are initially treated medically. The majority of patients with anal fissures respond to stool softeners, bulking agents, and topical anesthetics. An increase in dietary fiber intake by at least 15 g/day, along with topical lidocaine therapy, is often effective in healing acute fissures. Topical nitroglycerine or diltiazem may also be used in an effort to relax the internal anal sphincter and increase blood flow. Failure of medical management and fissure recurrence are indications for surgical therapy. The main objective of surgery is to reduce the hyperactivity of the internal anal sphincter.

> The relapse rate after medical management of chronic anal fissures approaches 50% at 12 months.

PREOPERATIVE EVALUATION

I. **History:** Patients with fissures typically complain of pain and bleeding with defecation. Most patients report a history of chronic constipation.

II. **Physical Examination:** Fissures are usually evident on examination as "boat-shaped" defects with edematous margins. Transverse fibers of the internal anal sphincter are sometimes seen at the ulcer base. Digital examination may cause intense pain and is not recommended.

> Is your patient's fissure located at the midline?

III. **Endoscopy:** Before surgical therapy for the treatment of anal fissure, a complete examination under anesthesia should be undertaken. The sensitivity of this evaluation may be enhanced by proctosigmoidoscopy to rule out underlying anorectal pathology.

COMPONENTS OF THE PROCEDURE AND APPLIED ANATOMY

I. **Preoperative Considerations**
   A. Bowel preparation is sometimes administered preoperatively, particularly if the patient is to undergo endoscopic evaluation.
   B. Sphincterotomy may be performed under general or spinal anesthesia.

II. **Patient Positioning and Preparation:** The patient is placed in the prone jack-knife position. The perianal region is prepped and draped.

III. **Surgical Approach**
   A. The main objective of surgery for anal fissures is to reduce the hyperactivity of the internal anal sphincter through division of its fibers.
   B. Lateral subcutaneous internal sphincterotomy
      1. Lidocaine containing epinephrine is injected into the submucosal and intersphincteric planes.
      2. The surgeon's index finger is placed into the anal canal.
      3. A small blade is inserted laterally into the intersphincteric groove, and the hypertrophied fibers of the internal sphincter are divided, avoiding division of the anal mucosa (Fig. 17-8).
   C. Open internal sphincterotomy
      1. Lidocaine containing epinephrine is injected into the submucosal and intersphincteric plane of the anal wall.
      2. The lateral aspect of the anal canal is exposed with a speculum.

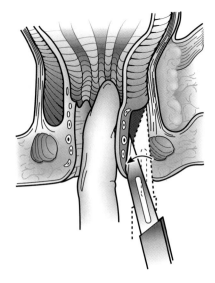

Figure 17-8
Lateral subcutaneous internal sphincterotomy. The fibers of the internal sphincter are sharply divided against an index finger without dividing the anal mucosa. *(From Cameron J: Current Surgical Therapy, 8th ed. Philadelphia, Mosby, 2004.)*

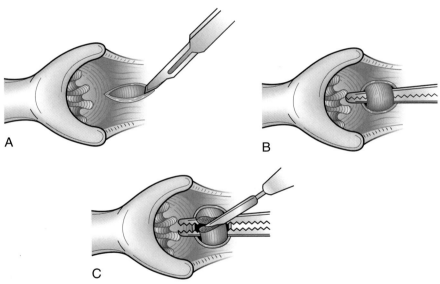

Figure 17-9
Open lateral sphincterotomy. The anoderm is incised, exposing the fibers of the internal sphincter (**A** and **B**). The fibers are sharply divided (**C**). *(From Cameron J: Current Surgical Therapy, 8th ed. Philadelphia, Mosby, 2004.)*

3. A 1- to 1.5-cm incision is made through the anoderm below the dentate line.
4. The anal mucosa is dissected away from the internal sphincter.
5. The fibers of the internal sphincter are divided (Fig. 17-9).

> POSTERIOR SPHINCTEROTOMY AND FISSURE EXCISION ARE NEVER WARRANTED BECAUSE THIS APPROACH IS ASSOCIATED WITH CHRONIC INCONTINENCE.

POSTOPERATIVE COURSE

Surgery for anal fissures is typically performed in the outpatient setting. Patients are prescribed analgesics, local anesthetics, and stool softeners before discharge.

COMPLICATIONS

I. **Bleeding** occurs in 2% to 3% of patients after surgery for anal fissures.
II. **Fecal incontinence** occurs in 3% to 5% of patients and can last for up to 2 or 3 months, but is usually self-limited.

SUGGESTED READINGS

Cameron JL: Current Surgical Therapy, 8th ed. Philadelphia, Mosby, 2004, pp 245–261.

Kleighley MRB: Anorectal disorders. In Fischer JE, Bland KI (eds): Mastery of Surgery, 5th ed. Philadelphia, Lippincott Williams & Wilkins, 2007, pp 1609–1627.

Nelson H: Anus. In Townsend CM, Beauchamp RD, Evers BM, Mattox KL (eds): Sabiston Textbook of Surgery: The Biological Basis of Modern Surgical Practice, 17th ed. Philadelphia, Saunders, 2004, pp 1483–1512.

CHAPTER 18

Splenectomy

Paul J. Foley, Thomas A. Wixted, and Donna J. Barbot

Case Study

A 20-year-old female with immune (idiopathic) thrombocytopenic purpura (ITP) is referred by her hematologist to a general surgeon for refractory thrombocytopenia despite treatment with corticosteroids and intravenous immune globulin (IVIG). Her platelet count is 20,000/mm^3, and she notes heavy menstrual periods, bruising, and gingival bleeding.

BACKGROUND

The spleen plays a central role in a variety of physiologic processes, including (1) hematopoiesis in early fetal development, (2) the maintenance of normal erythrocyte morphology and function, and (3) the generation of germinal center reactions. This diversity in function is reflected by the similarly diverse group of pathologic processes that sometimes affect the spleen and require surgical intervention. Indications for, and approaches to, splenectomy are the topics of this chapter.

INDICATIONS FOR SPLENECTOMY

I. **Platelet-Associated: ITP** is the most common indication for elective splenectomy. ITP is caused by circulating autoantibodies that bind to platelet membrane antigens and facilitate phagocytosis in the spleen and elsewhere.

A. Patients with ITP commonly present with a history of bruising, epistaxis, and gingival bleeding. Life-threatening complications, such as gastrointestinal or intracranial hemorrhage, are much less common. Women are affected more often than are men; however, in children, ITP affects both sexes equally. ITP in children is typically characterized by a more rapid onset and a more severe course than in adults. Spontaneous remission occurs in approximately 80% of affected children, and splenectomy should be reserved for cases of severe refractory ITP lasting longer than 1 year in this patient population.

B. Therapy for ITP is aimed at achieving sustained remission. In patients with asymptomatic disease, treatment is indicated for platelet counts between 20,000/mm^3 and 30,000/mm^3 or for platelet counts less than 50,000/mm^3 with additional risk factors for bleeding, such as hypertension and peptic ulcer disease. Initial treatment consists of glucocorticoids. In patients with platelet counts less than 20,000/mm^3 or with life-threatening bleeding, hospitalization is indicated. IVIG plays an important role in the management of acute bleeding as well as in the surgical preparation of patients with platelet counts of less than 20,000/mm^3. Splenectomy is indicated in patients with thrombocytopenia refractory to steroids and IVIG, steroid-associated side effects, or recurrent thrombocytopenia after steroid treatment.

C. Approximately 75% of patients respond to splenectomy and maintain a normal platelet count 2 months after surgery. Patients who do not respond to splenectomy or who experience a relapse should be evaluated for the presence of an accessory spleen, which is present in up to 10% of cases.

II. **Erythrocyte-Associated**

A. **Hereditary spherocytosis (HS):** HS is an autosomal dominant hemolytic anemia caused by a deficiency of spectrin, a protein that gives red blood cells their shape, strength, and flexibility. Erythrocytes that are deficient in spectrin lose surface area and deformability and have a characteristic spherical shape. Spherocytes are sequestered in the microcirculation of the spleen and destroyed. Patients with HS most commonly present with anemia, jaundice, and splenomegaly. Splenectomy significantly improves the anemia by eliminating the predominant site of red cell destruction. Splenectomy should be delayed until after 4 years of age to preserve immunologic function and reduce the risk of overwhelming postsplenectomy infection (see Complications). Given the high incidence of bilirubin gallstones in patients with this disorder, an abdominal ultrasound should be performed before splenectomy. If cholelithiasis is present, cholecystectomy should be performed at the time of splenectomy.

B. **Hemoglobinopathies:** Inherited disorders of hemoglobin synthesis, such as sickle cell disease and the thalassemias, are associated with increased erythrocyte destruction and anemia.

1. **Sickle cell disease** results from a genetic mutation in the beta globin chain that causes an abnormal hemoglobin tetramer (hemoglobin S). Deoxygenated hemoglobin S polymerizes within erythrocytes, leading to the characteristic sickle shape. These red blood cells can occlude capillaries and lead to microinfarction within various organ systems. Repeated vaso-occlusive insults cause the spleen to infarct and atrophy. **Splenic sequestration crisis** is characterized by a marked decrease in the hemoglobin concentration, hypovolemia, and splenomegaly. Patients may experience severe pain and require multiple blood transfusions. Splenectomy is indicated after a first episode of acute splenic sequestration and in patients with hypersplenism.

2. The **thalassemias** are a group of disorders resulting from abnormal synthesis of one of the hemoglobin chains. Patients with these disorders present with varying degrees of anemia and splenomegaly. Transfusions and iron chelation are the hallmarks of long-term treatment. Splenectomy is indicated in patients with increasing transfusion requirements and symptomatic splenomegaly.

C. **Autoimmune hemolytic anemia (AIHA):** *AIHA* is a term that describes a group of disorders characterized by the presence of autoantibodies that bind to the surface of erythrocytes and lead to hemolysis.

1. In warm-antibody AIHA, so named because the predominant IgG antibodies preferentially bind at 37°C, tissue macrophages within the spleen recognize antibody-bound erythrocytes and remove them from the circulation. Initial treatment consists of steroid therapy or other immunosuppressive agents. Splenectomy eliminates the major site of hemolysis and should be performed in patients in whom medical therapy is unsuccessful and in those who cannot receive corticosteroids.

2. Hemolysis in cold-antibody AIHA, so named because the predominant IgM antibodies preferentially bind at 4°C, is largely mediated by complement activation. Because the spleen is not a major site of erythrocyte destruction in this type of AIHA, splenectomy is generally not helpful.

III. **Leukocyte-Associated**

A. **Hodgkin's lymphoma:** Hodgkin's lymphoma is a malignancy that predominantly affects young adults. Historically, the staging of Hodgkin's lymphoma required laparotomy and splenectomy. Improvements in computed tomography (CT) scanning and other imaging modalities have made surgical staging far less important in directing treatment. Splenectomy is indicated for symptomatic splenomegaly.

Splenomegaly = Enlargement of the spleen

Hypersplenism = Increased or overactive hemolytic activity of the spleen

---

Splenic sequestration crises are recurrent in 50% of patients with sickle cell disease and fatal in 10% to 15% of patients.

B. **Non-Hodgkin's lymphoma (NHL):** NHL constitutes a diverse group of primary malignancies of the lymphoreticular tissue. Splenectomy is indicated in patients with hypersplenism resulting in anemia, thrombocytopenia, neutropenia, or symptomatic splenomegaly. NHL limited to the spleen is an additional indication for splenectomy.

C. **Hairy cell leukemia (HCL):** HCL is characterized by splenomegaly, pancytopenia, and evidence of cell membrane projections on microscopy. Purine analogues constitute first-line treatment. Splenectomy is reserved for patients with disease refractory to medical therapy and those with symptomatic splenomegaly.

D. **Chronic lymphocytic leukemia:** Chronic lymphocytic leukemia is a lymphoproliferative disorder characterized by the accumulation of functionally incompetent lymphocytes of monoclonal origin. Splenectomy is indicated for symptomatic splenomegaly and for hypersplenism.

E. **Chronic myelogenous leukemia (CML):** CML is a myeloproliferative disorder characterized by clonal proliferation of myeloid cells at all stages of maturation. A chromosomal translocation between chromosomes 9 and 22 (Philadelphia chromosome), which leads to the elaboration of a novel fusion protein (Bcr-Abl), is critical to the pathogenesis of this disease. Treatment of CML includes tyrosine kinase inhibitors and hematopoietic stem cell transplantation. Splenectomy may be performed for symptomatic splenomegaly or hypersplenism.

IV. **Nonhematologic Abnormalities of the Spleen**

A. **Tumors:** Primary nonlymphoid tumors of the spleen are uncommon. **Hemangiomas** are the most common benign primary tumor of the spleen and are sometimes associated with splenic rupture and thrombocytopenia when large. Splenectomy is indicated for symptomatic lesions. Splenic **hamartomas** and **lymphangiomas** are benign tumors and are rarely associated with symptoms. Splenectomy is sometimes performed for diagnostic purposes. **Angiosarcomas** are highly aggressive tumors with a poor prognosis. Patients may present with splenomegaly, hemolytic anemia, or spontaneous splenic rupture. Splenectomy is indicated, but is most often palliative. Metastases to the spleen are uncommon and are usually indicative of disseminated disease. Splenectomy may be appropriate if the spleen is the site of an isolated metastasis.

B. **Splenic cysts**
   1. **True (epithelium-lined) splenic cysts** may be parasitic or nonparasitic. In the United States, nonparasitic cysts are much more common. These are typically discovered incidentally, but may cause symptoms such as abdominal pain, nausea, and early satiety when large. Splenectomy is indicated for patients with symptomatic cysts. Parasitic cysts are rare in the United States and are most commonly due to infection with *Echinococcus granulosus*. Associated liver involvement is common. Cyst rupture and spillage of scoleces can be catastrophic; therefore, splenectomy is indicated for the treatment of all parasitic cysts.
   2. **Splenic pseudocysts** (i.e., those with no epithelial lining) are the most common type of splenic cysts and are typically post-traumatic. Splenectomy is indicated for symptomatic cysts and those larger than 10 cm.

C. **Splenic abscess:** Splenic abscesses may result from hematogenous spread of infection from a remote site, such as the heart (endocarditis) or bone (osteomyelitis), or from bacteremia (most commonly, in the setting of intravenous drug use). Other risk factors include malignancy, previous trauma, poor nutritional status, and immunocompromise. Patients may present with fever, vague abdominal pain, or pleuritic pain. Treatment consists of intravenous antibiotic therapy and control of the infectious source. Percutaneous drainage may be attempted for a unilocular splenic abscess. Multilocular abscesses typically require splenectomy. Failure of percutaneous drainage and clinical deterioration are additional indications for splenectomy.

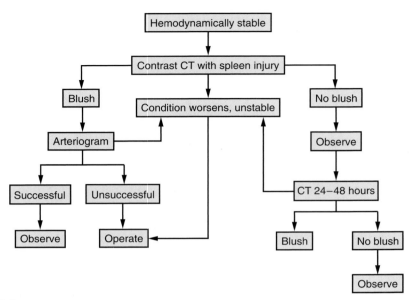

Figure 18-1

Algorithm for the management of splenic trauma. *(Modified from Townsend CM, Beauchamp RD, Evers BM, Mattox KL [eds]: Sabiston Textbook of Surgery: The Biological Basis of Modern Surgical Practice, 17th ed. Philadelphia, Saunders, 2004.)*

D. **Sinistral hypertension:** Pancreatitis is sometimes associated with splenic vein thrombosis and the development of sinistral (left-sided) portal hypertension, which may be complicated by gastric varix formation. Symptomatic hypersplenism and gastrointestinal bleeding from varices are indications for splenectomy.

E. **Infectious mononucleosis:** Infectious mononucleosis is rarely complicated by splenic rupture. Patients typically present with abdominal pain or hemodynamic compromise and require urgent splenectomy.

V. **Trauma**

A. Splenic injuries are most commonly caused by rapid deceleration, puncture from adjacent rib fractures, penetrating trauma, or high-energy transfer through the posterolateral aspect of the chest wall. Given the extensive arterial supply of the spleen, it is not surprising that such injuries can result in extensive hemorrhage. Current modalities for evaluating splenic injury include helical CT scanning and ultrasound. CT scanning is particularly useful in that it allows for the rapid evaluation of multiple abdominal organs and the retroperitoneum. The Focused Abdominal Sonography for Trauma (FAST) examination can identify fluid in the peritoneum. A positive finding on FAST examination in a hemodynamically unstable patient warrants emergent laparotomy.

B. Nonoperative management of splenic injuries is appropriate in certain situations. If a patient is hemodynamically stable without additional abdominal injuries requiring exploration and there is no blush (i.e., extravasation of contrast) from the spleen on CT scan, splenic injuries may be observed without immediate operative intervention (Fig. 18-1). Evidence of a hilar injury, hemodynamic instability after resuscitation, and persistent transfusion requirements are indications for operative exploration in patients with evidence of a splenic injury.

PREOPERATIVE EVALUATION

I. **Imaging Studies:** Preoperative imaging of the abdomen commonly includes CT. The need for additional imaging is largely dictated by the diagnosis.

II. **Vaccination:** All patients undergoing elective splenectomy should receive vaccines for the encapsulated organisms *Streptoccus pneumoniae, Neisseria meningiditis,* and *Haemophilus influenzae* type B 2 or more weeks before the planned operation. After urgent or emergent splenectomy, patients should be vaccinated before discharge.

ALL PATIENTS UNDERGOING SPLENECTOMY SHOULD RECEIVE VACCINES FOR *STREPTOCOCCUS PNEUMONIAE*, *NEISSERIA MENINGIDITIS*, AND *HAEMOPHILUS INFLUENZAE* TYPE B.

COMPONENTS OF THE PROCEDURE AND APPLIED ANATOMY

See Figures 18-2 and 18-3.

Open Splenectomy

I. **Patient Positioning and Preparation**
  A. The patient is placed in the supine position with the arms extended.
  B. The surgical preparation should extend to the nipples superiorly, the inguinal regions inferiorly, and the midaxillary lines laterally.

II. **Preoperative Considerations**
  A. **Antibiotics** are administered within 1 hour before the skin incision.
  B. A **urinary catheter** is inserted to allow for monitoring of intraoperative fluid status and to decompress the bladder.
  C. A **nasogastric tube** is inserted to decompress the stomach, allowing for better exposure.
  D. Long-term steroid use can lead to suppression of the hypothalamic-pituitary-adrenal axis. Patients receiving long-term steroid therapy may require **stress-dose steroids** before and after the operation.

III. **Incision:** A left subcostal incision can be used if the spleen is of normal size. A midline approach should be used in patients with splenomegaly and for the exploration of traumatic injuries.

IV. **Exposure and Splenectomy**
  A. The lesser sac is entered through an avascular window in the gastrocolic ligament.

Has your patient received the appropriate vaccinations? Should your patient receive stress-dose steroids in the perioperative period?

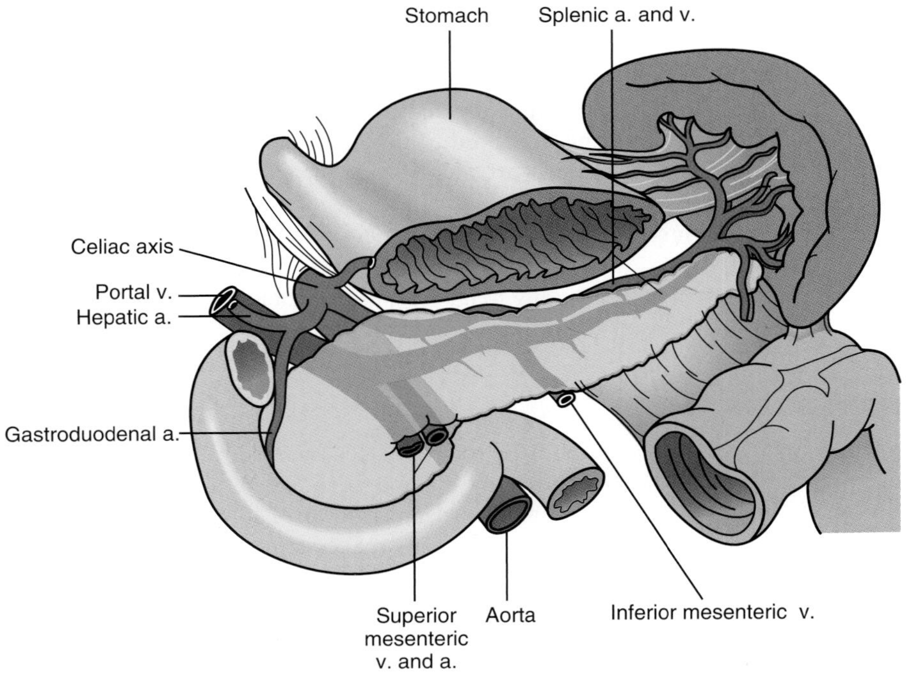

Figure 18-2

The spleen and its blood supply. The spleen is fed by the splenic artery, a branch of the celiac trunk that typically runs along the superior border of the pancreas. The splenic vein lies inferior to the artery and posterior to the pancreas and joins with the superior mesenteric vein to form the portal vein. (*From Townsend CM, Beauchamp RD, Evers BM, Mattox KL [eds]: Sabiston Textbook of Surgery: The Biological Basis of Modern Surgical Practice, 17th ed. Philadelphia, Saunders, 2004.*)

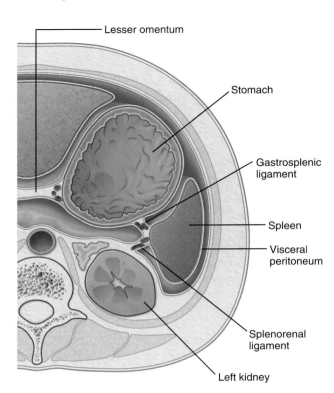

Lesser omentum

Stomach

Gastrosplenic
ligament

Spleen

Visceral
peritoneum

Splenorenal
ligament

Left kidney

Figure 18-3
Splenic ligaments. The spleen is
connected to surrounding structures
by several ligaments. The greater
curvature of the stomach and the
spleen are connected by the
gastrosplenic ligament, which contains
the short gastric and gastro-omental
vessels. The splenorenal ligament
connects the spleen to the left kidney
and contains the splenic vessels. *(From
Drake RL, Vogl W, Mitchell AWM:
Gray's Anatomy for Students.
Philadelphia, Churchill Livingstone,
2005.)*

B. The gastrosplenic ligament, which extends from the greater curvature of the stomach to the spleen and contains the short gastric vessels, is then divided. The most superior short gastric vessels are divided first, followed by the more inferior vessels, until a connection is made with the gastrocolic window.

C. Medial traction is applied to the spleen to expose the lateral peritoneal attachments, which are divided with electrocautery. The plane posterior to the spleen and the tail of the pancreas is then developed bluntly.

D. The splenocolic ligament is ligated and divided. The spleen is mobilized toward the midline and delivered to the level of the subcutaneous tissues.

E. The splenic artery and vein are identified at the splenic hilum and are individually ligated and divided.

F. Any remaining peritoneal attachments are divided, and the spleen is removed.

G. The abdomen is thoroughly irrigated and inspected for hemostasis. The fascia and skin are closed according to surgeon preference.

CARE MUST BE TAKEN TO AVOID INJURING THE TAIL OF THE PANCREAS DURING HILAR DISSECTION.

Laparoscopic Splenectomy

The laparoscopic approach may be used for most elective splenectomies. Absolute contraindications to laparoscopic splenectomy include cirrhosis, pregnancy, and severe cardiopulmonary disease. The laparoscopic approach is also probably ill advised in the setting of splenic trauma. The presence of splenomegaly makes laparoscopic splenectomy more challenging, but is not an absolute contraindication. The basic components of the laparoscopic operation are similar to those of the open approach. Dissection of the vascular and peritoneal attachments surrounding the spleen is followed by ligation of the hilar vessels.

I. **Patient Positioning and Preparation**

A. The patient is placed supine on the operating table in the modified lithotomy position. Alternatively, the patient can be placed in the right lateral decubitus position, with the iliac crest over the break in the table (Fig. 18-4).

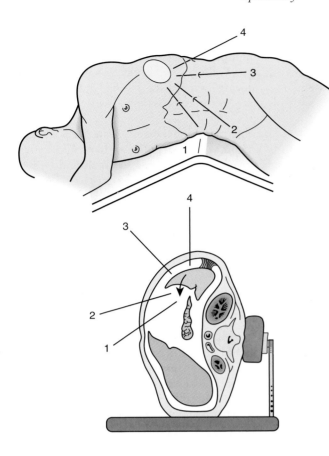

Figure 18-4
Patient positioning and port placement for laparoscopic splenectomy in the right lateral decubitus approach. Arrows 1 to 4 indicate the positions for ports in the left abdomen and flank. *(From Townsend CM, Beauchamp RD, Evers BM, Mattox KL [eds]: Sabiston Textbook of Surgery: The Biological Basis of Modern Surgical Practice, 17th ed. Philadelphia, Saunders, 2004.)*

B. If placed in the right lateral decubitus position, the patient should be placed on a bean bag to facilitate positioning. The left arm is supported across the body.

C. The surgical preparation should extend to the nipples superiorly and the inguinal regions inferiorly.

II. Port Placement

A. The camera is inserted through either an umbilical port or a port placed between the umbilicus and the left costal margin.

B. Three to four additional working ports are placed in the left abdomen and flank (see Fig. 18-4).

III. Technical Points

A. The abdomen is insufflated to a pressure of approximately 15 mm Hg. The camera is inserted, and a thorough exploration of the abdomen is undertaken to exclude the presence of accessory spleens.

B. The head of the table is tilted up, shifting the abdominal contents away from the left upper quadrant.

C. The splenocolic ligament is divided.

D. The short gastric vessels are divided and the stomach is rotated to the right, exposing the splenic hilum.

E. The splenic artery and vein are identified and divided with a stapler.

F. Remaining peritoneal attachments are divided, and the spleen is placed in an endoscopic bag. The spleen is then removed through one of the larger port sites, after morcellation with ring forceps. Alternatively, one of the port incisions can be extended to allow for the intact removal of the spleen.

G. The splenic bed and staple lines are irrigated, and hemostasis is confirmed.

H. All ports except for the camera port are removed under laparoscopic visualization. The camera port is then removed, and fascial defects from ports greater than 5 mm in diameter are closed.

Additional Operative Considerations

I. **Splenorrhaphy:** Splenic salvage is sometimes possible after low-grade splenic injuries. Topical hemostatic agents, such as Gelfoam or Surgicel, as well as argon beam coagulation can be useful in achieving hemostasis. Higher-grade injuries may sometimes be repaired with pledgeted sutures or wrapped with absorbable mesh.

II. **Drainage:** Some surgeons advocate routine placement of a drain in the operative bed to survey for the development of a pancreatic leak in the early postoperative period. If a pancreatic injury is suspected intraoperatively, a drain should be left to control pancreatic drainage.

III. **Partial Splenectomy:** The segmental blood supply to the spleen allows for the treatment of some traumatic injuries and splenic lesions (nonparasitic cysts and pseudocysts) with partial splenectomy. Partial splenectomy can be performed using an open or a laparoscopic approach.

POSTOPERATIVE COURSE

The nasogastric tube may be removed on the first postoperative day if the output is low. Once the nasogastric tube is removed, patients can be started on a clear liquid diet and advanced as tolerated. The Foley catheter should be removed early in the postoperative period as well. Early ambulation and regular use of an incentive spirometer should be encouraged. If stress-dose steroids are administered at the time of the operation, they should be tapered quickly in the postoperative period. Blood counts should be routinely monitored, especially in patients undergoing splenectomy for hematologic abnormalities. Leukocytosis and thrombocytosis are common and can persist for several months. Aspirin therapy should be started if platelet counts are greater than $1 \times 10^6/mm^3$ because of the associated risk of thrombosis.

COMPLICATIONS

I. **Hemorrhage:** Patients should be closely monitored for signs of postoperative bleeding; however, hemorrhage requiring reoperation is unusual.

II. **Iatrogenic Injuries:** Injury to the pancreatic tail may result from dissection around the splenic hilum. If recognized in the operating room, a closed-suction drain can be placed in the surgical bed. Alternatively, some surgeons leave a drain in place routinely. Unrecognized pancreatic injury may lead to a **pancreatic leak,** which can manifest with abdominal pain, nausea, vomiting, fever, or intra-abdominal abscess. CT of the abdomen may show a collection in the region of the pancreatic tail. Percutaneous drainage is typically sufficient to control pancreatic leaks, which are usually self-limited. Injury to the diaphragm is an uncommon complication of laparoscopic splenectomy and can lead to an effusion or pneumothorax.

III. **Infection:** Postoperative infections can include pneumonia, surgical site infections, urinary tract infection, and subphrenic abscess. **Overwhelming postsplenectomy infection (OPSI)** describes the onset of fulminant sepsis in asplenic patients. OPSI is caused by bacteremia from encapsulated organisms, most commonly *S. pneumoniae*. The risk is lifelong, but is highest in the first several years after splenectomy. The estimated incidence is 0.2% in adults and slightly higher in children. OPSI should be suspected in any asplenic patient presenting with fever. Broad-spectrum antibiotics should be initiated without delay because patients can deteriorate rapidly. Immunizations against encapsulated organisms are crucial in preventing OPSI. Daily antibiotic prophylaxis is recommended in children, although the optimal duration of therapy is unclear.

SUGGESTED READINGS

Beauchamp RD, Holzman MD, Fabian TC: Spleen. In Townsend CM, Beauchamp RD, Evers BM, Mattox KL (eds): Sabiston Textbook of Surgery: The Biological Basis of Modern Surgical Practice, 17th ed. Philadelphia, Saunders, 2004, pp 1679–1704.

Dente CJ, Parry NG, Rozycki GS: Splenic salvage procedures: therapeutic options. In Cameron JL (ed): Current Surgical Therapy, 8th ed. Philadelphia, Mosby, 2004, pp 539–543.

McKinlay R, Park AE: Splenectomy for hematologic diseases. In Cameron JL (ed): Current Surgical Therapy, 8th ed. Philadelphia, Elsevier Mosby, 2004, pp 533–536.

CHAPTER 19

Adrenalectomy

E. Carter Paulson   and   Rachel R. Kelz

Case Study

A 38-year-old female presents to an endocrinologist for evaluation of suspected hyperaldosteronism. Three years earlier, she was diagnosed with hypertension that remains poorly controlled on four antihypertensive medications. She is taking supplemental potassium chloride for recalcitrant hypokalemia. She reports increased fatigue, muscle weakness, and frequent urination.

Physical examination reveals a well-appearing 135-lb woman with a blood pressure of 151/85 mm Hg. Findings on abdominal examination are unremarkable. No masses or striae are appreciated.

She undergoes laboratory testing, which reveals a serum potassium level of 3.1 mEq/L, a serum renin level of 1.31 ng/mL/hr (normal range, 0.15–3.39 ng/mL/hr), and a serum aldosterone level of 82 ng/dL (normal range, 1–16 ng/dL). A computed tomography (CT) scan of the abdomen shows a 2-cm left adrenal mass and a normal-appearing right adrenal gland (Fig. 19-1).

BACKGROUND

The adrenal glands are bilateral, retroperitoneal endocrine glands that are located above the kidneys. Each gland consists of a **medulla** and surrounding **cortex.** The chromaffin cells of the medulla, which are derived from the neural crest, are the body's main source of the catecholamine hormones epinephrine and norepinephrine. The adrenal cortex is a site of steroid hormone synthesis. Three distinct regions of the adrenal cortex, the zona glomerulosa, zona fasciculata, and zona reticularis, are responsible for the production of mineralocorticoids (e.g., aldosterone), glucocorticoids (e.g., cortisol), and

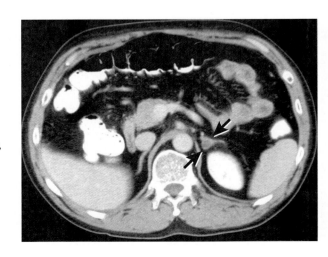

Figure 19-1
CT scan of the abdomen. A left adrenal mass (*arrows*) is seen. (*From Mettler F: Essentials of Radiology, 2nd ed. Philadelphia, Saunders, 2004.*)

TABLE 19-1 Studies Frequently Obtained in the Evaluation of Functional Adrenal Tumor

Tumor	Secreted Hormone	Clinical Syndrome	Biochemical Test (Typical Findings)	Additional Studies
Aldosteronoma	Alderosterone	Hyperaldosteronism (Conn's syndrome)	Serum aldosterone level (elevated) Aldosterone:renin ratio (elevated) Serum potassium level (low)	Abdominal CT scan Abdominal MRI Adrenal vein sampling
Cortisol-producing adenoma	Cortisone	Cushing's syndrome	24-hour urine cortisol level (elevated) Dexamethasone suppression test (little suppression of serum cortisol)	Abdominal CT scan Abdominal MRI
Pheochromocytoma	Adrenaline	Pheochromocytoma	Serum metanephrine level (elevated) 24-hour urine vanillylmandelic acid and metanephrine levels (elevated)	Abdominal MRI ^{131}I-MIBG scan

CT, computed tomography; ^{131}I-MIBG, iodine-131-metaiodobenzylguanidine; MRI, magnetic resonance imaging.

androgens (e.g., dehydroepiandrosterone), respectively. The cortex is regulated by neuroendocrine hormones secreted by the pituitary gland and hypothalamus and the renin–angiotensin axis.

Tumors arising within the adrenal gland are broadly categorized as either **functioning** or **nonfunctioning.** The former secrete one of a number of hormones (Table 19-1). The indications for adrenalectomy, the subject of this chapter, include the treatment of functioning adrenal tumors, suspected primary adrenal malignancies, and in select cases, isolated metastases from extra-adrenal malignancies.

> Does your patient have a *functioning* or *nonfunctioning* adrenal mass?

INDICATIONS FOR ADRENALECTOMY

I. **Aldosteronoma**
   A. Aldosteronomas are the most common functional adrenal tumor and the most common cause of primary hyperaldosteronism (see Table 19-1). Patients classically present with hypertension refractory to multiple medications and hypokalemia. Other symptoms include headaches, polyuria, nocturia, muscle weakness, and cramping.
   B. The presence of a unilateral adrenal lesion with biochemical evidence of primary hyperaldosteronism (see Table 19-1) is an indication for adrenalectomy. When imaging shows either bilateral normal glands or bilateral adrenal nodules, adrenal vein sampling may be used to establish the laterality of the lesion. Patients with lateralizing venous sampling benefit from adrenalectomy. Laparoscopic adrenalectomy is the procedure of choice because these lesions are generally small and benign. In contrast, bilateral aldosterone hypersecretion is managed medically (typically with spironolactone).

II. **Cortisol-Producing Adenoma**
   A. Cortisol overproduction (**Cushing's syndrome**) can result from increased adrenocorticotropic hormone (ACTH) production by the pituitary gland (**Cushing's disease**) or an ectopic source, or from increased adrenal production of cortisol itself. Cushing's syndrome may present with central obesity,

glucose intolerance, hypertension, excess hair growth, osteoporosis, kidney stones, menstrual irregularity, and emotional lability.

Cushing's syndrome refers to the signs and symptoms of hypercortisolism. When caused by a pituitary adenoma, this syndrome is known as *Cushing's disease*.

B. The presence of a unilateral adrenal tumor in patients with biochemical evidence of Cushing's syndrome (see Table 19-1) is an indication for adrenalectomy. Patients with bilateral adrenal hyperplasia and Cushing's syndrome require bilateral adrenalectomy. Bilateral adrenalectomy is also indicated in patients in whom trans-sphenoidal surgery for Cushing's disease is unsuccessful and in some patients with ectopic Cushing's syndrome when the ACTH-secreting tumor cannot be removed.

III. **Pheochromocytoma**

A. Pheochromocytomas are rare catecholamine-secreting tumors. The symptoms classically associated with these tumors are attributable to excess adrenaline production and include recurrent episodes of sweating, headache, and anxiety. Excessive catecholamine secretion can also precipitate life-threatening hypertension or cardiac arrhythmias.

Pheochromocytoma is known as the 10% tumor: 10% malignant, 10% multiple, 10% bilateral, 10% familial, 10% extra-adrenal, 10% in children.

B. More than 90% of pheochromocytomas are located within the adrenal glands. Extra-adrenal pheochromocytomas, which develop in the paraganglion chromaffin tissue of the sympathetic nervous system, may occur anywhere from the base of the brain to the urinary bladder. Common locations include the organ of Zuckerkandl (at the origin of the inferior mesenteric artery), the bladder wall, the heart, the mediastinum, and the carotid and glomus jugular bodies.

C. The presence of an adrenal tumor with biochemical evidence of a pheochromocytoma (see Table 19-1) is an indication for adrenalectomy. Manipulation of a pheochromocytoma during surgery can result in the release of large amounts of catecholamines and hemodynamic instability. All patients should receive α- and β-antagonists and volume replacement before surgery. α-Blockade must be initiated before β-blockade because hypertensive crises can result from unopposed alpha stimulation.

α-BLOCKADE MUST BE STARTED BEFORE β-BLOCKADE TO AVOID HYPERTENSIVE CRISES.

IV. **Adrenocortical Carcinoma**

A. Adrenocortical carcinoma is a rare tumor, affecting one to two persons per 1 million. The median age at diagnosis is 44 years. Between 60% and 80% of these tumors are functional. Nonfunctional tumors often present with symptoms related to local invasion or mass effect, such as abdominal or flank pain. Only 30% of these malignancies are confined to the adrenal gland at the time of diagnosis.

B. Cross-sectional imaging (CT scan and magnetic resonance imaging [MRI]) often localizes the tumor. Radiographic findings that suggest malignancy include large size (most adrenal carcinomas are larger than 6 cm at the time of diagnosis), irregular borders, and invasion into surrounding structures. Radical surgical excision, generally performed using an open approach, is the treatment of choice for patients with localized malignancies and remains the only therapy with which long-term disease-free survival can be achieved.

V. **Adrenal Metastases.** The adrenal glands are relatively common sites of metastases. Breast, lung, and renal cell cancers; melanomas; and lymphomas may metastasize to the adrenal glands. Surgical resection of solitary adrenal metastases in patients with a long previous disease-free interval and no evidence of extra-adrenal disease results in prolonged survival. Imaging, including positron emission tomography scanning to rule out the presence of other metastatic disease and appropriate laboratory testing to determine the functionality of the lesion, should be performed before resection. If pheochromocytoma is ruled out, fine-needle aspiration under CT or ultrasound guidance may also be useful in making a definitive diagnosis.

FINE-NEEDLE ASPIRATION OF AN UNDIAGNOSED PHEOCHROMOCYTOMA CAN RESULT IN A HYPERTENSIVE CRISIS BECAUSE OF CATECHOLAMINE RELEASE.

VI. **Incidentalomas.** The term *incidentaloma* refers to an asymptomatic mass or lesion discovered on routine imaging. Adrenal incidentalomas are noted on up to 5% of all abdominal CT scans. In the absence of a history of malignancy, nonfunctioning lesions smaller than 4 to 5 cm are typically followed with serial imaging (CT scan or MRI). Adrenalectomy is usually recommended for nonfunctioning adrenal

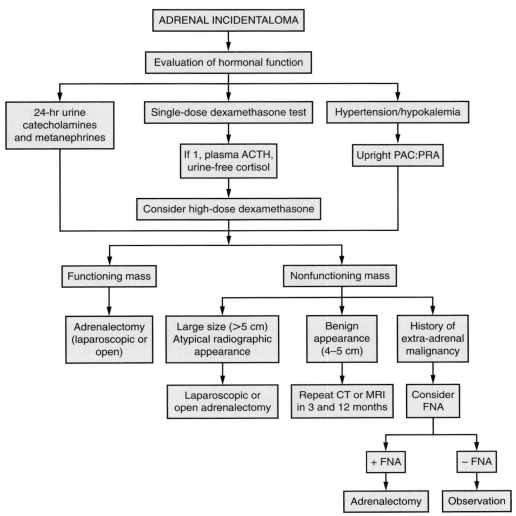

Figure 19-2

Algorithm for the evaluation and management of adrenal incidentalomas. ACTH, adrenocorticotropic hormone; CT, computed tomography; FNA, fine-needle aspiration; MRI, magnetic resonance imaging; PAC, plasma aldosterone concentration; PRA, plasma renin activity. *(Adapted from Cameron J: Current Surgical Therapy, 7th ed. Philadelphia, Mosby, 2001.)*

masses larger than 5 cm because of the elevated risk of malignancy associated with larger lesions. All functioning incidentalomas should be resected (Fig. 19-2).

PREOPERATIVE EVALUATION

I. **Tests of endocrine function** include 24-hour urine catecholamines, metanephrines, and cortisol; plasma ACTH, aldosterone, and renin; serum potassium; and dexamethasone suppression tests. These tests distinguish functioning from nonfunctioning masses.

II. **Cross-Sectional Imaging.** CT scanning and MRI may aid in the localization of adrenal masses and the identification of malignant characteristics. Adrenal lesions that are large (>5 cm in diameter) and have irregular borders are more likely to be malignant. Invasion into surrounding structures is diagnostic of malignancy. These modalities also allow for identification of extra-adrenal disease (e.g., extra-adrenal pheochromocytomas or extra-adrenal metastatic disease).

III. **Iodine-131-Metaiodobenzylguanidine (MIBG) Scanning.** ^{131}I-MIBG selectively accumulates in chromaffin cells and may aid in the identification of small, recurrent, or extra-adrenal pheochromocytomas that cannot be localized with CT scanning and MRI.

Does your patient's adrenal lesion have radiographic features suggesting malignancy?

IV. **Adrenal vein sampling** is primarily used to differentiate between unilateral hyperaldosteronism and bilateral adrenal hypersecretion. Aldosterone and cortisol levels are measured in venous blood samples from both adrenal veins and the inferior vena cava.

COMPONENTS OF THE PROCEDURE AND APPLIED ANATOMY

See Figure 19-3.

There are multiple operative approaches to adrenalectomy. Traditionally, adrenal resections were performed in an open fashion through one of four approaches: transabdominal, lateral flank, posterior retroperitoneal, and thoracoabdominal. The laparoscopic approach has largely supplanted the lateral flank and posterior retroperitoneal approaches and is described in detail. The retroperitoneal laparoscopic and open approaches are briefly reviewed.

Preoperative Considerations

I. **Urinary catheterization** is indicated to decompress the bladder and monitor intraoperative and postoperative volume status.
II. Manipulation of pheochromocytomas can result in the release of catecholamines, which may be accompanied by wide and unpredictable fluctuations in blood pressure. An **arterial line,** to allow for continuous blood pressure monitoring, should therefore be inserted before resection of a pheochromocytoma.

Patient Positioning and Preparation

I. The patient is placed in the lateral decubitus position, with the side opposite the lesion down (Fig. 19-4).

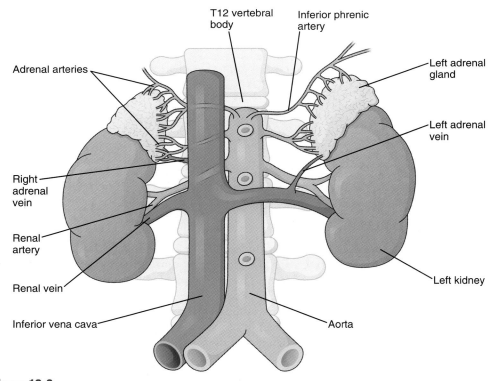

Figure 19-3

Anatomy of the adrenal glands. The adrenal gland receives blood supply from branches of the inferior phrenic arteries (superior suprarenal arteries) and branches of the aorta (middle and inferior suprarenal arteries). The right adrenal vein drains directly into the vena cava, whereas the left adrenal vein drains into the left renal vein. *(From Becker JM, Stucchi AF [eds]: Essentials of Surgery. Philadelphia, Saunders, 2006.)*

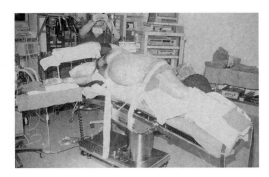

Figure 19-4
Lateral decubitus position. The patient is placed on a padded mattress. The table is flexed, and the patient is placed in a reverse Trendelenburg position. *(From Townsend CM, Beauchamp RD, Evers BM, Mattox KL [eds]: Sabiston Textbook of Surgery: The Biological Basis of Modern Surgical Practice, 17th ed. Philadelphia, Saunders, 2004.)*

II. The table is flexed and the patient is placed in a slight reverse Trendelenburg position.

III. The anterior and posterior axillary lines are useful landmarks for port placement and should be marked before the patient is prepped.

IV. The abdomen is prepped to the nipples superiorly, to the anterior superior iliac crest inferiorly, to the umbilicus anteriorly, and to the vertebral column posteriorly.

Port Placement

I. In general, left adrenalectomy is performed through three operative ports and right adrenalectomy is performed through four operative ports. The additional port on the right side allows for the placement of a liver retractor.

II. Initial access to the abdomen is obtained just medial to the anterior axillary line and lateral to the rectus muscle. This can be accomplished using a "blind" percutaneous technique using a Veress needle or an open technique; the latter is more commonly used.

III. **Open Technique for Placement of the First Port**
A. A small transverse incision is made just medial to the anterior axillary line five fingerbreadths below the costal margin.
B. The external oblique fascia is exposed after blunt dissection of the subcutaneous soft tissue. The fascia is incised.
C. The three muscle layers underlying the fascia are bluntly dissected to reveal the transversalis fascia.
D. The posterior fascia and underlying peritoneum are divided under direct vision.
E. Sutures are placed in the fascia to secure the port and to minimize CO_2 leakage and loss of pneumoperitoneum.
F. The port is inserted through the incision using a blunt-tipped trocar.
G. CO_2 is insufflated through the port. The abdomen should distend symmetrically and become uniformly tympanic. If this does not happen, extraperitoneal port placement should be suspected.
H. The laparoscope is inserted through the port, and the peritoneal cavity is surveyed.

IV. **Placement of the Remaining Ports**
A. The remaining ports are inserted under direct intra-abdominal visualization. Cutting (sharp) introducers are used to penetrate the fascia and enter the peritoneal cavity.
B. The additional ports are placed, evenly spaced at least 5 cm apart, along the costal margin (Fig. 19-5).
C. On the left side, the splenic flexure of the colon is mobilized before insertion of lateral ports to reduce the risk of colonic injury.

> **THE VERESS NEEDLE APPROACH SHOULD NOT BE USED IN PATIENTS WHO HAVE HAD PREVIOUS ABDOMINAL SURGERY.**

Figure 19-5
Port placement for laparoscopic adrenalectomy.
*(From Cameron J: Current Surgical Therapy, 7th ed.
Philadelphia, Mosby, 2001.)*

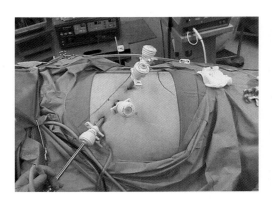

Right Adrenalectomy

I. **Exposure**
   A. The right triangular ligament of the liver is divided using electrocautery to allow for retraction of the right liver lobe and exposure of the inferior vena cava (IVC) and right adrenal gland (Fig. 19-6).
   B. A liver retractor is inserted through the most medial port to retract the right lobe of the liver medially.
   C. An atraumatic grasper is used to apply lateral traction to the adrenal gland.
   D. Electrocautery is used to create a plane between the medial edge of the gland and the lateral border of the IVC, exposing the right adrenal vein.

II. **Isolation and Division of the Right Adrenal Vein**
   A. A dissector is used to expose the right adrenal vein circumferentially.
   B. Three surgical clips, two placed proximally on the IVC side and one placed distally, are applied to the vein.
   C. The vein is divided sharply between the proximal and distal clips.

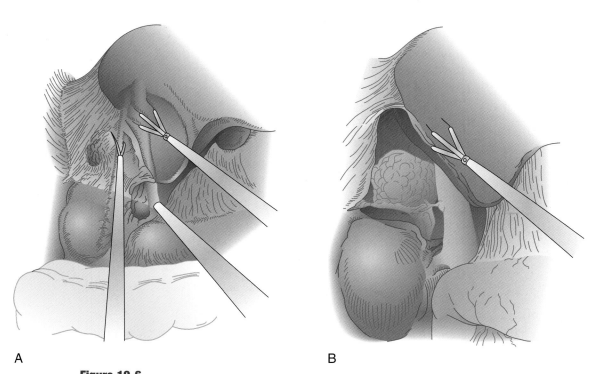

A   B

Figure 19-6
A, The right triangular ligament of the liver is divided to allow for medial rotation of the right lobe. **B,** The medial border of the adrenal is dissected to expose the inferior vena cava and right adrenal vein. *(From Brunt LM: Laparoscopic adrenalectomy. In Eubanks WS, Swanstrom LL, Soper NJ [eds]: Mastery of Endoscopic and Laparoscopic Surgery. Philadelphia, Lippincott Williams & Wilkins, 2000, p 325.)*

III. **Mobilization of the Right Adrenal Gland**
    A. Dissection is continued along the edge of the gland inferiorly and superiorly.
    B. Most small arteries entering the gland can be cauterized; however, larger branches should be clipped.
    C. The inferior dissection proceeds in a medial to lateral direction. Care should be taken to stay close to the edge of the adrenal gland to avoid injuring branches of the renal vessels.
    D. Superiorly, dissection continues in the relatively avascular plane between the superior pole of the gland and the musculature of the diaphragm.
    E. Posteriorly, the avascular attachments to the back muscles and retroperitoneal fat can be divided with electrocautery.
    F. Once it is fully mobilized, the specimen is placed in an impermeable bag.
    G. The retroperitoneum is irrigated and inspected for hemostasis.

IV. **Specimen Extraction**
    A. The specimen is extracted through one of the port sites.
    B. For large tumors, a separate incision (umbilical or suprapubic) may facilitate specimen removal.
    C. In general, malignant tumors or metastatic lesions should be removed intact to allow for thorough pathologic evaluation.

Left Adrenalectomy

I. **Exposure**
    A. The splenic flexure of the colon is mobilized by dividing the splenocolic ligament, allowing retraction of the colon away from the left kidney and the inferior pole of the spleen (Fig. 19-7).

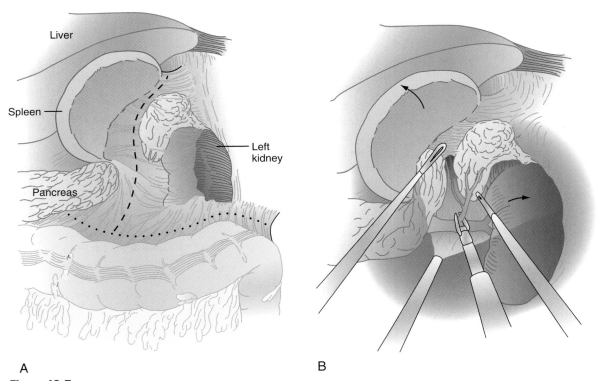

A   B

Figure 19-7
A, The splenocolic ligament is divided (*dotted line*), followed by division of the splenorenal ligament (*dashed line*). **B,** The spleen is rotated medially, and the kidney is retracted laterally. The adrenal vein is ligated at the inferomedial border of the adrenal with endoscopic clips. (*From Brunt LM: Laparoscopic adrenalectomy. In Eubanks WS, Swanstrom LL, Soper NJ [eds]: Mastery of Endoscopic and Laparoscopic Surgery. Philadelphia, Lippincott Williams & Wilkins, 2000, pp 326, 327.*)

DURING DISSECTION OF THE LEFT ADRENAL GLAND, CARE MUST BE TAKEN TO AVOID INJURIES TO THE LEFT RENAL VEIN AND THE TAIL OF THE PANCREAS.

    B. The splenorenal ligament (between the inferior pole of the spleen and the superior pole of the kidney) is divided close to the spleen to allow medial rotation of the spleen and access to the left retroperitoneum.

    C. The medial and lateral borders of the adrenal gland are defined using electrocautery dissection.

    D. Dissection is continued inferiorly to identify the left adrenal vein, a branch of the left renal vein, which exits the gland in an inferiomedial position.

II. **Isolation and Division of the Left Adrenal Vein**

    A. A dissector is used to expose the left adrenal vein circumferentially.

    B. The vein is doubly clipped and divided.

III. **Mobilization and Detachment of the Left Adrenal Gland**

    A. Dissection is continued along the medial and lateral edges of the gland.

    B. The superior and posterior attachments to the diaphragm and retroperitoneal fat are divided.

    C. Once the dissection is complete, the specimen is placed in an impermeable bag and the retroperitoneum is irrigated and inspected for hemostasis.

IV. **Specimen Extraction**

    A. The specimen is extracted in the same manner described for the right adrenal gland.

    B. Of note, care should be taken to inspect the tail of the pancreas. If there is concern that the parenchyma of the pancreas was injured, a closed-suction drain should be left in place.

Other Operative Approaches

I. The **posterior retroperitoneal laparoscopic approach** is useful for bilateral adrenalectomy or in patients who have had previous abdominal surgery. The procedure is performed with the patient in prone position. The initial port is placed just inferior to the tip of the 12th rib into the retroperitoneum. A balloon dissector is used to expose the retroperitoneal space. Two additional trocars are placed: one at the edge of the erectus spinus muscle and one at the posterior axillary line. The adrenal gland is identified above the kidney. Exposure and dissection of the adrenal glands proceed in the same fashion as for the transabdominal lateral laparoscopic approach.

II. The **open transabdominal approach,** which allows access to both adrenal glands and the entire abdominal cavity, is the preferred method for tumors too large to be removed laparoscopically and for all invasive adrenal tumors. This approach may be performed through a subcostal or midline incision. Exposure and dissection proceed as described for laparoscopic adrenalectomy.

III. The **open posterior retroperitoneal approach,** performed through a hockey-stick incision on the back (Fig. 19-8), has been almost entirely supplanted by laparoscopic approaches. This approach allows for visualization of both adrenal glands, but provides limited working space. Furthermore, the incision is not well tolerated by patients.

IV. The **open lateral retroperitoneal approach** is sometimes preferred in obese patients or patients with large tumors. As with the lateral laparoscopic approach, the patient is placed in the lateral decubitus position, with the table flexed. A subcostal or intercostal incision centered at the midaxillary line is used. Like the posterior open method, this approach has been largely supplanted by laparoscopic resection.

V. The **open thoracoabdominal approach** is performed through an incision that extends from the abdominal wall to the eighth intercostal space and provides exposure to both the abdominal and chest cavities. This exposure allows for control of the vena cava, which is sometimes necessary for the safe resection of large adrenal tumors or those that involves the vena cava.

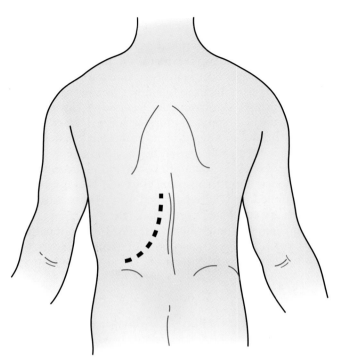

Figure 19-8
Incision for open posterior approach to adrenalectomy (*dashed line*). The incision is extended inferiorly and laterally from the tenth rib to the posterior iliac crest. (*From Townsend CM, Beauchamp RD, Evers BM, Mattox KL [eds]: Sabiston Textbook of Surgery: The Biological Basis of Modern Surgical Practice, 17th ed. Philadelphia, Saunders, 2004.*)

Additional Operative Considerations

I. The role of laparoscopic adrenalectomy in the setting of **large or malignant adrenal tumors** remains controversial. From a technical standpoint, removing large lesions laparoscopically is challenging. Furthermore, tumor fragmentation, excess manipulation, laparoscopic dissection, and even pneumoperitoneum have been implicated in tumor spread. Occasionally, a laparoscopic approach combined with a hand port can be used with less morbidity than a traditional open approach for large tumors.

II. Occasionally, **identification of the adrenal gland** can be challenging, particularly in obese patients. If, after careful and appropriate dissection, the gland is not evident, intraoperative ultrasound may be used to identify the appropriate landmarks as well as the gland itself.

III. **Conversion to open adrenalectomy** is sometimes required because of bleeding or difficulty identifying the gland, or to safely resect invasive tumors.

NORMAL POSTOPERATIVE COURSE

After an uncomplicated laparoscopic adrenalectomy, patients frequently feel well with limited analgesia, and can quickly tolerate a regular diet. If a patient is hemodynamically stable, the urinary catheter is removed on the morning of the first postoperative day. If a drain is left in place at the time of surgery, it is removed on the morning of the first postoperative day as well, assuming minimal, nonbloody drainage. Often, patients can be discharged from the hospital on the first or second postoperative day.

Patients who undergo open adrenalectomy generally have a more prolonged postoperative course. They often experience significant postoperative pain and require intravenous analgesia for several days after surgery.

Additional Postoperative Considerations

I. Spironolactone is discontinued immediately after adrenalectomy in patients with **aldosteronomas** to prevent hyperkalemia. Other antihypertensive medications are continued. Appropriate hormone replacement therapy must be initiated before discharge in patients who undergo bilateral adrenalectomy.

II. Patients with **Cushing's syndrome** are exposed to chronically elevated levels of steroid hormones, which suppress normal adrenal function in the contralateral gland. After the removal of a hyperfunctioning gland, patients often have transient adrenal insufficiency requiring steroid therapy. Patients are maintained on stress-dose steroids for 24 to 72 hours after surgery and are monitored for signs of adrenal insufficiency. Oral maintenance steroid therapy is initiated before discharge and continued until adrenal function recovers. Most often, antihypertensive medications are continued postoperatively.

III. In patients who undergo uneventful resection of a **pheochromocytoma,** close monitoring of blood pressure is necessary in the postoperative period. Antihypertensive medications are usually discontinued postoperatively.

Complications

Bleeding is the most common complication after laparoscopic adrenalectomy. **Wound infections** and intra-abdominal abscesses are relatively rare. As in all types of laparoscopic surgery, **bowel injury** can occur during port placement. Thermal injuries from the electrocautery device can occur at sites distant from the operative field. Other complications associated with adrenalectomy include:

I. **Pancreatic tail injury,** which can occur during either laparoscopic or open left adrenalectomy. If such an injury is suspected intraoperatively, closed-suction drainage is usually sufficient treatment. Patients who have an unidentified pancreatic injury often have a fluid collection in the region of the pancreatic tail. Presenting signs and symptoms may include greater than anticipated output from a surgical drain, vague abdominal complaints, leukocytosis, and fever. If a drain is left in place, a fluid amylase level can be obtained. In the absence of a drain, suspected pancreatic injuries should be evaluated with a CT scan. If a fluid collection is present, a drain can be placed percutaneously by an interventional radiologist.

> Pancreatic exocrine secretions are clear and rich in amylase.

II. Pancreatic injury can also lead to **pancreatitis.** Patients present with persistent and often severe epigastric abdominal pain. Laboratory testing shows elevated serum amylase and lipase levels. A CT scan should be obtained to determine if concomitant pancreatic leak and fluid collection are present.

III. **Diaphragmatic injuries** that are recognized intraoperatively should be repaired. If the pleura adjacent to the diaphragm is injured, a pneumothorax may develop. In extremely rare instances, injuries to the diaphragm are large enough to allow herniation of abdominal contents into the chest. Patients with atypical upper abdominal or chest pain after adrenalectomy should initially be evaluated with a chest radiograph or a CT scan of the chest. Such injuries typically require operative repair.

SUGGESTED READINGS

Brunt LM: Minimal access adrenal surgery. Surg Endosc 20:351–361, 2006.

Cobb WS, Kercher KW, Sing RF, Heniford BT: Laparoscopic adrenalectomy for malignancy. Am J Surg 189:405–411, 2005.

Gumbs AA, Gagner M: Laparoscopic adrenalectomy. Best Pract Res Clin Endocrinol Metab 20:483–499, 2006.

Mitchell IC, Nwariaku FE: Adrenal masses in the cancer patient: surveillance or excision. Oncologist 12:168–174, 2007.

Thyroidectomy and Parathyroidectomy

Giorgos C. Karakousis and Douglas L. Fraker

THYROIDECTOMY

Case Study

A 48-year-old female presents to her primary care physician with a palpable mass in her right neck just lateral to the trachea. She denies neck pain, dysphagia, recent weight loss or gain, diaphoresis, palpitations, and previous radiation exposure.

Physical examination reveals a 3-cm nodule in the right thyroid lobe of her neck that moves with swallowing. There is no cervical or supraclavicular adenopathy. An ultrasound of the thyroid shows a dominant 2.6-cm nodule in the right lobe (Fig. 20-1). Results of thyroid function tests, including triidothyronine (T_3), thyroxine (T_4), and thyroid-stimulating hormone (TSH) levels, are all within normal limits. A fine-needle aspiration biopsy (FNA) of the nodule demonstrates cytology consistent with a follicular neoplasm.

BACKGROUND

The thyroid gland is a bilobed structure that develops from **endoderm** and descends during development into the neck from the base of the tongue. The thyroid gland is located anterior to the trachea, to which it is attached by the **ligament of Berry,** and below the thyroid cartilage. The thyroid receives its blood supply from the superior thyroid arteries (branches of the external carotid arteries) and the inferior thyroid arteries (branches of the thyrocervical trunks). Thyroid ima arteries, branches of the aorta, provide additional blood supply to the gland inferiorly. Venous drainage is via the superior, inferior, and middle thyroid veins. The bridge of tissue connecting the two thyroid lobes

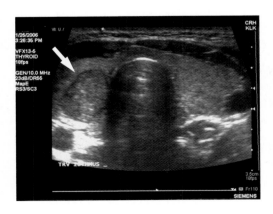

Figure 20-1

Thyroid ultrasound showing a large right thyroid nodule. (*From Townsend CM, Beauchamp RD, Evers BM, Mattox KL [eds]: Sabiston Textbook of Surgery: The Biological Basis of Modern Surgical Practice, 18th ed. Philadelphia, Saunders, 2008.*)

and overlying the trachea is called the **isthmus.** In some patients, thyroid tissue extends superiorly from the isthmus or the medial aspects of the thyroid lobes to form a **pyramidal lobe.**

The thyroid parenchyma consists of **follicular cells,** which store and are responsible for the organification of iodide, and **parafollicular cells,** derived from the neural crest, which produce the short-chain polypeptide **calcitonin.** Thyroid follicular cells couple inorganic iodide with tyrosine moieties to produce the more biologically active T_3 hormone and the more abundant T_4 hormone. Production and release of thyroid hormone is regulated by the **hypothalamo-pituitary-thyroid axis** through a negative feedback system. The principal stimulant of thyroid production is **TSH,** produced by the anterior pituitary. TSH production is inhibited by circulating thyroid hormone and stimulated by thyrotropin-releasing hormone from the hypothalamus.

> The half-life of T_3 hormone is approximately 3 days, whereas the half-life of T_4 hormone is approximately 1 week.

INDICATIONS FOR THYROID SURGERY

I. **Suspicious or Symptomatic Thyroid Nodule:** The workup of a solitary thyroid nodule typically includes an ultrasound, a thyroid scan, thyroid function tests, and **FNA.** In the vast majority of cases (70%), FNA reveals benign pathology (e.g., adenomatoid or hyperplastic lesions or colloid cysts). In approximately 15% of cases, FNA will be nondiagnostic. In the remaining 15% of cases, FNA is suspicious in 10% and consistent with malignancy (either primary thyroid cancer or metastatic disease) in 5%. Thyroid lobectomy is indicated after nondiagnostic or suspicious FNA findings in a patient with a symptomatic nodule or a concerning clinical history (e.g., a rapidly growing nodule or a significant radiation history). Importantly, 80% of patients with **follicular neoplasms** (i.e., suspicious lesions) are ultimately found to have benign adenomas; the remaining 20% are found to have follicular carcinomas. Typically, a thyroid lobectomy is performed after the diagnosis of a follicular neoplasm. If **capsular or vascular invasion** is present on the final pathology, establishing the diagnosis of a carcinoma, a completion thyroidectomy is performed. In a patient already receiving thyroid replacement hormone preoperatively, a total thyroidectomy is often recommended as the initial treatment.

> Follicular adenoma and follicular adenocarcinoma cannot be distinguished by fine-needle aspiration biopsy.

II. **Thyroid Cancer:** Thyroid cancer types include **papillary, follicular, medullary, and anaplastic.** Thyroid lymphomas and metastatic disease to the thyroid are less common diagnoses. Papillary thyroid cancer is the most common type (80%–90%) in the United States and has an excellent prognosis (10-year survival rate, 90%–95%); it is characterized histologically by the presence of **psammoma bodies** (microscopic rounded collections of calcium) and **optically clear nuclei** ("Orphan Annie eyes"). Unlike papillary carcinoma, which when metastatic, usually spreads through the lymphatics to regional lymph nodes, follicular thyroid cancer metastasizes hematogenously to the lung and, less frequently, to bone. Generally, the management of these cancers includes total thyroidectomy followed by **radioactive iodine ablation.** En bloc resection of clinically palpable nodes and ipsilateral modified radical neck dissection, if these lymph nodes contain metastases, are also indicated. **Medullary thyroid cancer** develops from parafollicular cells and is often associated with **MEN IIA, MEN IIB, and non-MEN** familial syndromes. Treatment includes thyroidectomy with central lymph node dissection. **Anaplastic thyroid cancer** has a very poor prognosis, with a median survival of several months. Surgery has a limited role; radiation and chemotherapy are typically the primary treatment modalities.

> MEN IIA: Pheochromocytoma, medullary thyroid cancer, and parathyroid hyperplasia
> MEN IIB: Pheochromocytoma, medullary thyroid cancer, and paragangliomas
> Non-MEN familial medullary thyroid cancer: Only medullary thyroid cancer

> Older age is associated with a poorer prognosis in patients with well-differentiated thyroid cancers (i.e., papillary and follicular carcinoma).

III. **Goiter:** The term *goiter* refers to benign enlargement of the thyroid gland. Surgery is generally reserved for patients with symptomatic or rapidly growing goiters.

IV. **Toxic Nodule and Toxic Multinodular Goiter (TMG):** Toxic nodules are most often follicular adenomas and are distinguished by the higher than normal uptake of radioactive tracer on thyroid scan (i.e., a *hot nodule*). Toxic multinodular goiters are characterized by the presence of several *hot nodules.* The descriptor *toxic* indicates excessive production of thyroid hormone. Although radioactive iodine is usually effective for the treatment of toxic nodules or TMG, surgery is indicated if radioactive iodine is contraindicated, or for the treatment of large symptomatic TMGs.

V. **Graves' Disease:** Graves' disease is a disorder caused by autoantibodies that bind the TSH receptor and stimulate excessive thyroid hormone secretion and hyperthyroidism. Symptoms include tachycardia, hypertension, diaphoresis, and weight loss. Additional manifestations of the disease include **exopthalmos,** which frequently does not improve with treatment, and **pretibial myxedema.** Initial treatment includes antithyroid medications, such as **propylthiouracil** and **methimazole,** which restore euthyroidism. Radioactive iodine therapy is then used to ablate the diseased thyroid gland. Surgery may be indicated in pregnant patients (in whom radioactive iodine is contraindicated), in children (in whom medical therapy is frequently ineffective), in patients who have been unsuccessfully treated with radioiodine, and when an underlying malignancy cannot be excluded. Typically, a near-total thyroidectomy is the procedure of choice. The remaining thyroid tissue protects against hypothyroidism, but may be associated with disease recurrence.

> **METHIMAZOLE AND RADIOACTIVE IODINE ARE CONTRAINDICATED IN PREGNANCY.**

PREOPERATIVE EVALUATION

I. **Thyroid function tests** include T_3, T_4, and TSH levels. These tests allow for the diagnosis of hyperthyroidism or hypothyroidism.

II. **Thyroid Ultrasound:** Thyroid ultrasound is routinely obtained to better characterize thyroid nodules and help guide FNA of nodules that are not clinically evident.

III. **Thyroid scan** is a nuclear medicine study that can be used to characterize thyroid nodules on the basis of their functional activity. Radioactive tracer (99m-technetium pertechnetate, 123-iodine, or 131-iodine) is administered and is taken up by the thyroid gland. Nodules are characterized as *hot* (if they take up tracer at higher levels than normal thyroid tissue), *cold* (if they take up tracer at lower levels than normal thyroid tissue), or *warm* (if they take up iodine at levels similar to normal thyroid tissue).

COMPONENTS OF THE PROCEDURE AND APPLIED ANATOMY

Thyroidectomy and thyroid lobectomy are performed similarly, except that in the case of the latter, the isthmus is divided and only one thyroid lobe is removed. The basic goals of lobectomy and thyroidectomy include removal of the diseased thyroid and identification and preservation of the recurrent laryngeal nerves and parathyroid glands. Total thyroidectomy is discussed below.

I. **Preoperative Considerations**

A. Thyroidectomy is typically performed under **general anesthesia;** however, regional anesthesia (superficial cervical plexus block) and local anesthesia are alternatives in selected patients.

B. Preoperative preparation of patients with hyperthyroidism, including a **medical regimen** to achieve euthyroidism (propylthiouracil or methimazole) and control tachycardia and hypertension (β-blockade), significantly enhances the safety of surgery. In patients with ongoing symptomatic hyperparathyroidism, β-blockade should be continued throughout the perioperative period.

II. **Patient Positioning and Preparation**

A. The patient is placed in the **supine position** with the neck hyperextended; typically, a rolled sheet or other support is placed under the shoulders. The head is supported with a foam cushion that also serves to stabilize and prevent movement during the procedure.

B. The entire neck is prepped to the chin and mandibles superiorly and past the clavicles inferiorly.

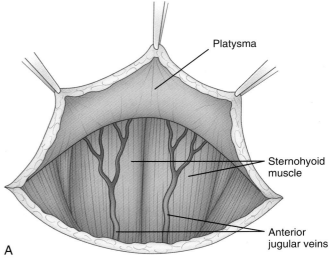

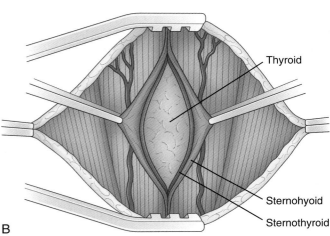

Figure 20-2
Exposure for thyroidectomy showing the creation of subplatysmal flaps (**A**) and the division of the median raphe between the strap muscles (**B**). *(From Osborn C, Parangi S: Partial thyroidectomy: Illustrated reflections for surgical residents. Curr Surg 63:39–43, 2006.)*

III. **Incision:** An incision is made one to two fingerbreadths above the sternal notch following **Langer's lines,** centered in the midline. The length of the incision is influenced by the patient's body habitus and the size of the thyroid gland.

IV. **Exposure**
   A. Dissection is carried down through the subcutaneous tissue and the platysma muscle. Flaps are raised superiorly and inferiorly in the avascular plane, just beneath the platysma muscle, superficial to the anterior jugular veins.
   B. The vertical plane between the strap muscles (**sternohyoid and sternothyroid muscles**) is developed up to the thyroid cartilage and down to the sternal notch. The strap muscles are retracted laterally. The loose areolar tissue just deep to the sternothyroid muscles is dissected using electrocautery to expose the thyroid gland (Fig. 20-2).

V. **Dissection**
   A. Mobilization of the thyroid gland is begun by dividing one of the middle thyroidal veins.
   B. Gentle medial traction is placed on the ipsilateral gland, allowing for exposure of the vessels to the superior pole. Care is taken when dividing these vessels to dissect in a medial to lateral direction to minimize potential injury to the external branch of the superior laryngeal nerve.

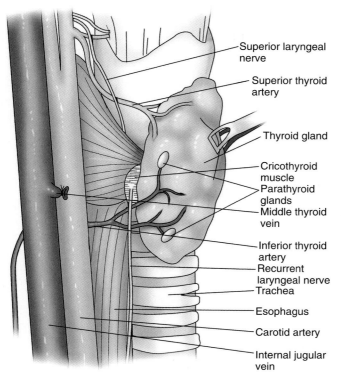

Figure 20-3

Relation of the recurrent laryngeal nerve and parathyroid glands to adjacent structures. *(From Cameron JL [ed]: Current Surgical Therapy, 8th ed. Philadelphia, Mosby, 2004.)*

Labels in figure:
- Superior laryngeal nerve
- Superior thyroid artery
- Thyroid gland
- Cricothyroid muscle
- Parathyroid glands
- Middle thyroid vein
- Inferior thyroid artery
- Recurrent laryngeal nerve
- Trachea
- Esophagus
- Carotid artery
- Internal jugular vein

C. After division of the superior pole vessels, the gland is retracted further medially, allowing for improved exposure of the inferior pole. The recurrent laryngeal nerve (RLN), which typically resides in the tracheoesophageal groove, just posterior to the inferior thyroid artery, is identified.

D. The RLN is followed along its entire course to its entry into the larynx superiorly (Fig. 20-3).

E. During dissection, the parathyroid glands are identified and preserved if possible. This is particularly important during total thyroidectomy, in which the risk of postoperative hypoparathyroidism is increased. Reimplantation of inadvertently removed parathyroid glands into the sternocleidomastoid muscle may help to reduce the incidence of this complication.

F. After mobilization of the lower pole, medial traction is again placed on the thyroid gland as it is sharply dissected off of the trachea, dividing the ligament of Berry.

G. The contralateral lobe is then mobilized in a similar fashion.

VI. **Closure:** The wound is thoroughly irrigated and hemostasis is confirmed. The strap muscles and platysma are reapproximated. The skin is closed using a running suture.

VII. **Additional Operative Considerations**

A. **Drainage:** Closed-suction drainage is often unnecessary following thyroid lobectomy. Although it is not a substitute for achieving meticulous hemostasis following resection, placement of a drain may be helpful in patients after total thyroidectomy, particularly for large goiters, to limit seroma formation.

B. **Intraoperative Nerve Monitoring:** Use of a specialized endotracheal tube with probes that sense motion in the larynx may be helpful during reoperative thyroid surgery, in which scar tissue makes identification of the recurrent laryngeal nerve more difficult.

> **DISSECTION WITH ELECTROCAUTERY SHOULD BE AVOIDED NEAR THE RECURRENT LARYNGEAL NERVE.**

POSTOPERATIVE COURSE

After thyroid surgery, pain is typically well controlled with oral analgesics. In the early postoperative period, patients are monitored closely for the development of neck swelling, suggesting hematoma formation. Patients who undergo total thyroidectomy are given thyroid replacement therapy within 24 hours of surgery. Serum calcium levels are checked after total thyroidectomy as well, and calcium supplementation is initiated if hypocalcemia is noted. If placed intraoperatively, surgical drains are typically removed the morning after surgery, assuming low volume output.

COMPLICATIONS

I. Although significant **bleeding** after thyroid surgery is relatively uncommon (<1%), patients should be closely monitored for signs of hematoma formation. An expanding **neck hematoma** associated with dyspnea or stridor suggests impending airway compromise. In the presence of these signs and symptoms, the neck incision should be opened at the bedside, the hematoma evacuated, and the patient promptly returned to the operating room.

II. **Injury to the RLN** is a rare complication of thyroid surgery (<1). Unilateral RLN injury may lead to vocal cord paresis and medialization of the cord (clinically manifested as **voice hoarseness**). After total thyroidectomy, bilateral RLN injury can lead to **airway occlusion.**

III. **The superior laryngeal nerve** has two branches: the **internal** (which provides sensory innervation to the larynx) and the **external** (which provides motor innervation to the cricothyroideus muscle). The external branch of the nerve is closely associated with the superior thyroid artery and may be injured during mobilization of the upper thyroid poles. Injury may result in loss of vocal projection, particularly at higher pitches.

IV. **Hypoparathyroidism** with associated hypocalcemia may result from removal or devascularization of the parathyroid glands. Hypocalcemia may be detected clinically by tapping on the facial nerve in the preauricular area to elicit facial twitching (**Chvostek's sign**) or inflating a blood pressure cuff to elicit carpal spasm (**Trousseau's sign**). Hypocalcemia should be treated with calcium supplementation.

V. **Thyroid storm** is a rare complication of thyroid surgery in patients with hyperthyroidism (e.g., Graves' disease). In the anesthetized patient, thyroid storm may manifest as tachycardia or cardiac arrhythmias and hyperthermia. Immediate cessation of the operative procedure is indicated, in conjunction with β-blockade (propanolol), antithyroid medications (propylthiouracil), corticosteroids, and iodine.

PARATHYROIDECTOMY

Case Study

A 54-year-old female presents to the surgical clinic after an evaluation by her primary care physician for symptoms of depression and a recent visit to the emergency room for kidney stones.

Findings on physical examination are unremarkable. No cervical masses or lymphadenopathy are appreciated. Laboratory evaluation is remarkable for a serum calcium level of 11.5 mg/dL and a parathyroid hormone (PTH) level of 186 pg/mL, and 24-hour urine calcium levels are found to be elevated.

A sestamibi scan is obtained and shows increased uptake in the left side of the neck (Fig. 20-4).

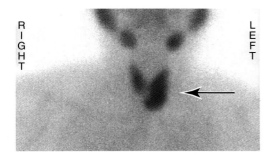

Figure 20-4
Sestamibi scan showing increased uptake in the left neck area. *(From Kumar V, Abbas A, Fausto N: Robbins and Cotran Pathologic Basis of Disease, 7th ed. Philadelphia, Saunders, 2005.)*

BACKGROUND

The normal parathyroid glands typically are ovoid and red-brown in color and weigh 30 to 50 mg. Most often there are four glands (one superior gland and one inferior gland on each side of the neck), although **supernumerary** glands are present in up to 13% of individuals. Although the superior glands are usually located posterior to the thyroid gland, just above the inferior thyroid arteries, the location of the inferior glands can be quite variable. All four parathyroid glands receive their blood supply via the **inferior thyroid artery.** Parathyroid glands produce **PTH**, which increases serum calcium levels by stimulating: (1) osteoclastic release of calcium stores in bone, (2) increased renal absorption of calcium, and (3) increased renal production of 1,25-dihydroxyvitamin D_3 [1,25-$(OH)_2D_3$] which, in turn, increases intestinal absorption of calcium.

   Primary hyperparathyroidism is characterized by excessive production of parathyroid hormone, resulting in dysregulation of calcium homeostasis. Patients with primary hyperparathyroidism typically have elevated serum calcium and PTH levels; serum phosphorus levels are usually low. Classic symptoms are summarized by the phrase *stones, bones, moans, groans, and psychiatric overtones*; this refers to the increased incidence of renal calculi, osteopenia, bone pain, gastrointestinal symptoms, and psychiatric disturbances in patients with primary hyperparathyroidism. **Secondary hyperparathyroidism** occurs in patients with renal failure who have elevated PTH levels as a result of increased calcium loss from the kidneys; such patients generally have elevated phosphorus levels. **Tertiary hyperparathyroidism** occurs in patients with renal failure who have undergone successful renal transplantation, but continue to have laboratory values consistent with hyperparathyroidism.

INDICATIONS FOR PARATHYROID SURGERY

  I. **Primary Hyperparathyroidism**
     A. Most cases of primary hyperparathyroidism (80%–85%) are due to **single adenomas;** the remaining cases are due to **multiglandular hyperplasia** (10%–15%) or **double adenomas** (5% to 10%). Although most often sporadic, multiglandular disease can be associated with familial syndromes, such as MEN I and MEN IIA. Parathyroidectomy is indicated in patients with **symptomatic** primary hyperparathyroidism or in **asymptomatic** patients who meet the following criteria (per the 2002 National Institutes of Health consensus guidelines):
        1. Serum calcium > 1.0 mg/dL above the upper limit of normal
        2. Urine calcium > 400 mg/day
        3. Bone density with T-score < −2.5
        4. Creatinine clearance < 30% that of age-matched control subjects
        5. Age < 50 years
        6. Poor follow-up
     B. Surgical resection of aberrant parathyroid tissue cures primary hyperparathyroidism. In patients with single or double adenomas, surgery consists of the removal of the abnormal gland(s). In patients with multiglandular hyperplasia, surgery involves either a subtotal (3.5 glands) parathyroidectomy or total parathyroidectomy with autotransplantation of parathyroid tissue into the sternocleidomastoid muscle or brachioradialis muscle of the forearm.

MEN I: Pituitary adenomas, parathyroid hyperplasia, and pancreatic neuro-endocrine tumors

II. **Secondary Hyperparathyroidism:** The majority of patients with secondary hyperparathyroidsim are treated medically. Occasionally, patients require surgery for refractory bone pain or fractures and generally undergo a subtotal parathyroidectomy or total parathyroidectomy with autotransplantation of parathyroid tissue.

III. **Tertiary Hyperparathyroidism:** Patients with tertiary hyperparathyroidism almost invariably have multiglandular disease and frequently benefit from surgery with either a subtotal parathyroidectomy or total parathyroidectomy with autotransplantation.

IV. **Parathyroid cancer** accounts for fewer than 0.1% of cases of primary hyperparathyroidism and is often associated with extremely high calcium levels or, in some instances, **hypercalcemic crisis** (characterized by severe neurologic, gastrointestinal, and renal symptoms). Treatment of severe hypercalcemia involves intravenous fluid resuscitation, loop diuretics, bisphosphonates, calcitonin, and occasionally dialysis, if other measures prove unsuccessful. The finding of a **palpable neck mass** in a patient with primary hyperparathyroidism should raise suspicion for the diagnosis of parathyroid carcinoma. Treatment of a parathyroid carcinoma includes excision of the tumor with en bloc thyroid lobectomy and removal of associated cervical lymph nodes.

PREOPERATIVE EVALUATION

I. **Serum calcium levels** are typically checked on at least two occasions to verify hypercalcemia. Frequently, either an ionized calcium level or a calculated calcium level corrected for the patient's serum albumin level is also obtained.

II. **Serum PTH level** is typically elevated, or higher than anticipated for the corresponding calcium level, in patients with primary hyperparathyroidism.

III. **Vitamin D (1,25-dihydroxyvitamin D$_3$ [1,25-(OH)$_2$D$_3$]) level** can help to identify patients with mild hyperparathyroidism and vitamin D deficiency who may benefit from vitamin D supplementation.

IV. **Twenty-four-hour urine calcium levels** help to determine whether an asymptomatic patient meets the criteria for parathyroid surgery and exclude the diagnosis of **familial hypercalcemic hypocalciuria (FHH)**. Patients with FHH will typically have a normal PTH level, with mildly elevated calcium levels and paradoxically low urinary calcium levels. Such patients do not benefit from parathyroidectomy.

V. **Technetium-99m sestamibi scanning** can localize an abnormal parathyroid gland (distinguished on the basis of enhanced tracer uptake). The sensitivity of the scan is limited (60%–90%), although a negative finding is associated with a higher incidence of multiglandular disease.

VI. **High-resolution ultrasound** can be helpful in identifying an enlarged parathyroid gland and has a sensitivity of 60% to 80%. In combination with sestamibi scanning, the specificity of abnormal parathyroid gland localization is greater than 90%.

VII. **Computed tomography (CT) scan and magnetic resonance imaging (MRI)** are not routinely obtained before parathyroid surgery, although they may be helpful in patients who require reoperative parathyroid surgery.

VIII. **Selective venous sampling of PTH levels** is not routinely performed before parathyroid surgery, but may be helpful in reoperative cases in which other imaging modalities do not localize the abnormal gland. Blood from both jugular veins at multiple levels is sampled, and the concentration gradient of PTH may help to localize the lesion.

Familial hypercalcemic hypocalciuria results from an abnormality in the renal parathyroid hormone receptor.

COMPONENTS OF THE PROCEDURE AND APPLIED ANATOMY

I. **Preoperative Considerations:** Conventional parathyroidectomy involves bilateral neck exploration with visualization of all four parathyroid glands (and sometimes biopsy of normal-appearing glands to exclude multiglandular disease). Increasingly, surgeons are adopting **minimally invasive parathyroidectomy (MIP).** In this approach, a unilateral dissection is performed on the side of the localized abnormal gland. This approach is associated with shorter operative times and a decreased risk of recurrent laryngeal nerve injury. **Intraoperative parathyroid hormone monitoring** with the rapid PTH immunoassay has emerged as an important adjunct to this approach. Because of the short half-life of PTH (approximately 3 minutes), a PTH level can be sent 10 to 15 minutes after resection of the suspected abnormal gland. A drop by more than 50% from the baseline level (i.e., serum PTH level before dissection and gland manipulation) and to the normal range suggests curative resection. Conversely, failure of PTH levels to normalize after resection of an abnormal gland should raise suspicion for the presence of additional disease and prompt further exploration.

II. **Patient Positioning and Preparation**
   A. Positioning and preparation of the patient for parathyroidectomy are similar to those used for thyroidectomy.
   B. Parathyroid surgery is typically performed under **general anesthesia,** although **regional** or **local anesthesia** may be sufficient in selected cases if a parathyroid adenoma has been localized preoperatively.

III. **Incision:** Parathyroidectomy is performed through a cervical collar incision following the Langer's lines 1 to 2 cm above the sternal notch. Small skin incisions of 2 to 4 cm are the hallmark of minimally invasive parathyroidectomy.

IV. **Exposure**
   A. Dissection is carried down through the subcutaneous tissue and the platysma muscle. Flaps are raised superiorly and inferiorly in the avascular plane, just beneath the platysma muscle, superficial to the anterior jugular veins.
   B. The vertical plane between the strap muscles (**sternohyoid and sternothyroid muscles**) is developed up to the thyroid cartilage and down to the sternal notch. The strap muscles are retracted laterally. The loose areolar tissue just deep to the sternothyroid muscles is dissected using electrocautery to expose the thyroid gland (Fig. 20-5).

V. **Dissection**
   A. The position of the superior parathyroid glands is more predictable than that of the inferior glands; they are usually located just superior to the inferior parathyroid artery. After identification, the gland is dissected free from the thyroid and other adjacent tissue. The gland's vascular pedicle is then clipped or ligated and divided.
   B. The inferior parathyroid glands are more variable in position, although they are most commonly found at the inferolateral aspect of the thyroid in the region of the thyrothymic ligament. As with the superior gland, great care should be taken to dissect the gland free without injuring the recurrent laryngeal nerve.

VI. **Closure:** The neck wound is thoroughly irrigated, and hemostasis is confirmed. The strap muscles and platysma are reapproximated. The skin is then closed using a running suture.

VII. **Additional Operative Considerations: Ectopic parathyroid glands** may be located within the thymus gland, in the carotid sheath, in the thyroid gland, low in the tracheoesophageal groove, or elsewhere in the mediastinum (Fig. 20-6). Intraoperative ultrasound is sometimes helpful in the identification of ectopic glands, including those that are intrathyroidal. When an abnormal gland cannot be identified during neck exploration, transcervical thymectomy may be considered. If exhaustive efforts to locate the abnormal gland are unsuccessful, the patient should undergo cross-sectional imaging studies (e.g., CT scan or MRI). In some cases, reoperation through a sternotomy is necessary to remove a mediastinal ectopic parathyroid gland.

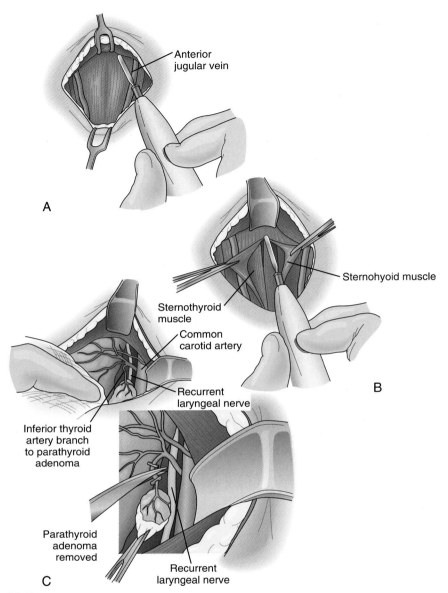

Figure 20-5
Exposure and dissection of a parathyroid adenoma. **A,** Subplatysmal flaps are developed. **B,** The strap muscles are retracted laterally and the thyroid gland is retracted medially to expose the parathyroid adenoma. **C,** The vascular pedicle to the adenoma is clipped and divided. *(From Udelsman R: Unilateral neck exploration under local or regional anesthesia. In Gagner M, Inabnet W [eds]: Textbook of Minimally Invasive Endocrine Surgery. Philadelphia, Lippincott Williams & Wilkins, 2002.)*

POSTOPERATIVE COURSE

After parathyroidectomy for primary hyperparathyroidism, pain is generally well controlled with oral analgesics, and patients may be discharged the same day. After subtotal parathyroidectomy or total parathyroidectomy with autotransplantation for secondary or tertiary hyperparathyroidism, patients are generally observed in the hospital. Serum calcium levels are checked serially until they can be maintained at adequate levels without the need for intravenous supplementation.

Oral calcium supplementation is usually prescribed before discharge. Patients are also instructed to take additional supplemental calcium and to contact the surgeon's office if they have symptoms of hypocalcemia (e.g., perioral parasthesias and muscle weakness).

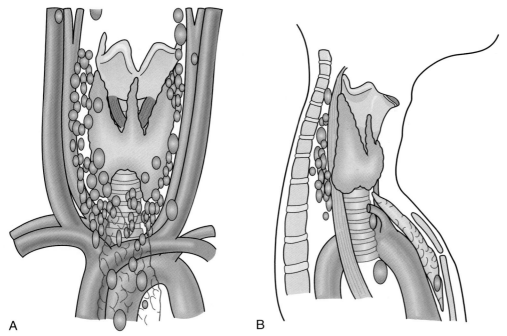

A   B

Figure 20-6
Variable location of abnormal parathyroid glands. **A**, Anterior view. **B**, Lateral view. *(From Udelsman R, Donovan PI: Remedial parathyroid surgery: Changing trends in 130 consecutive cases. Ann Surg 244:471–479, 2006.)*

COMPLICATIONS

I. The risk of **bleeding and neck hematoma** is relatively low after parathyroid surgery (<1%).

II. **Injury to the recurrent laryngeal nerve** is a very rare complication of parathyroidectomy. A benefit of MIP surgery for localized parathyroid disease is that dissection is limited to one side of the neck, precluding the possibility of bilateral RLN injury.

III. Temporary **hypocalcemia** may be seen in up to 30% of patients after parathyroidectomy. After total parathyroidectomy and autotransplantation, rarely, patients have refractory hypocalcemia requiring long-term intravenous calcium supplementation. Cryopreservation of parathyroid tissue at the time of parathyroidectomy, if feasible, may allow for subsequent reautotransplantation.

SUGGESTED READINGS

Mittendorf EA, McHenry CR: Thyroid cancer. In Cameron JL (ed): Current Surgical Therapy. Philadelphia, Mosby, pp 580–592.

Weigel RJ: Thyroid. In Norton JA, Bollinger RR, Chang AE, et al (eds): Essential Practice of Surgery. New York, Springer, 2003, pp 379–387.

Mastectomy

Robert E. Roses   and   Brian J. Czerniecki

Case Study

A 52-year-old female presents to her physician's office after palpating a firm mass in her right breast. She has no history of breast disease. She was 12 years of age at the time of menarche and is premenopausal. She has no children, nor has she ever been pregnant. Her last screening mammogram, 2 years earlier, was normal. An older sister was diagnosed with breast cancer at the age of 55 years and underwent a mastectomy.

On physical examination, a firm, irregular mass is noted just above the areola in the right breast. No overlying skin changes or axillary lymphadenopathy is appreciated.

A mammogram is obtained, which shows a stellate mass in the right breast (Fig. 21-1). A core needle biopsy is obtained and shows poorly differentiated invasive ductal carcinoma.

Figure 21-1
Mammogram. Craniocaudal view of the right breast shows a stellate mass. *(From Townsend CM, Beauchamp RD, Evers BM, Mattox KL [eds]: Sabiston Textbook of Surgery: The Biological Basis of Modern Surgical Practice, 17th ed. Philadelphia, Saunders, 2004.)*

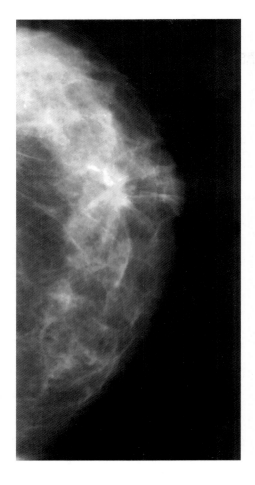

BACKGROUND

Breast cancer is the most common malignancy in women, excluding cancers of the skin. Fortunately, the majority of breast cancers are diagnosed as early-stage lesions and are therefore amenable to surgical intervention with good anticipated outcomes (for current staging, see Box 21-1). The surgical management of breast cancer has undergone a dramatic transformation over the past several decades. Until the mid-1970s, **radical mastectomy,** a procedure that involved removal of breast tissue, the underlying pectoralis muscles, and regional axillary nodes, was the procedure of choice for the treatment of breast cancers. This operation was subsequently replaced by the **modified radical mastectomy** (which spares the pectoralis muscles) and the **total or simple mastectomy** (a pectoralis-sparing mastectomy without axillary lymphadenectomy). Over the past 2 decades, breast-conserving therapy, consisting of **partial mastectomy** (lumpectomy) and radiation therapy,

Risk factors for breast cancer include age, history of breast cancer, atypical ductal hyperplasia, atypical lobular hyperplasia, LCIS, family history, *BRCA1* or *BRCA2* mutation, early menarche, late menopause, nulliparity, exogenous hormone usage, and thoracic radiation.

BOX 21-1 Joint Committee on Cancer Staging System for Breast Cancer

TNM Definitions

Primary Tumor (T)

- Tx: Primary tumor cannot be assessed
- T0: No evidence of primary tumor
- Tis: Ductal carcinoma in situ (DCIS), lobular carcinoma in situ (LCIS), or Paget's disease of the nipple with no tumor
- T1: Tumor not larger than 2 cm in greatest dimension
- T2: Tumor larger than 2 cm but not larger than 5 cm in greatest dimension
- T3: Tumor larger than 5 cm in greatest dimension
- T4: Tumor of any size with direct extension to chest wall or skin

Regional Lymph Nodes (N)

- Nx: Regional lymph nodes cannot be assessed
- N0: No regional lymph node metastasis
- N1: Metastasis to movable ipsilateral axillary lymph nodes
- N2: Metastasis to ipsilateral fixed or matted axillary lymph nodes or to ipsilateral internal mammary nodes in the absence of clinically evident axillary node metastasis
- N3: Metastasis in ipsilateral infraclavicular or supraclavicular lymph nodes or to ipsilateral internal mammary nodes in the presence of clinically evident axillary node metastasis

Distant Metastasis (M)

- Mx: Cannot be assessed
- M0: No distant metastasis
- M1: Distant metastasis

AJCC Stage Groupings

- 0: Tis, N0, M0
- 1: T1, N0, M0
- IIa: T0–T1, N1, M0; T2, N0, M0
- IIb: T2, N1, M0; T3, N0, M0
- IIIa: T0–T2, N2, M0; T3, N1–N2, M0
- IIIb: T4, N0–N2, M0
- IIIc: Any T, N3, M0
- IV: Any T, Any N, M1

From Singletary SE, Allred C, Ashley P, et al: Revision of the American Joint Committee on Cancer staging system for breast cancer. J Clin Oncol 20:3628–3636, 2002. Reprinted with permission from the American Society of Clinical Oncology.

has assumed a prominent role in the treatment paradigm for increasing numbers of breast cancers. More recently, **sentinel lymph node biopsy** has greatly reduced the number of axillary lymph node dissections performed on patients without clinically evident nodal metastases.

This chapter focuses on partial mastectomy and total mastectomy, which remain important components of the management of in situ and invasive breast cancers. Sentinel lymph node biopsy is addressed in detail in Chapter 23, as is **axillary lymphadenectomy,** which is sometimes performed in conjunction with total mastectomy.

INDICATIONS FOR MASTECTOMY

I. **Invasive Breast Cancer:** Most early breast cancers are treated with partial mastectomy and radiation (breast-conserving therapy) (Fig. 21-2). Contraindications to this approach include: large tumor burden relative to small breast size, previous radiation therapy or other contraindications to radiation therapy (e.g., pregnancy), and multicentric disease (cancer foci in multiple quadrants of the breast). Sentinel lymph node biopsy is performed in conjunction with partial or total mastectomy for most invasive and some in situ cancers. Axillary lymphadenectomy is indicated in patients with sentinel lymph nodes containing metastases or clinically positive axillary nodes.

II. **Ductal Carcinoma in Situ (DCIS):** DCIS is a premalignant lesion characterized by clustered malignant cells confined by a basement membrane. Most often, DCIS is diagnosed by screening mammography. Microcalcifications are the most common associated mammographic finding. DCIS is most often treated with breast-conserving therapy. In patients with extensive or diffuse disease, however, mastectomy is sometimes performed.

III. **Lobular Carcinoma in Situ (LCIS):** LCIS is characterized by the presence of neoplastic cells that distend the breast acini (blind sacs that empty into the ductal system of the breast) without disrupting the breast's lobular architecture. Because it is not palpable and is not associated with radiographic abnormalities, LCIS is typically an incidental finding on biopsy performed for other indications. It is important to note that LCIS is not a preinvasive lesion; rather, it is a risk factor

Figure 21-2
Algorithm for the evaluation and treatment of suspected breast cancer.

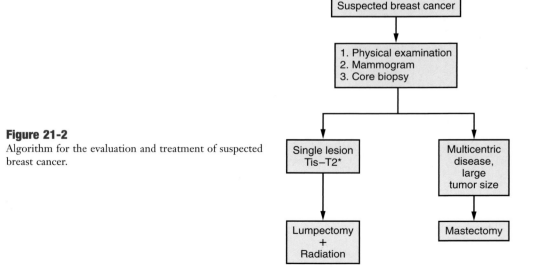

*American Joint Committee on Cancer Staging System for Breast Cancer, 2002; see Box 21-1.

for the subsequent development of ductal carcinoma of the breast. Both breasts are at equal risk, which is estimated to be slightly lower than 1% per year. Close clinical follow-up, consisting of biannual breast examinations and annual mammography, is indicated after diagnosis. Bilateral prophylactic mastectomy is an alternative option and may be considered in women with a strong family history of breast cancer or with mutations of the *BRCA1* or *BRCA2* gene.

IV. **Family History and Genetic Factors:** The risk of breast cancer is increased by a factor of two to three in first-degree relatives (mothers, sisters, and daughters) of patients with breast cancer. In families with multiple affected members with bilateral and early-onset cancers, the absolute risk to first-degree relatives approaches 50%. Genetic factors, such as mutations in the *BRCA1* and *BRCA2* genes, are responsible for an estimated 5% to 10% of breast cancers and may account for 25% of breast cancers in women younger than 30 years of age. *BRCA1* mutations are also associated with an increased risk of ovarian cancer (15%–45%), whereas *BRCA2* mutations are associated with an increased risk of breast cancer in men. Women with a mutation in *BRCA2* also have a 20% to 30% lifetime risk of ovarian cancer. Bilateral prophylactic mastectomy should be given serious consideration in such high-risk patients.

V. **Other indications** for partial or total mastectomy include a number of other primary tumors of the breast.

   A. The often indolent **phyllodes tumor** and the frequently aggressive **angiosarcoma** are both treated with wide resection to achieve negative margins. The former can often be treated with partial mastectomy. Treatment of the latter often necessitates mastectomy. Unlike adenocarcinoma of the breast, malignant phyllodes tumors and angiosarcomas spread hematogenously. Therefore, axillary dissection is not indicated for their treatment.

   B. **Paget's disease of the breast,** a condition characterized by erythema, scaling, and ulceration of the nipple, is associated with an underlying breast carcinoma in 97% of patients. After evaluation with mammography or magnetic resonance imaging (MRI) to identify an underlying malignancy or multicentric disease, patients may undergo either partial mastectomy, including excision of the nipple–areolar complex, or total mastectomy, with or without axillary lymphadenectomy.

PREOPERATIVE EVALUATION

I. **Mammography:** Standard mammography consists of craniocaudal and mediolateral oblique views. Diagnostic mammography, obtained to further evaluate a recognized breast abnormality, may include additional magnification and compression views. Mammography remains an important component of the preoperative evaluation of a breast lesion and may aid in determining the extent of disease and identifying additional lesions in the ipsilateral or contralateral breast.

II. **Breast Biopsy:** A variety of biopsy techniques are used in evaluating breast lesions. **Core needle biopsy** has become the most prevalent. Patients with an inconclusive finding on core needle biopsy or discordance between core needle histology and mammographic findings should undergo **excisional surgical biopsy.** Surgical biopsy for nonpalpable findings is facilitated by preoperative imaging-guided placement of a localizing wire (needle localization) and specimen radiographic confirmation at surgery (Fig. 21-3).

III. **Additional diagnostic modalities** sometimes used in the evaluation of breast lesions include ultrasound and MRI. Ultrasound is helpful in distinguishing solid from cystic masses. MRI is highly sensitive in detecting breast cancers and is increasingly used in the evaluation of breast lesions and in screening high-risk patients for occult breast cancers.

Is your patient a candidate for breast-conserving therapy?

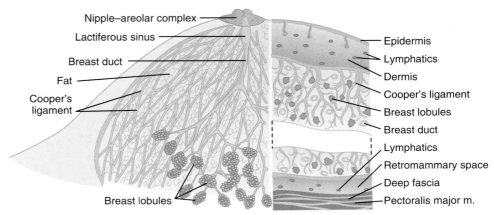

Figure 21-3
Breast tissue is surrounded by the subcutaneous fat of the overlying skin and the pectoralis muscle. The suspensory ligaments of the breast, known as *Cooper's ligaments*, are continuous with the superficial fascia deep to the dermis and are divided during mastectomy. The breast lobules, the milk-forming glandular units of the breast, are made up of acini (milk-forming glands) and their small efferent ducts. These small ducts join others, forming successively larger ducts that ultimately join to form the lactiferous sinuses, which empty at the nipple–areolar complex. *(From Townsend CM, Beauchamp RD, Evers BM, Mattox KL [eds]: Sabiston Textbook of Surgery: The Biological Basis of Modern Surgical Practice, 17th ed. Philadelphia, Saunders, 2004.)*

COMPONENTS OF THE PROCEDURE AND APPLIED ANATOMY

Preoperative Considerations

   I. Prophylactic **antibiotics** are rarely indicated for isolated breast procedures, although some surgeons advocate their administration if the patient has had previous breast surgery (i.e., reoperative breast surgery). Antibiotics are frequently administered before axillary lymph node dissection and, therefore, before modified radical mastectomy.
  II. **Urinary catheter** placement before mastectomy is usually unnecessary. Obvious exceptions to this rule include combined mastectomy and autologous breast reconstruction procedures, which are frequently lengthy.

Patient Positioning and Preparation

   I. The patient is placed in the supine position.
  II. The sterile preparation should include the entire breast and extend several inches past the midline to the contralateral breast, above the clavicle and below the inframammary fold. Laterally, the preparation should extend to the posterior axillary line.
 III. Breast procedures are often performed in conjunction with sentinel lymph node biopsy or axillary lymphadenectomy. Therefore, it is often necessary to position the patient with one or both arms at 90 degrees. The axilla and upper arm on the side of surgery should be included in the preparation.

Partial Mastectomy

Partial mastectomy involves segmental excision of the lesion with a limited margin of surrounding breast tissue. Several principles should be adhered to in performing a partial mastectomy. These include the following:
   I. Incisions should generally be oriented along lines of minimal skin tension. Central lesions may be approached through periareolar incisions, whereas radial incisions are sometimes used for peripheral breast lesions (Fig. 21-4).
  II. Incisions should overlie the lesion to avoid tunneling through unaffected breast tissue.

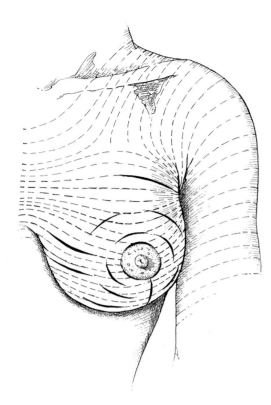

Figure 21-4
Incision choices for partial mastectomy. *(From Roses DF [ed]: Breast Cancer, 2nd ed. Philadelphia, Churchill Livingstone, 2005.)*

III. Microscopically, tumor-free margins of at least 2 to 3 mm should be achieved.
IV. The specimen should be labeled at a minimum of two points to facilitate histologic analysis and guide further resection if the margins obtained are not adequate.
V. Microclips may be placed in the resection cavity after removal of the specimen to guide subsequent radiation therapy and aid in the interpretation of future mammograms.

Total Mastectomy

I. A transverse elliptical incision is made to include the nipple–areolar complex (Fig. 21-5). If a previous surgical biopsy was performed, the ellipse should include the scar. Incisions may be modified when mastectomy is combined with a reconstructive procedure.
II. Skin flaps are raised sharply (usually with electrocautery), separating breast tissue from overlying skin and subcutaneous fat and dividing Cooper's ligaments. This plane is relatively avascular.
III. Flaps are developed to the clavicle superiorly, the sternum medially, the rectus abdominis muscle inferiorly, and the latissimus dorsi muscle laterally (Fig. 21-6).

> What is the best site for the partial mastectomy incision in your patient?

> **THE CREATION OF OVERLY THIN OR LONG FLAPS MAY RESULT IN FLAP NECROSIS.**

> Mastectomy flaps should extend to the clavicle superiorly, the sternum medially, the rectus abdominis muscle inferiorly, and the latissimus dorsi muscle laterally.

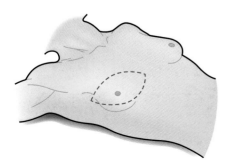

Figure 21-5
Skin incisions are generally transverse and surround the central breast and nipple–areolar complex. *(From Townsend CM, Beauchamp RD, Evers BM, Mattox KL [eds]: Sabiston Textbook of Surgery: The Biological Basis of Modern Surgical Practice, 17th ed. Philadelphia, Saunders, 2004.)*

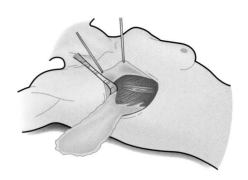

Figure 21-6
Skin flaps are raised sharply, separating the gland from the overlying skin, and underlying muscle. *(From Townsend CM, Beauchamp RD, Evers BM, Mattox KL [eds]: Sabiston Textbook of Surgery: The Biological Basis of Modern Surgical Practice, 17th ed. Philadelphia, Saunders, 2004.)*

IV. Superiorly and medially, the plane of dissection is carried down to the underlying pectoralis muscles. Breast tissue with the pectoralis muscle fascia is dissected off of the underlying muscle, beginning medially and ending at the latissimus dorsi.

V. After removal of the specimen, the wound is irrigated and hemostasis is achieved. A closed-suction drain is placed between the underlying muscle and flaps and brought through the skin lateral to the incision.

VI. The wound is closed.

Skin-Sparing Mastectomy

Increasingly, mastectomies are performed in conjunction with breast reconstruction procedures. Skin-sparing mastectomy, performed by removing the breast tissue and nipple–areolar complex through a small incision around the areola, may allow for improved cosmetic results.

POSTOPERATIVE COURSE

Partial mastectomy is most often performed on an outpatient basis. Postoperative pain is usually well controlled with oral analgesics. Total mastectomy, on the other hand, may require intravenous analgesia in the early postoperative period. Patients are most often discharged with a surgical drain in place on the first or second postoperative day.

COMPLICATIONS

In addition to **bleeding** (hematoma formation) and **surgical site infections,** complications of mastectomy include **seroma formation** (accumulation of serous fluid under the skin flaps) and **skin flap necrosis.**

I. **Seroma formation:** Some serous accumulation under the skin flaps is anticipated after mastectomy and may be controlled through maintenance of closed-suction drainage for approximately 1 week after surgery.

II. **Skin flap necrosis** may result from the creation of overly thin or long flaps, with resultant compromise of the skin microcirculation. This problem may be exacerbated in smokers.

SUGGESTED READINGS

Iglehart JD, Kaelin CM: Diseases of the breast. In Townsend CM, Beauchamp RD, Evers BM, Mattox KL (eds): Sabiston Textbook of Surgery: The Biological Basis of Modern Surgical Practice, 17th ed. Philadelphia, Saunders, 2004, pp 867–927.

Roses DF, Giuliano AE: Surgery for breast cancer. In Roses DF (ed): Breast Cancer, 2nd ed. Philadelphia, Churchill Livingstone, 2005, pp 401–460.

Singletary SE, Allred C, Ashley P, et al: Revision of the American Joint Committee on Cancer staging system for breast cancer. J Clin Oncol 20:3628–3636, 2002.

CHAPTER 22

Breast Reconstruction

Suhail K. Kanchwala   and   Joseph M. Serletti

Case Study

A 38-year-old female undergoes genetic testing after her sister is diagnosed with breast cancer and is found to have a BRCA2 mutation. She is 5 feet 11 inches tall and weighs 120 pounds. She has decided to undergo bilateral prophylactic mastectomy and presents to your office to discuss options for breast reconstruction.

BACKGROUND

Breast reconstruction has become an essential component of the care of women with breast cancer. The goals of modern breast reconstruction are to recreate a natural-appearing breast mound that matches the opposite breast in size, contour, and degree of ptosis (i.e., droopiness). This chapter discusses a variety of alloplastic (implant-based) and autologous techniques for breast reconstruction after mastectomy.

Autologous reconstruction is defined as any form of breast reconstruction that uses a patient's own tissues to recreate the breast mound. A variety of donor sites can be used for autologous breast reconstruction, including the lower abdomen, buttocks, and back. **Alloplastic** reconstruction refers to any form of breast reconstruction in which an implant is used. Implant-based reconstruction is typically performed in stages. The first stage involves placement of an inflatable tissue expander that permits the recruitment of additional skin and soft tissue. Subsequently, the expander is replaced with a permanent prosthesis.

Delayed breast reconstruction is defined as reconstruction that occurs after a patient has undergone a mastectomy. Delayed breast reconstruction is most commonly performed for patients who require postoperative radiation therapy. **Immediate breast reconstruction,** on the other hand, refers to any reconstruction that begins at the time of mastectomy.

> Immediate reconstruction is performed at the time of mastectomy. Delayed reconstruction is performed after the mastectomy is completed.

INDICATIONS FOR BREAST RECONSTRUCTION

I. **Total Mastectomy Defect:** Breast reconstruction most often follows total mastectomy (i.e., removal of the nipple–areolar complex as well as the complete removal of breast tissue) for the treatment of malignancy or a premalignant condition. Genetic screening for mutations within the *BRCA* gene loci has led to a dramatic rise in the frequency with which bilateral prophylactic mastectomy is performed. Such procedures are often coupled with bilateral reconstruction.

II. **Partial Mastectomy Defect:** Lumpectomy deformities after "breast-conserving" therapies are sometimes significant enough to justify reconstruction.

PREOPERATIVE EVALUATION

I. **History:** A number of factors influence the choice of a reconstruction technique. A history of **radiation therapy** or planned postmastectomy radiation therapy significantly influences the timing and choice of a reconstruction approach. Specifi-

> Will your patient require postoperative radiation therapy?

cally, implant-based techniques are contraindicated in patients who are likely to receive radiation therapy.

II. Current **smoking** adversely affects wound healing after surgery for breast reconstruction. Patients should be encouraged to stop smoking several weeks before surgery.

III. The presence of **diabetes** can have an adverse effect on wound healing. Appropriate perioperative management of blood sugar is essential.

IV. Patient **age** can influence the choice of reconstructive technique. Elderly patients are at slightly higher risk for complications after autologous reconstruction. Conversely, autologous reconstruction is often favored in younger patients.

V. The lower abdomen is the most common source of autologous tissue for breast reconstruction. Patients must, therefore, have sufficient lower abdominal tissue to allow for autologous reconstruction. Very thin patients are often better served by implant-based reconstruction. Although obese patients have sufficient tissue, they are also at greater risk of developing wound complications.

> What is your patient's body mass index?

COMPONENTS OF THE PROCEDURE AND APPLIED ANATOMY

There are various techniques for reconstructing the breast mound after mastectomy. The most common procedures involve using either autologous tissues (e.g., transverse rectus abdominis myocutaneous [TRAM] flap), tissue expander placement followed by a silicone gel prosthetic implantation, or some combination of the two (e.g., latissimus dorsi flap with implant).

Preoperative Considerations

Autologous reconstruction procedures are typically lengthy and require the placement of a **urinary catheter** for bladder decompression and monitoring of urine output.

Patient Positioning and Preparation

I. The patient is placed **supine** on the operating room table. The patient should be placed with the hips at the break in the table to facilitate sitting upright.

II. The sterile preparation is applied to both breasts, the entire abdomen, and the bilateral groin area.

Skin-Sparing Mastectomy

Mastectomy techniques have a significant effect on the outcome of autologous breast reconstruction. Since 1996, the skin-sparing mastectomy has been increasingly used in conjunction with immediate autologous breast reconstruction. A skin-sparing mastectomy is typically performed with a periareolar incision and is so named because the skin envelope of the breast is kept intact during the procedure (Fig. 22-1). Thus, the reconstructive surgeon must simply replace the volume of the mastectomy specimen with either autologous tissue or an implant. This approach avoids the challenges associated with shaping the breast during traditional delayed reconstruction.

Autologous Reconstruction: TRAM Flap

I. **Pedicled TRAM Flap Technique**

A. The pedicled TRAM flap was first described by Hartrampf in 1982 and is the most common form of autologous reconstruction performed today. The TRAM flap transfers the lower abdominal skin and fat using the ipsilateral rectus muscle as a conduit for the blood supply (superior epigastric vessels) (Fig. 22-2).

B. In most cases, the reconstruction procedure begins simultaneously with the mastectomy and is carried out by a separate surgical team.

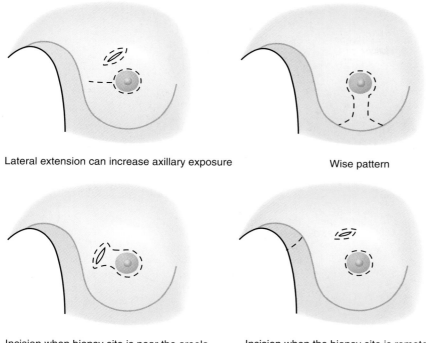

Lateral extension can increase axillary exposure

Wise pattern

Incision when biopsy site is near the areola

Incision when the biopsy site is remote
from the areola with axillary incision for
lymphadenectomy

Figure 22-1

Incisions for skin-sparing mastectomy. *(From Townsend CM, Beauchamp RD, Evers BM, Mattox KL [eds]: Sabiston Textbook of Surgery: The Biological Basis of Modern Surgical Practice, 18th ed. Philadelphia, Saunders, 2008.)*

C. An elliptical incision is drawn on the lower abdomen preoperatively while the patient is in the upright position. The area of excision should not be too large to close without tension (Fig. 22-3).

D. The skin and subcutaneous fat are incised, and the abdominal fascia is exposed circumferentially.

E. The upper abdominal flap is developed up to the costal margin in the plane immediately superficial to the abdominal wall fascia.

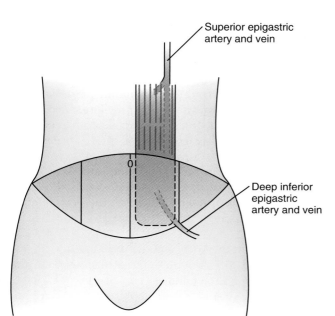

Superior epigastric
artery and vein

Deep inferior
epigastric
artery and vein

Figure 22-2

Vascular territories of the abdominal wall supplied by a unilateral transverse rectus abdominis myocutaneous flap. In a standard pedicled TRAM flap, the skin island is based on the superior epigastric vessels. *(From Townsend CM, Beauchamp RD, Evers BM, Mattox KL [eds]: Sabiston Textbook of Surgery: The Biological Basis of Modern Surgical Practice, 18th ed. Philadelphia, Saunders, 2008.)*

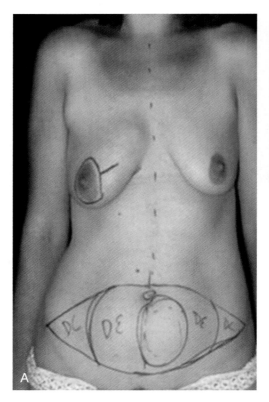

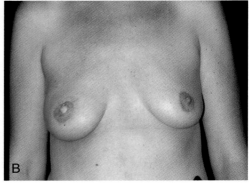

Figure 22-3
A, Patient with a large cancer of the right breast marked preoperatively for a pedicled transverse rectus abdominis myocutaneous reconstruction. **B,** The final result after nipple–areolar reconstruction. *(Courtesy of L.P. Bucky, MD.)*

   F. Most often, the rectus muscle contralateral to the mastectomy site is used for reconstruction. The flap is elevated in a lateral to medial fashion until the medial edge (i.e., linea alba) and the lateral edge (i.e., linea semilunaris) of the rectus sheath are exposed.

   G. The rectus sheath is then incised medially and laterally up to the costal margin. The rectus muscle is elevated off of the posterior rectus sheath. The flap, consisting of muscle and anterior sheath, is then transected inferiorly.

   H. A subcutaneous tunnel is developed at the inframammary crease to allow passage of the flap from the abdomen to the breast. The flap is then tunneled up to the breast and sutured to the chest wall.

   I. The TRAM flap is then shaped, excess tissue is trimmed, and any abdominal wall skin that will be buried underneath the mastectomy flaps is de-epithelialized.

   J. The abdominal fascia is repaired with prosthetic mesh.

 II. **Free TRAM Flap Technique**

   A. The lower abdominal tissue can also be transferred without preserving the superior epigastric vessels. The inferior epigastric vessels provide a more robust blood supply to the lower abdomen compared with the superior epigastric vessels and can be anastomosed to the thoracodorsal or internal mammary vessels.

   B. The free TRAM flap procedure is performed in much the same way as the pedicled TRAM flap procedure except that the deep inferior epigastric vessels are dissected out. A section of the rectus muscle containing the deep inferior epigastric vessels, as well as any perforators to the overlying fat and skin, is excised.

   C. The free TRAM flap is detached from the body, and the deep inferior epigastric vessels are then re-anastomosed to either the internal mammary or the thoracodorsal vessels using microsurgical techniques (Fig. 22-4).

   D. Because free TRAM flaps have a more robust blood supply, this procedure can be performed in patients at higher risk for complications with pedicled TRAM

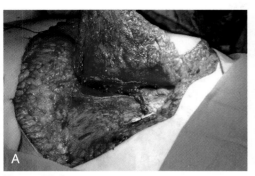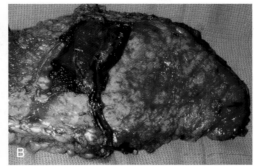

Figure 22-4
A, The abdominal tissue has been raised off of the fascia, the lateral rectus sheath has been entered, and the inferior epigastric vessels have been dissected from the iliac vessels. **B,** An example of a free transverse rectus abdominis myocutaneous flap before anastomosis in the chest. *(Courtesy of J.M. Serletti, MD.)*

surgery (i.e., smokers and obese patients). Additionally, because less of the rectus muscle can be taken with the free flap, the donor site morbidity of the TRAM flap is minimized.

Implant Reconstruction

The principal advantage of implant-based reconstruction is the avoidance of donor site morbidity. Furthermore, implant-based reconstruction may be the only option in patients without sufficient abdominal tissue for reconstruction. Implant reconstruction should not be performed in patients requiring radiation therapy because of the high associated complication rate (primarily capsular contracture and fibrosis).

I. **Technique**
   A. The anatomic boundaries of the breast are marked preoperatively in the upright position.
   B. The pectoralis fascia is incised immediately lateral to the border of the pectoralis major muscle through the incision made for the mastectomy. The plane between the pectoralis major muscle and the chest wall is developed until the medial insertion of the pectoralis major muscle on the sternum is identified.
   C. Frequently, portions of the inferior pectoralis insertion must be released to allow appropriate placement of the tissue expander.
   D. An appropriately sized temporary tissue expander is placed in the subpectoral plane. The serratus anterior muscle can be mobilized to cover any exposed expander laterally. The wound is then closed (Fig. 22-5).

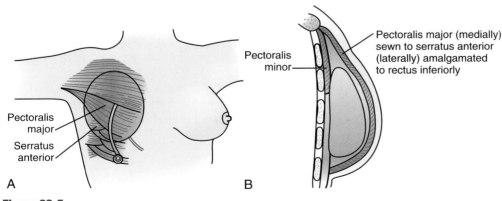

Figure 22-5
Tissue expander placed underneath the pectoralis major muscle. **A,** Anterior view. **B,** Cross-section view. *(From Townsend CM, Beauchamp RD, Evers BM, Mattox KL [eds]: Sabiston Textbook of Surgery: The Biological Basis of Modern Surgical Practice, 18th ed. Philadelphia, Saunders, 2008.)*

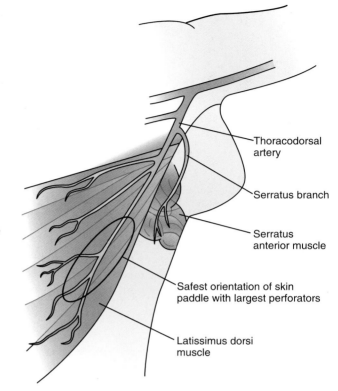

Figure 22-6

Anatomy of latissimus dorsi muscle reconstruction. *(From Townsend CM, Beauchamp RD, Evers BM, Mattox KL [eds]: Sabiston Textbook of Surgery: The Biological Basis of Modern Surgical Practice, 18th ed. Philadelphia, Saunders, 2008.)*

Thoracodorsal artery

Serratus branch

Serratus anterior muscle

Safest orientation of skin paddle with largest perforators

Latissimus dorsi muscle

  E. Expansion with sterile saline is typically performed in the office 3 to 4 weeks after surgery and at weekly intervals thereafter until the final volume of expansion is reached.

  F. Once full expansion has been achieved, the patient undergoes a second surgery to replace the tissue expander with a permanent implant prosthesis.

 II. **Combined Techniques: Latissimus Dorsi Flap**

  A. When there is insufficient abdominal tissue for a TRAM flap, the latissimus dorsi flap can be used as an alternative (Fig. 22-6). In modern breast reconstruction, the latissimus dorsi flap is most commonly reserved for salvage of unsuccessful implant or autologous reconstructions.

  B. Technique

   1. The anatomic boundaries of the breast are marked preoperatively in the upright position.

   2. An incision is made over the lateral border of the latissimus dorsi muscle to create an appropriately sized skin paddle. The incision is sharply carried down to the fascia overlying the latissimus dorsi muscle.

   3. The muscle is harvested through this incision. The humeral insertion of the latissimus dorsi is often released through a separate counterincision to allow full rotation of the muscle.

   4. The muscle and skin paddle is then positioned in the mastectomy defect through a subcutaneous tunnel between the back and the breast.

   5. Typically, an implant prosthesis is placed under the flap.

Nipple–Areolar Reconstruction

Nipple–areolar reconstruction is usually the final stage of either autologous or implant-based breast reconstruction. Typically, the nipple and areola are fashioned from local tissues. Numerous techniques exist for recreating a nipple. The most commonly performed procedure is the star flap shown in Figure 22-7. The areola can be recreated with either a skin graft taken from the lower abdominal incision or postoperative tattooing.

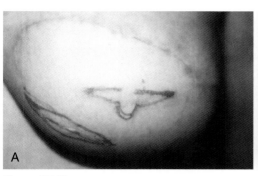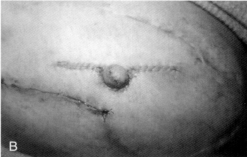

Figure 22-7
The star flap design for nipple reconstruction. **A,** The breast is marked preoperatively. **B,** The completed reconstruction is shown. *(From Townsend CM, Beauchamp RD, Evers BM, Mattox KL [eds]: Sabiston Textbook of Surgery: The Biological Basis of Modern Surgical Practice, 18th ed. Philadelphia, Saunders, 2008.)*

POSTOPERATIVE COURSE

  I. **Autologous Reconstruction:** The postoperative care of patients after autologous reconstruction focuses on monitoring the integrity of the flap, wound care for the donor site, and pain control. After a free TRAM flap in particular, hourly vascular checks are especially important during the first 48 postoperative hours; loss of a flap pulse requires urgent revision. Patients are encouraged to ambulate slowly in a hunched position over the course of several days and are typically discharged on the fifth postoperative day.

 II. **Implant Reconstruction:** Patients who undergo implant-based reconstruction have a recovery similar to that of patients receiving mastectomy alone. Some patients do, however, have increased pain because of the tension placed on the pectoralis muscle. Muscle relaxants, such as diazepam, can provide significant relief and are commonly prescribed postoperatively.

COMPLICATIONS

  I. **Seroma formation** is the most common complication of breast reconstruction. Both autologous reconstruction and implant-based reconstruction involve the creation of tissue flaps under which fluid may accumulate. Postoperative drains are routinely used and minimize accumulation. Seroma formation after drain removal is typically managed conservatively with in-office aspiration or observation. Rarely, reoperation and replacement of a closed-suction drain are required.

 II. **Fat necrosis** may occur after autologous tissue reconstruction when the blood supply to a region of a TRAM or, less commonly, a latissumus dorsi flap is compromised. Patients present postoperatively with a firm mass in the breast. Small areas of fat necrosis are often observed; larger areas may need to be surgically excised.

III. Superficial **infections** after breast reconstruction with implants can pose a significant problem. Early readmission and treatment with intravenous antibiotics may be effective; however, patients with delayed presentation often require implant removal. After such an infection, further implant reconstruction is typically delayed for 6 months or longer.

SUGGESTED READINGS

Kanchwala SK, Bucky LP: Precision transverse rectus abdominis muscle flap breast reconstruction: A reliable technique for efficient preoperative planning. Ann Plast Surg 60:521–526, 2008.

Serletti JM: Breast reconstruction with the TRAM flap: pedicled and free. J Surg Oncol 94:532–537, 2006.

Sigurdson L, Lalonde DH: Breast reconstruction. Plast Reconstr Surg 121(1 Suppl):1–12, 2008.

Thorne CH, Beasley RW, Aston SJ, et al: Grabb and Smith's Plastic Surgery, 6th ed. Philadelphia, Lippincott Williams & Wilkins, 2007.

CHAPTER 23

Sentinel Lymph Node Biopsy and Axillary Dissection

Robert E. Roses

Case Study

A 55-year-old male presents for evaluation of a pigmented lesion on his upper mid-back. He notes that the lesion has increased in diameter, has become raised, and has changed coloration over the past several months. He is fair skinned, with blue eyes and blond hair. He reports a history of blistering sunburns as a teenager. An asymmetric lesion with a maximal diameter of 1 cm and variegated brown coloration is noted on his mid-back. He has multiple other pigmented lesions scattered over his trunk and extremities. No adenopathy in his axillae, neck, or groin is appreciated. A punch biopsy shows a malignant melanoma with a thickness of 2.9 mm.

BACKGROUND

Lymph node staging is an important component of the surgical management of both **malignant melanoma** and **breast cancer.** Until the 1990s, complete regional lymphadenectomy represented the standard approach to achieving this goal. The development of sentinel lymph node biopsy has allowed for the more limited, selective treatment of regional lymph nodes and has decreased the number of complete regional dissections performed in patients without nodal metastases. This procedure, as it is currently performed, maps the lymphatic drainage from the skin or breast to a primary lymph node or nodes, using a **vital blue dye** or a **radioisotope-labeled tracer.** Surgical excision and pathologic evaluation of these nodes for metastases allows for reliable staging and the prediction of additional lymph node metastases. Generally, patients found to have metastases in the sentinel node or nodes (i.e., positive sentinel node biopsy) undergo completion lymphadenectomy. In contrast, patients with negative findings on sentinel lymph node biopsy can safely forgo lymphadenectomy in view of the very low risk of nonsentinel nodal involvement. Sentinel lymph node biopsy also allows a meticulous histologic evaluation of multiple sections augmented by immunohistochemical staining for melanoma-related antigens and cytokeratins for breast cancer. This, not infrequently, allows more precise staging of both diseases.

With few exceptions, the axillary lymph nodes represent the first site of metastasis from melanomas of the upper extremities and upper trunk and cancers of the breast. This chapter focuses on axillary lymph node biopsy; however, the techniques described are applicable to sentinel lymph node biopsy performed at other sites (e.g., the groin for lower extremity melanomas and the cervical, parotid, and occipital lymph nodes for head and neck melanomas). Axillary dissection, which remains an important component of the management of breast cancer and melanoma and typically follows a positive finding on sentinel lymph node biopsy, is also described.

INDICATIONS FOR SURGERY

I. **Breast Cancer**

    A. Patients with invasive breast cancer who can safely undergo surgery benefit from lymph node staging. This is generally achieved through sentinel lymph node biopsy. Exceptions include patients with axillary lymphadenopathy suspicious for metastatic disease and patients who have had previous breast or chest wall irradiation, which may disrupt the lymphatics and preclude accurate lymphatic mapping. Such patients should forgo sentinel lymph node biopsy in favor of axillary dissection. Elderly patients or those with significant comorbidities, with favorable stage I tumors, also may forgo sentinel lymph node biopsy.

    B. Although patients with in situ breast cancers should not, theoretically, have nodal metastases, invasive foci in the area of the in situ disease is present in 10% to 30% of patients. A number of indications for sentinel lymph node biopsy in patients with **ductal carcinoma of the breast (DCIS)** have, therefore, emerged. Sentinel lymph node biopsy is indicated in patients with multicentric or broad areas of high-grade DCIS, as well as in those undergoing total mastectomy (which precludes subsequent nodal staging without axillary dissection).

II. **Melanoma** is the eighth most common cancer in the United Stated and the most common cause of skin cancer–related deaths. Tumor thickness is the dominant prognostic factor and is correlated with the risk of regional metastasis. Generally, sentinel lymph node biopsy is offered to patients with melanomas exceeding 1 mm in thickness. Completion lymphadenopathy is performed if the sentinel node is found to contain metastatic disease. Patients with "intermediate-thickness" melanomas (1–4 mm) are at relatively higher risk of having nodal metastases compared with patients with thinner lesions, but they are at lower risk, compared with patients with thicker lesions, of having distant metastases. Notably, the therapeutic utility of sentinel lymph node biopsy in patients with such lesions was recently evaluated in the **Multicenter Selective Lymphadenectomy Trial.** This trial compared wide local excision and sentinel lymph node biopsy with wide local excision alone for the treatment of intermediate-thickness melanomas and demonstrated a survival advantage for patients randomized to the former treatment group who had nodal micrometastases.

PREOPERATIVE EVALUATION

The components of the preoperative evaluation of patients with breast cancer and melanoma are distinct and are discussed separately.

I. **Breast Cancer**

    A. The **evaluation of a suspected breast cancer** typically includes **breast examination, mammography,** and **breast biopsy.** Additional diagnostic modalities increasingly used in the evaluation of breast lesions include **ultrasound** and **magnetic resonance imaging.** The goals of this evaluation are to: (1) establish a tissue diagnosis, (2) clinically stage patients, and (3) identify candidates for breast-conserving therapy versus patients who require mastectomy.

    B. An **assessment for regional metastases** should begin with a **physical examination** of the bilateral axillary and supraclavicular fossae. Adenopathy suggestive of metastatic disease may be further evaluated with **fine-needle aspiration;** malignant cells seen on cytologic evaluation or a high degree of suspicion for nodal metastases should prompt axillary dissection rather than sentinel lymph node biopsy.

II. **Melanoma**

    A. The **evaluation of a suspected melanoma** begins with a biopsy to both diagnose and microstage the lesion if proven to be a melanoma. **Excisional biopsy** (i.e., removal of the lesion with grossly negative margins) is the optimal technique for smaller lesions. A **punch biopsy** directed at the clinically thickest area is sufficient for larger lesions. Shave biopsies may preclude accurate assessment of tumor thickness and should be avoided. After biopsy, tumor thickness is characterized on the basis of anatomic level of invasion (**Clark level**) and, most importantly, by thickness in millimeters (**Breslow thickness**). Subsequent wide excision margins reflect the risk of recurrence and are determined by tumor thickness. Tumors less than 1 mm thick are best excised with 1-cm margins whereas lesions thicker than 1 mm may require initial margins of 2 cm.

B. As in breast cancer, an **assessment for regional metastases** should begin with a physical examination of the potential draining lymph node basins. In the absence of clinically evident nodal metastases, sentinel lymph node biopsy should be performed in conjunction with wide local excision of the primary tumor.

C. In patients with lesions thicker than 1 mm, a baseline chest radiograph and liver function tests as well as a lactate dehydrogenase level should be obtained. Patients with thicker lesions (≥4 mm) are at relatively high risk for distant metastases. A more rigorous evaluation for metastases, including computed tomography (CT) scans or positron emission tomography and CT scans of the chest, abdomen, and pelvis, should be obtained before surgery.

> What is the thickness of the melanoma?

APPLIED ANATOMY AND COMPONENTS OF THE PROCEDURE

See Figure 23-1.

Preoperative Considerations

I. **Prophylactic antibiotics** are not generally administered before sentinel lymph node biopsy. Most surgeons give antibiotics before axillary dissection. The chosen antibiotic should have activity against skin flora (i.e., gram-positive organisms) and should be administered within 1 hour before skin incision.

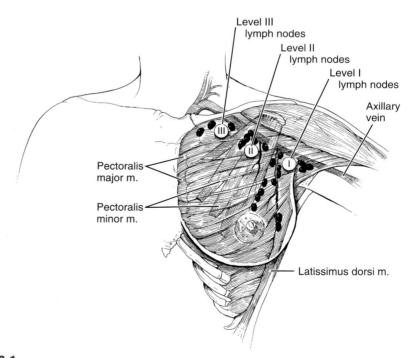

Figure 23-1

Schematic division of axillary lymph nodes. The axillary lymph nodes may be divided into three groups. Level I lymph nodes are located between the lateral border of the pectoralis minor muscle and the anterior border of the latissimus dorsi muscle. Level II lymph nodes underlie the pectoralis minor muscle. Level III lymph nodes lie medial to the pectoralis minor muscle. (*From Roses DF [ed]: Breast Cancer, 2nd ed. Philadelphia, Churchill Livingstone, 2005.*)

II. When performed in conjunction with wide local excision or mastectomy, sentinel lymph node biopsy is generally performed first, before surgical disruption of draining lymphatics from the primary tumor.

Patient Positioning and Preparation

I. The patient is placed in the supine position. The axilla is exposed by extending the arm at a 90-degree angle.
II. The sterile preparation should include the axilla and upper arm. When performed in conjunction with a mastectomy, the preparation should also include the ipsilateral breast, extending several inches past the midline, above the clavicle and below the inframammary fold. Laterally, the preparation should extend to the posterior axillary line.

Sentinel Lymph Node Biopsy

I. **Radioisotope-labeled tracer** (technetium-99m sulfur colloid) is injected 1 or more hours before sentinel lymph node biopsy. In patients with melanomas of the trunk or head and neck, particularly if near the midline, where lymphatic drainage may be ambiguous, **lymphoscintigraphy** should be performed in the nuclear medicine suite after the injection of tracer. This technique, which tracks the tracer with a scintiscanner as it travels from the injection site to the sentinel node, can be helpful in accurately identifying the laterality or bilaterality of the sentinel nodes (e.g., right vs. left axilla or bilateral axillae). In the operating room, minutes before making the incision, the surgeon injects **vital blue dye** 10 minutes or more before making the incision (Fig. 23-2). In the patient with melanoma, the tracer and dye are injected intradermally so that they may enter the dermal lymphatics draining the site. In patients with breast cancer, injection may be performed using a number of different approaches, with largely equivalent results; the most common sites for injection include the peritumoral breast parenchyma and the subareolar breast parenchyma.

> Lymphatics of the breast drain centripetally to the subareolar plexus and then to the axilla.

II. A gamma probe is calibrated and placed on the surgical field in a sterile sheath to allow for subsequent localization of the radioisotope-labeled tracer.
III. A transverse incision is made just below the hair-bearing area of the axilla.

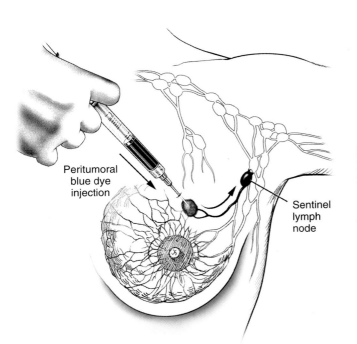

Peritumoral blue dye injection

Sentinel lymph node

Figure 23-2
Blue dye or radioisotope isotope injection at the site of cancer. *(From Roses DF [ed]: Breast Cancer, 2nd ed. Philadelphia, Churchill Livingstone, 2005.)*

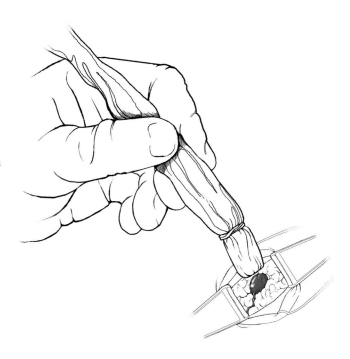

Figure 23-3
A blue-stained lymphatic and lymph node are identified with the aid of a gamma probe. *(From Roses DF [ed]: Breast Cancer, 2nd ed. Philadelphia, Churchill Livingstone, 2005.)*

IV. The incision is carried down to the clavipectoral fascia, which is divided.
V. Blue-stained lymphatics are identified. The gamma probe may be used to help direct the surgeon toward the area of maximal uptake (Fig. 23-3).
VI. Blue channels are traced proximally and distally to identify blue nodes with high radioisotope counts (as detected by the gamma probe).
VII. When identified, these "hot and blue" nodes are gently delivered into the field and excised.
VIII. The site of excision is examined with the gamma probe for the presence of residual radioactivity. Nodes with radioactivity greater than 10% of that measured in the sentinel node should be excised as well.
IX. The site is examined for any apparent or palpable lymphadenopathy.
X. Hemostasis is confirmed, and the incision is closed.

> Failure to identify a sentinel node should prompt axillary dissection.

Axillary Dissection

I. A curvilinear incision is made just below the hair-bearing area of the axilla, extending laterally to the posterior axillary line and medially no further than the lateral edge of the pectoralis major muscle.
II. Flaps are developed beneath the subcutaneous layer, extending medially to the edge of the pectoralis major muscle, superiorly to its tendinous insertion, inferiorly to the level of the sixth rib, and posteriorly to the edge of the latissimus dorsi (Fig. 23-4).
III. Medial retraction of the pectoralis major allows for the identification of the lateral edge of the pectoralis minor muscle. The medial pectoral nerve is identified lateral to the pectoralis minor muscle and preserved.
IV. The clavipectoral fascia, contiguous with the pectoralis minor fascia, is opened parallel to the lateral edge of the muscle, exposing the lymphadipose contents of the axilla.
V. Superior and medial retraction of the pectoralis muscle and inferior traction on the lymphadipose tissue allow for exposure of the axillary vein.
VI. Lymphatic dissection proceeds along the axillary vein, beginning medially beneath the pectoralis minor muscle (level II nodes) and proceeding laterally (Fig. 23-5).

> The medial pectoral nerve innervates the pectoralis minor muscle. Frequently, a branch also innervates the lateral pectoralis major muscle.

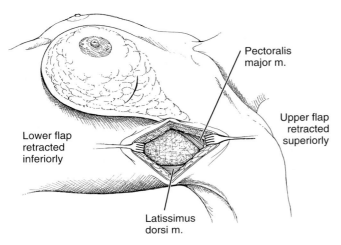

Figure 23-4
Flaps are elevated to expose the axilla. *(From Roses DF [ed]: Breast Cancer, 2nd ed. Philadelphia, Churchill Livingstone, 2005.)*

VII. As the dissection proceeds, the inferior axillary contents are dissected off the serratus anterior fascia.

VIII. The intercostobrachial nerve is identified as it exits the second intercostal space and is preserved, if possible.

IX. As the dissection is carried toward the junction of the serratus anterior and subscapularis muscles, lateral intercostal perforating vessels are divided and ligated.

X. The long thoracic nerve is identified as it courses superficial and lateral to the serratus anterior muscle, and is preserved.

XI. The thoracodorsal nerve and vessels are identified as they course over the subscapularis muscle and are preserved (Fig. 23-6). The remaining lateral axillary contents are dissected with the specimen, which is transected at the border of the latissimus dorsi muscle.

> **TRANSECTION OF THE INTERCOSTOBRACHIAL NERVE RESULTS IN PARESTHESIAS OF THE SKIN OF THE AXILLA AND MEDIAL ARM.**

> **INJURY TO THE LONG THORACIC NERVE RESULTS IN A WINGED SCAPULA DEFORMITY BECAUSE OF THE RESULTANT PARALYSIS OF THE SERRATUS ANTERIOR MUSCLE.**

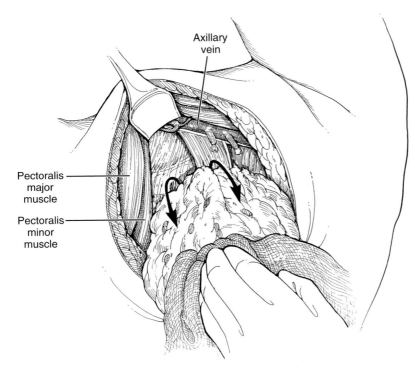

Figure 23-5
Axillary dissection proceeds from level II laterally. *(From Roses DF [ed]: Breast Cancer, 2nd ed. Philadelphia, Churchill Livingstone, 2005.)*

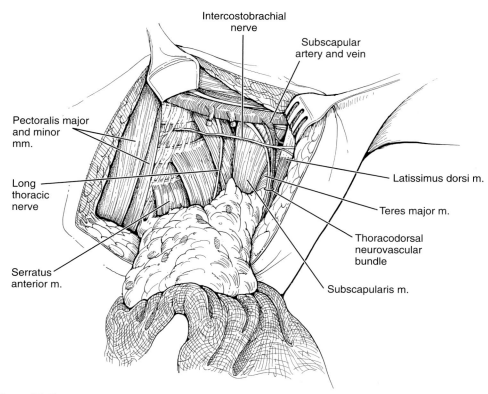

Figure 23-6
The intercostobrachial, long thoracic, and thoracodorsal nerves are identified and preserved as dissection proceeds laterally to the anterior border of the latissimus dorsi muscle. *(From Roses DF [ed]: Breast Cancer, 2nd ed. Philadelphia, Churchill Livingstone, 2005.)*

    XII. A closed-suction drain is placed within the axilla and brought out through a stab wound beneath the inferior flap.

   XIII. The incision is closed, typically in two layers (subcutaneous and subcuticular).

POSTOPERATIVE COURSE

Sentinel lymph node biopsy can be performed on an outpatient basis and is rarely associated with significant postoperative pain. Hospital admission, however, may be required when sentinel lymph node biopsy is performed in conjunction with a more extensive procedure to treat the primary tumor (e.g., total mastectomy). In contrast, axillary dissection may necessitate hospital admission to ensure early pain control and appropriate observation. Closed-suction drains are typically maintained for approximately 1 week. Many surgeons advocate continuation of antibiotic prophylaxis while the drain is maintained. In the immediate postoperative period, patients are encouraged to gently elevate the ipsilateral arm to maintain range of motion. Full range-of-motion exercises are usually delayed until the drain has been removed and the skin becomes adherent to the underlying axillary hollow because vigorous exercise may exacerbate seroma formation. Application of a blood pressure cuff and needle sticks are avoided on the ipsilateral arm, although the likelihood of promoting lymphedema with such interventions is low.

COMPLICATIONS

Complications of sentinel lymph node biopsy are unusual; surgical site infection, although rare, is the most common. Axillary dissection may be associated with several complications.

    I. **Seroma formation** is anticipated after axillary dissection. Accumulation may be minimized through maintenance of closed-suction drainage for the first week after surgery. Seroma formation after the drain is removed may be managed by aspiration.

II. **Lymphedema,** manifested by swelling or heaviness of the ipsilateral arm, is not uncommon after axillary dissection, with an incidence of 5% to 25%. In most cases, lymphedema is subtle; obvious or disabling enlargement is uncommon. Radiation therapy (for breast cancer) and obesity are contributory factors. Arm elevation, weight loss, and the use of elastic pressure-graded sleeves may be helpful.

III. **Lymphangiosarcoma** is a rare, but devastating, complication associated with chronic lymphedema, and is heralded by vascular-appearing nodules in the edematous extremity (Stewart-Treves syndrome). The mean interval between surgery and the diagnosis of lymphangiosarcoma is 10 years. Therapy may include wide local excision or even amputation. Unfortunately, the prognosis is very poor, with a median survival of 2 years.

IV. **Nerve injury** may result from axillary dissection. Nerves at risk include the intercostobrachial, long thoracic, thoracodorsal, and medial pectoral. Division of the **intercostobrachial nerve** results in numbness or paresthesias of the upper medial nerve and axilla. These symptoms often resolve over months because of the rich sensory innervation of the area. Division of the **long thoracic nerve** results in a winged scapula from paralysis of the serratus anterior muscle, whereas division of the **thoracodorsal** nerve results in limitation of backward motion of the extended arm from denervation of the latissimus dorsi muscle. Division of the **medial pectoral** nerve may result in atrophy of the lateral pectoralis major muscle.

SUGGESTED READINGS

Lange JR, Balch CM: Cutaneous melanoma. In Cameron JL (ed): Current Surgical Therapy, 8th ed. Philadelphia, Mosby, 2004.

Morton DL, Thompson JF: Sentinel-node biopsy or nodal observation in melanoma. N Engl J Med 355:1944, 2006.

Roses DF, Guiliano AE: Surgery for breast cancer. In Roses DF (ed): Breast Cancer, 2nd ed. Philadelphia, Churchill Livingstone, 2005.

CHAPTER 24

Carotid Endarterectomy and Carotid Stenting

Grace J. Wang and Ronald M. Fairman

Case Study

A 75-year-old male with a medical history significant for insulin-dependent diabetes, coronary artery disease, hypertension, hypercholesterolemia, and tobacco use presents to a vascular surgeon's office. He reports several recent episodes of visual changes that he describes as a "shade being pulled over my right eye," each of which lasted several seconds. On physical examination, a right carotid bruit is noted. On fundoscopic examination, small yellow plaque-like crystals are seen within the right retinal artery. A carotid duplex shows an 80% stenosis of the right internal carotid artery and a patent left internal carotid artery.

BACKGROUND

Stroke is the third leading cause of death in the United States. More than 700,000 strokes occur annually. Additionally, nonfatal strokes result in substantial morbidity and health care expenditures; the American Heart Association estimated this cost to be $18 billion annually in 1993. Strokes are broadly categorized as **hemorrhagic** (20%) or **ischemic** (80%); up to 30% of ischemic strokes attributable to carotid disease.

C. Miller Fisher, a neurologist, first recognized the relationship between atherosclerotic disease of the carotid bifurcation and symptoms of ipsilateral monocular blindness and contralateral hemiplegia in 1951. Atherosclerotic plaque formation in the carotid bulb may lead to embolization of friable plaque or thrombus and subsequent neurologic deficits. Rarely, a flow-limiting stenosis of the carotid artery results in symptomatic cerebral hypoperfusion. Because it is a manifestation of atherosclerosis, carotid disease is associated with hypertension, diabetes, hyperlipidemia, and tobacco use. Patients with carotid disease may present with transient ischemic attacks (TIAs), defined as neurologic deficits lasting less than 24 hours. These embolic events are often associated with focal motor or language and speech deficits. Alternatively, patients present with **amaurosis fugax** (monocular blindness secondary to embolization of the ophthalmic artery, a branch of the internal carotid artery). Physical examination of patients with carotid disease may reveal a carotid bruit, reflecting turbulent flow through a stenotic lesion. Importantly, the presence of a bruit does not reflect the severity of stenosis, and patients may have severe carotid stenoses in the absence of a bruit. Duplex examination is the most frequently used screening modality to assess carotid disease and has largely supplanted physical examination.

Carotid endarterectomy (CEA), the subject of this chapter, is a well-established mode of primary stroke prevention in patients with carotid disease. The use of carotid angioplasty and stenting has emerged as an alternative to CEA in selected patients and is discussed in brief.

INDICATIONS FOR SURGERY

I. **Symptomatic Stenosis of Greater than 70%:** Patients with a symptomatic stenosis of more than 70% and associated symptoms (e.g., TIAs) are offered CEA.

The benefit of surgery in this population was established by several randomized controlled trials, including the North American Symptomatic Carotid Endarterectomy Trial (**NASCET**). This trial compared rates of stroke in patients who received surgery and in those treated with aspirin alone and showed a benefit from surgery. This finding was corroborated by subsequent trials, including the European Carotid Surgery Trial (ECST).

II. **Asymptomatic Stenosis of Greater than 60%:** Asymptomatic stenosis is the most common indication for CEA. The benefit of surgery in patients with asymptomatic disease was established in the Asymptomatic Carotid Atherosclerosis Study (**ACAS**). This study showed that surgery was more effective than medical management in preventing strokes in patients with asymptomatic carotid stenoses of more than 60%.

III. **Unstable Symptoms:** An ulcerated atherosclerotic plaque may act as a nidus for fresh thrombus formation. Symptoms suggesting the presence of an unstable plaque and ongoing embolization are an indication for urgent CEA (within 24 hours). **Crescendo TIAs** are TIAs that occur at increasingly short intervals. Complete resolution of symptoms is noted between attacks. In contrast, patients with **stroke in evolution** have repeated TIAs and their symptoms only partially resolve between events.

> Does your patient have symptomatic or asymptomatic carotid disease?

PREOPERATIVE EVALUATION

I. **Carotid duplex ultrasonography** is the most commonly used modality for detecting carotid stenoses because of its widespread availability and high degree of accuracy (100% in some series). An internal carotid artery peak systolic velocity (PSV) of more than 220 cm/sec in conjunction with an internal carotid artery: common carotid artery PSV ratio of more than 4.0 suggests high-grade carotid stenosis. A peak end-diastolic velocity of more than 100 cm/sec is consistent with a stenosis of greater than 70%.

II. **Magnetic resonance angiography (MRA)** allows for evaluation of the origins of the great vessels, which are not well imaged with duplex ultrasound. MRA is particularly indicated if signs of subclavian artery occlusive disease, such as a disparity between right and left brachial blood pressures or a supraclavicular bruit, are noted. Symptoms associated with **subclavian steal syndrome,** such as arm claudication, lightheadedness, or near syncope, are likewise an indication for MRA.

III. **Computed tomography angiography (CTA)** can be used to delineate the extent of aortic and carotid disease in patients with normal renal function who cannot undergo MRA. CTA of the brain is also highly accurate for evaluating intracranial occlusive disease and aneurysms.

COMPONENTS OF THE PROCEDURE AND APPLIED ANATOMY

Preoperative Considerations

I. CEA can be performed under regional or general anesthesia. If the regional approach is chosen, the awake patient's neurologic function can be grossly assessed throughout the procedure. Changes in neurologic function after clamping of the carotid artery can be addressed with immediate placement of a temporary shunt to restore cerebral perfusion. The use of general anesthesia is typically coupled with either routine shunt placement or continuous electroencephalographic (EEG) monitoring and selective shunting.

II. Placement of an arterial catheter allows for continuous blood pressure monitoring during and after CEA.

III. Despite the low incidence of surgical site infection after carotid endarterectomy, antibiotic prophylaxis is indicated because of the morbidity associated with infections when they do occur. Most surgeons use a prosthetic patch to close the arte-

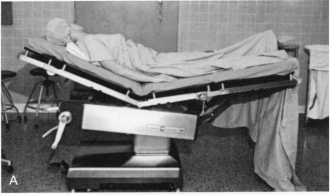

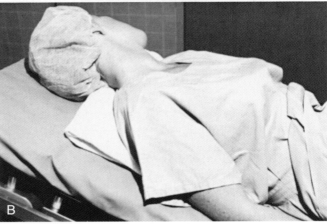

Figure 24-1
Patient positioning for carotid endarterectomy. **A,** The patient is placed in a semirecumbent position. **B,** The neck is mildly hyperextended, and the head is turned away from the operative side. *(From Rutherford RB: Vascular Surgery, 6th ed. Philadelphia, Saunders, 2005.)*

riotomy. Infection of the patch necessitates reoperation and patch excision. Antibiotics are administered within 1 hour before incision.

Patient Positioning and Preparation

I. Electroencephalographic leads are placed on the patient preoperatively.
II. The patient is placed in the supine position with an inflatable bag under the shoulders. This results in neck extension, which moves the carotid bifurcation downward and anteriorly, facilitating exposure.
III. The table is placed in "beach chair" position (i.e., the hips and knees are flexed), and the table is placed in reverse Trendelenburg position (Fig. 24-1).
IV. The sterile preparation should include the neck, ipsilateral earlobe, mandible, chin, sternal notch, and clavicle.

Incision and Exposure

I. The CEA procedure is frequently performed through an incision along the anterior border of the sternocleidomastoid muscle, with a slight posterior curve away from the greater auricular nerve superiorly (Fig. 24-2). Alternatively, a curvilinear or hockey stick incision is used, which may provide for better cosmesis.
II. The skin and the underlying platysma muscle are divided.
III. The sternocleidomastoid muscle is retracted laterally, exposing the internal jugular vein.
IV. The facial vein, a branch of the internal jugular vein that typically crosses over the carotid bifurcation, is identified and divided (Fig. 24-3). Care is taken to avoid injuries to the 12th cranial nerve (CN XII), which often lies immediately posterior to the facial vein.

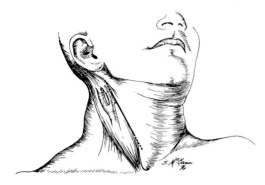

Figure 24-2
Incision for carotid endarterectomy and its relationship to the carotid bifurcation. *(From Rutherford RB: Vascular Surgery, 6th ed. Philadelphia, Saunders, 2005.)*

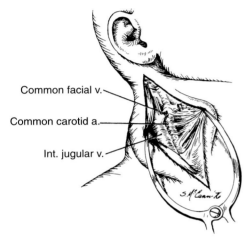

Common facial v.

Common carotid a.

Int. jugular v.

Figure 24-3
Division of the facial vein. The facial vein, a tributary to the internal jugular vein, is divided to allow access to the carotid bifurcation. *(From Rutherford RB: Vascular Surgery, 6th ed. Philadelphia, Saunders, 2005.)*

   V. The common, internal, and external carotid arteries are dissected free from surrounding tissues and encircled with vessel loops. The superior thyroid artery, which is the first branch of the external carotid, is likewise encircled with a vessel loop.

  VI. CN XII, which typically crosses over the external and internal carotid arteries approximately 1.5 cm above the carotid bulb, is identified and preserved. The vagus nerve (CN X) is identified within the carotid sheath; it usually resides posterior to the common carotid artery but can occasionally be identified more laterally or even anteriorly.

 VII. Aggressive retraction is avoided to prevent traction injuries to CN X, the hypoglossal nerve (CN XII), and the marginal mandibular branch of CN VII (Fig. 24-4).

Endarterectomy

   I. Systemic heparin is administered.

  II. The internal, common, and external carotid arteries are sequentially clamped. An abnormal EEG reading at this juncture is an indication for the use of a shunt.

 III. An arteriotomy is made at the carotid bifurcation and extended proximally and distally (into the internal carotid artery) beyond the area of gross disease. If appropriate, a shunt is placed in the lumen of the internal carotid artery distally and the common carotid artery proximally to allow for continuous blood flow during the endarterectomy.

 IV. Plaque is dissected off of the artery wall with a blunt dissector. The appropriate plane of dissection removes diseased intima from the media at the level of the internal elastic lamina. This plane is most easily established proximally, at the carotid bulb opposite the external carotid artery, where disease is typically most severe (Fig. 24-5).

> Blood vessels are composed of three layers: tunica intima, tunica media, and tunica adventitia.

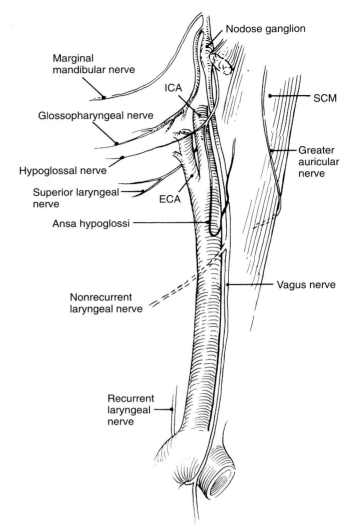

Figure 24-4
Relationship of structures
encountered during exposure of the
carotid bifurcation. ECA, external
carotid artery; ICA, internal carotid
artery; SCM, sternocleidomastoid
muscle. *(From Moore WS [ed]:
Vascular and Endovascular Surgery:
A Comprehensive Review, 7th ed.
Philadelphia, Saunders, 2006.)*

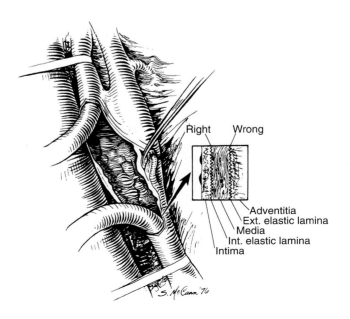

Figure 24-5
The endarterectomy dissection plane.
The proper plane of dissection lies
between the intima and the media at
the level of the internal elastic
lamina. *(From Rutherford RB: Vascular
Surgery, 6th ed. Philadelphia, Saunders,
2005.)*

V. The distal aspect of the plaque is visualized and separated from the intima of the adjacent, normal artery, leaving a smooth residual surface. Occasionally, the endarterectomy leaves behind a flap of intima, which, if left alone, may serve as a nidus for postoperative thrombus formation. Fine suture may be used to tack down a residual intimal flap.

Arterial Reconstruction and Wound Closure

I. The arteriotomy is closed with a patch of polyester, polytetrafluoroethylene, bovine pericardium, or autogenous vein. The edges of the arteriotomy are sewn to the patch with a running suture.

II. Before completion of the arteriotomy closure, the clamps on the external, internal, and common carotid arteries are sequentially released briefly to flush out debris and air. The arterial reconstruction is then completed.

III. The surgical site is inspected for hemostasis, and a pulse in the internal carotid artery is confirmed.

IV. A closed-suction drain is placed in the surgical bed.

V. The platysma muscle layer and the skin are closed.

VI. Before extubation, neurologic function is grossly assessed. Once the patient is extubated, a more extensive neurologic examination is performed to exclude contralateral motor or sensory disturbances. An attempt is made to elicit signs associated with injuries to CN X (vocal weakness), CN XII (tongue deviation), and the marginal mandibular branch of CN VII (lip droop).

> Synthetic patches are readily available but carry a small risk of infection. Autologous vein patches are less likely to become infected but require vein harvest though a separate incision.

> **A NEW NEUROLOGIC DEFICIT IMMEDIATELY AFTER CAROTID ENDARTERECTOMY GENERALLY MANDATES OPERATIVE RE-EXPLORATION.**

POSTOPERATIVE COURSE

In the early postoperative period, patients' systolic blood pressure is maintained between 100 and 140 mm Hg. Hypertension is avoided to prevent bleeding complications and reperfusion injury. Hypotension is avoided to prevent thrombus formation. Antiplatelet agents and cholesterol-lowering agents are restarted postoperatively and continued indefinitely. Drains are typically removed on the first postoperative day. Patients are discharged when their blood pressure is well controlled and they can ambulate independently.

The rate of carotid restenosis after endarterectomy is estimated at 1% per year. There is a bimodal distribution of recurrence, with 40% of cases occurring within 2 years (secondary to intimal hyperplasia) and the rest of cases occurring at more than 5 years postoperatively (presumably because of recurrent atherosclerosis). Duplex scanning is performed at 1 month, at 6 months, and then annually to detect recurrent stenosis and monitor disease in the contralateral carotid artery. Continued risk modification with antiplatelet agents and lipid-lowering drugs is emphasized during follow-up visits.

COMPLICATIONS

I. Perioperative **stroke** occurs in a small, but finite number of patients. Etiologies include embolization of debris during dissection, thrombosis resulting from creation of an intimal flap or other technical errors, and reperfusion injury. If the patient emerges from anesthesia with a neurologic deficit or has a deficit within 24 hours of surgery, operative re-exploration is typically performed to exclude the presence of an intimal flap and correct technical problems. If the findings on exploration are negative, a thromboembolic event is more likely. A CT of the head is performed to rule out a hemorrhagic stroke. In the absence of intracranial hemorrhage, heparin therapy is initiated.

II. **Reperfusion injury** is believed to result from rupture of chronically dilated small vessels and capillaries after restoration of blood flow. Such injuries are often heralded by the clinical triad of ipsilateral headache, seizure, and intracerebral edema or hemorrhage, and are most often seen between 48 and 72 hours after surgery. Hypertension may contribute to the pathogenesis of these injuries, and blood pressure should therefore be tightly controlled postoperatively. Patients with contralateral internal carotid artery occlusion are at elevated risk for reperfusion injuries.

III. **Neck hematoma** may occur in the face of inadequate hemostasis or systolic hypertension during emergence from anesthesia. Large neck hematomas may cause airway compromise. Stridor or difficulty breathing should prompt emergent exploration of the neck incision and evacuation of the hematoma.

IV. **Cranial nerve injuries** occur in 1% to 5% of patients who undergo CEA. The most commonly affected nerves are the hypoglossal and vagus. Injuries are most often traction related and usually resolve within 6 weeks.

V. **Myocardial infarction** is the most common cause of death in patients with carotid disease and the most common non-neurologic complication of CEA.

CAROTID ANGIOPLASTY AND STENTING

The indications for carotid angioplasty and stenting (CAS) are the same as those for open endarterectomy. However, the use of CAS instead of CEA remains somewhat controversial. In general, CAS is offered to patients with severe medical comorbidities, difficult anatomy (e.g., a high carotid bifurcation above the level of the second cervical vertebra), restenosis after CEA, or a previously irradiated neck. Important aspects of the procedure and perioperative care are summarized.

| Has your patient had previous neck irradiation? |

I. The CAS procedure is performed under local anesthesia with the patient awake.

II. The patient rests supine on a table compatible with angiography.

III. Arterial access is obtained through placement of an arterial sheath, usually into the right common femoral artery.

IV. A series of wire and catheter manipulations is used to position a shuttle sheath into the mid-common carotid artery. An angiogram is performed to help delineate the anatomy. A distal embolic protection device is positioned in the distal internal carotid artery.

V. Stents are deployed across the lesion and across the carotid bifurcation, covering the external carotid artery.

VI. Balloon angioplasty of the stent is then performed. Manipulation of the carotid bulb may result in profound bradycardia, which is effectively treated with atropine.

VII. A completion angiogram is performed to confirm adequate treatment of the lesion and restoration of flow. The embolic protection device is removed under fluoroscopic guidance. All catheters and wires are removed, and the sheath is pulled back into the external iliac artery and secured in place.

VIII. The sheath is removed from the groin once the patient's coagulation parameters have normalized.

IX. The patient's neurologic function and blood pressure are monitored overnight. Patients are typically discharged on aspirin and clopidogrel bisulfate (Plavix) as well as a lipid-lowering agent.

SUGGESTED READINGS

Endarterectomy for asymptomatic carotid artery stenosis. Executive Committee for the Asymptomatic Carotid Atherosclerosis Study. JAMA 173:1421–1428, 1995.

Ferguson GG, Eliasziw M, Barr HW, et al: The North American Symptomatic Carotid Endarterectomy Trial: Surgical results in 1415 patients. Stroke 30:1751–1758, 1999.

Krupski WC, Moore WS: Indications, surgical technique and results for repair of extracranial occlusive lesions. In Rutherford RB (ed): Vascular Surgery, 6th ed. Philadelphia, Saunders, 2005.

Moore WS: Extracranial cerebrovascular: the carotid artery. In Moore WS (ed): Vascular and Endovascular Surgery: A Comprehensive Review, 7th ed. Philadelphia, Saunders, 2006.

CHAPTER 25

Abdominal Aortic Aneurysm Repair

Benjamin M. Jackson   and   Jeffrey P. Carpenter

Case Study

A 70-year-old female with a medical history of coronary artery disease, hypertension, and tobacco use presents to the emergency department complaining of 10 hours of severe abdominal and back pain. Physical examination shows a pulsatile, tender epigastric mass. A computed tomography (CT) scan is performed without contrast and shows a 7-cm abdominal aortic aneurysm (AAA) (Fig. 25-1).

BACKGROUND

Abdominal aortic aneurysms, defined as focal dilations of the abdominal aorta to a 50% or greater increased diameter, are the most common true aneurysms. Mortality from AAAs results from aneurysm rupture; half of all patients with ruptured AAAs die before arrival at a hospital and those patients who do reach a hospital alive have a 50% in-hospital mortality rate. In the United States, ruptured AAAs are the 15th leading cause of death, accounting for 15,000 fatalities per year. In contrast, elective open (as opposed to endovascular) AAA repair has a surgical mortality rate of less than 5%. Most deaths from AAAs are, therefore, preventable with prophylactic surgery.

> True aneurysms involve all layers of the arterial wall, whereas pseudoaneurysms do not.

The majority of AAAs are **infrarenal** (i.e., they involve the aorta below the renal arteries). Approximately 5% of AAAs also involve the suprarenal aorta, and are termed **suprarenal** AAAs. A higher percentage of aneurysms are **juxtarenal.** Approximately 25% of AAAs also involve one or both iliac arteries (aortoiliac aneurysms). Aneurysm morphology may be described as **fusiform** (i.e., relatively symmetric and spindle-shaped) or **saccular** (i.e., focal asymmetric outpouching). Atherosclerotic ulcers or "blebs" sometimes involve the AAA, and this may increase the risk of rupture.

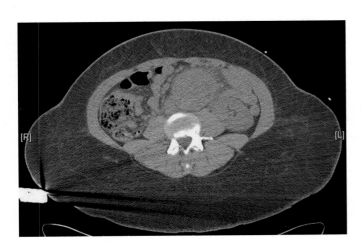

Figure 25-1
Noncontrast computed tomography scan of a symptomatic 7-cm abdominal aortic aneurysm.

Most AAAs are degenerative (sometimes described as *atherosclerotic*). Other, much less common, etiologies are infection (mycotic aneurysms), arteritis, cystic medial necrosis (as in Marfan's disease), trauma, and inherited connective tissue disorders. Risk factors for the development of degenerative AAAs include smoking history, male sex, age greater than 50 years, and family history of aneurysm disease.

Aneurysm size is the most significant determinant of the risk of aneurysm rupture. Aneurysms that are between 5 and 6 cm in diameter have a yearly rupture risk of approximately 10%. In addition, chronic obstructive pulmonary disease (COPD) and hypertension confer an increased rupture risk. Female sex is sometimes considered a risk factor for rupture as well, most likely because aneurysms of the same diameter are larger in comparison to the normal diameter of the abdominal aorta in women than in men.

> Abdominal aortic aneurysms may be associated with popliteal aneurysms, femoral artery aneurysms, and thoracic aortic aneurysms.

INDICATIONS FOR ELECTIVE SURGERY

Indications for elective AAA repair include:
I. **Asymptomatic AAAs:** Asymptomatic aneurysms 5 to 5.5 cm or greater in diameter and those that are expanding by 1 cm or more in diameter per year are repaired because of the relatively high associated risk of rupture.
II. **Symptomatic AAAs:** Symptoms of abdominal or back pain without other evident etiology in the presence of an AAA suggest imminent rupture and are an indication for expeditious aneurysm repair.
III. **Symptomatic embolism** of an aneurysm thrombus.

PREOPERATIVE EVALUATION

Most AAAs are asymptomatic and are diagnosed on the basis of physical examination findings or, more often, are incidental findings on abdominal imaging performed for another reason. Patients with symptomatic but nonruptured aneurysms most often present with pain, suggesting expansion of the aneurysm. Patients with ruptured aneurysms present with some combination of abdominal or back pain, hypotension, syncope, or a pulsatile abdominal mass. Because morbidity and mortality rates after aneurysm surgery are significantly increased in patients with coronary artery disease and COPD, evaluation of patients before elective AAA repair commonly includes **stress testing, echocardiography** and, if pulmonary disease is suspected, **pulmonary function testing.** In addition, patients frequently undergo **carotid ultrasound** to exclude carotid stenoses, which would predispose to stroke in the perioperative period.
I. **Ultrasound** is an excellent imaging modality for the diagnosis and surveillance of aortoiliac aneurysms; however, it does not provide sufficient objective anatomic information to enable operative planning and cannot reliably identify aneurysm rupture. Moreover, the presence of bowel gas and an obese body habitus may decrease the sensitivity of a sonographic evaluation.
II. **Magnetic resonance imaging (MRI) and magnetic resonance arteriography (MRA)** have been used frequently as diagnostic modalities and in operative planning, especially in the evaluation of patients with chronic renal insufficiency. The incidence of nephrogenic systemic fibrosis in patients with impaired renal function after gadolinium exposure and the frequency of other contraindications to MRI (e.g., pacemakers and defibrillators), however, limit the utility of this modality.
III. **Arteriography** is not sensitive in detecting AAAs or in measuring aneurysm extent or diameter because of the frequent presence of thrombus in the aneurysm sac, which narrows the lumen through which blood can flow. Angiography, however, is useful for delineating the anatomy and patency of aortic branches, including the celiac, superior and inferior mesenteric, renal, and hypogastric arteries.
IV. **Computed tomography** and, in particular, **computed tomography arteriography (CTA)** are extremely useful for both diagnosis and operative planning. They also are highly sensitive for the detection of rupture. Most surgeons use CT or CTA as their imaging modality of choice.

V. **Three-dimensional modeling** of aortic aneurysms after cross-sectional imaging (MRI or CT scan) has become more popular with the increased application of stent grafting for the treatment of AAAs. Such modeling allows for the detailed evaluation and measurement of segments of the aorta and aortic branches. In addition, center-line lengths along the course of the aorta and iliac arteries can be measured, obviating the geometric corrections necessary when grafts are sized or designed with axial imaging. Some software even allows insertion of a virtual stent graft and visualization of the projected completed repair.

COMPONENTS OF THE PROCEDURE AND APPLIED ANATOMY

The standard treatment for patients with AAA is open **endoaneurysmorrhaphy.** This has traditionally been undertaken either through a **transperitoneal** (anterior) approach or a **retroperitoneal** approach. Since its introduction in 1991, **endovascular AAA repair (EVAR)** has largely supplanted open aneurysm repair for the treatment of infrarenal AAAs. These operative approaches, along with their attendant advantages, are addressed in the next section.

Preoperative Considerations

I. **Open AAA Repair**
   A. Patients undergo open AAA repair under **general endotracheal anesthesia,** almost exclusively. Frequently, this is supplemented with epidural anesthesia to ensure intraoperative and postoperative analgesia. Some studies suggest a decrease in cardiac complication rates with the use of epidural anesthesia.
   B. Open aneurysmorrhaphy requires aortic cross-clamping. The associated hemodynamic variability necessitates continuous arterial line blood pressure monitoring with a **radial artery catheter.** Furthermore, obligate blood loss (from lumbar arteries arising from the aortic sac) calls for **large-bore intravenous access** for resuscitation.
   C. Any repair that will require a suprarenal (or more proximal) aortic clamp entails a period of renal, and possibly visceral, ischemia, frequently resulting in oliguria at some stage of a patient's intraoperative or early postoperative course. A **pulmonary artery catheter** may facilitate monitoring of intravascular volume and resuscitation.
   D. **Urinary catheter** placement allows continuous monitoring of urine output, and placement of a **nasogastric tube** allows for gastric decompression during, and after, aneurysm repair.

II. **Endovascular AAA Repair**
   A. An EVAR procedure can be undertaken with **general anesthesia, epidural or spinal anesthesia,** or even **sedation with local analgesia**.
   B. Because EVAR does not require aortic cross-clamping and because blood loss in uncomplicated EVAR is frequently minimal, the requirements for intra- and postoperative monitoring are fewer. **Foley catheter placement, large-bore intravenous access,** and **continuous arterial pressure monitoring** are recommended. Because arterial access is integral to this approach to AAA repair, sheaths for delivery and manipulation of grafts can be transduced intraoperatively and sometimes postoperatively in place of radial arterial catheterization.

Operative Approach

I. **Anterior Approach:** The anterior or transperitoneal approach to open aneurysmorrhaphy provides excellent exposure for the repair of infrarenal AAAs. Advantages of this approach include easy access to the bilateral iliac and, if necessary, femoral arteries. An aortic clamp site proximal to the renal arteries, however, is generally more difficult to obtain compared with the retroperitoneal approach. In

Are there contraindications to transperitoneal abdominal aortic aneurysm repair?

In approximately 50% of patients, repair can be accomplished with a tube graft; in the remainder, a bifurcated graft sewn to the bilateral iliac arteries is required because the aortic bifurcation is aneurysmal or severely calcified.

HEPARIN IS ADMINISTERED BEFORE THE APPLICATION OF AORTIC AND ILIAC CLAMPS.

addition, previous abdominal surgery and the presence of a stoma are relative contraindications to this approach. Because it is most useful for infrarenal aortic aneurysms, the transperitoneal approach is undertaken more infrequently in the era of EVAR.

A. The patient is positioned **supine** on the operating room table.

B. The abdomen is entered and explored, and the transverse colon is retracted superiorly. The ligament of Treitz is divided to allow retraction of the small intestine to the right side of the abdomen.

C. The parietal peritoneum overlying the aneurysm is incised and opened from the crossing of the left renal vein superiorly down to the aortic bifurcation and then down each iliac artery. Care is taken to protect the ureters as they cross anterior to the iliac bifurcations.

D. If access to the left iliac bifurcation is required (e.g., in the case of aneurysmal degeneration throughout the extent of the common iliac artery), it is most easily accessed by reflecting the sigmoid mesocolon medially to allow a separate retroperitoneal counterincision. The left limb of a bifurcated graft can subsequently be tunneled within the unopened portion of the left common iliac artery directly beneath the mesentery (Fig. 25-2).

E. Clamp sites are identified immediately distal to the renal arteries and on the bilateral iliac arteries. The superior clamp is placed as close to the renal arteries as possible, so that the graft can be sewn to exclude as much proximal aorta as possible, thereby preventing subsequent aneurysmal degeneration of the juxtarenal segment.

F. Most surgeons systemically heparinize the patient (50–150 units/kg) before clamping the aorta and iliac arteries to prevent thrombosis of the arteries of the legs.

G. Some surgeons clamp the bilateral iliac arteries first, then the aortic neck, to prevent embolization of thrombus at the proximal clamp site to the legs and pelvis. Others clamp the proximal aorta and then open the aneurysm, allowing the iliac arteries to back-bleed to flush out any thrombus, before clamping or occluding the iliac arteries with balloons (Fig. 25-3). In either case, the anesthesia team must be kept informed of the sequence and timing of clamping, and blood pressure should be pharmacologically lowered to avoid severe hypertension with proximal aortic clamping.

H. The aneurysm is opened longitudinally, with care taken to avoid injuring the origin of the inferior mesenteric artery (IMA), so that it can be reimplanted if necessary. Thrombus is removed manually to expose back-bleeding lumbars and the IMA. The lumbars are suture ligated from within the sac.

I. If the IMA is chronically occluded, it need not be identified or interrogated. However, if it is patent, it should be locally heparinized and clamped just outside the sac, to allow interrogation after re-establishment of in-line aortic flow.

J. Dacron or polytetrafluoroethylene (PTFE) grafts are used for aneurysmorrhaphy. The surgeon must decide at this juncture whether a bifurcated graft, sewn to the bilateral iliac arteries, or a tube graft, sewn to the distal aorta, will be required.

K. The proximal anastomosis is prepared by dividing the aneurysm from the healthy proximal aorta transversely around the anterior 180 degrees of its circumference. The back wall of the aorta is not disturbed to prevent disruption of the veins lying posterior to the aorta. The anastomosis incorporates a double layer of the posterior aortic wall. If a bifurcated graft is to be used, the main body is kept short, and the limbs long, to allow flexibility in completing the repair and to prevent kinking of either limb.

L. The proximal anastomosis is performed in a running fashion.

M. The graft is clamped, and the proximal clamp is released to test the proximal anastomosis; if intact, the aortic clamp is left in place, but loosened to allow for rapid reclamping, if necessary.

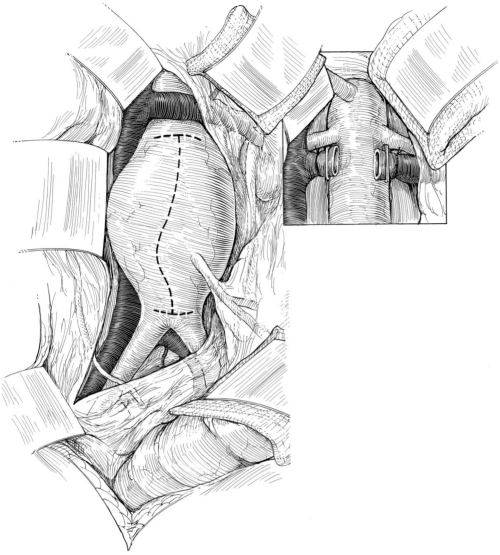

Figure 25-2
Anterior (transperitoneal) exposure of an abdominal aortic aneurysm. *(From Ouriel K, Rutherford RB: Atlas of Vascular Surgery: Operative Procedures. Philadelphia, Saunders, 1998.)*

N. If a tube graft is indicated, the distal anastomotic ring is fashioned in a similar manner to that used for the proximal anastomosis, leaving the posterior wall of the aorta and iliac arteries intact and encompassing both iliac orifices in the sewing ring. Alternatively, in the case of a bifurcated graft, one anastomosis is performed to the distal common iliac artery initially. This limb is opened to allow back-bleeding through the still open contralateral limb. Aortic flow can be re-established to one leg while the contralateral anastomosis is performed.

O. The anesthesia team must be informed again about the unclamping of each iliac artery. Hypotension can result from reperfusion of the pelvis and legs. Usually, this hypotension is easily treated with volume resuscitation, but reclamping one iliac limb, or partially clamping the aortic graft in the case of a tube graft, may be transiently necessary to allow the anesthesiologist to "catch up."

P. At the conclusion of the distal anastomosis, the IMA should be assessed. If pulsatile back-bleeding is encountered, the IMA may be sacrificed. However, if a patent IMA is not bleeding or is bleeding slowly, if the patency of one or

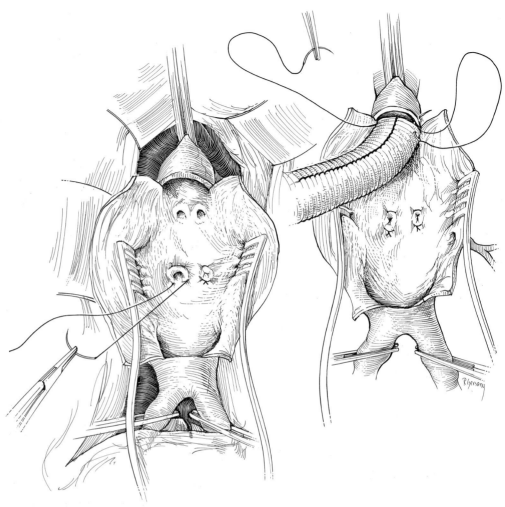

Figure 25-3
With the aneurysm clamped proximally and distally, the sac is opened and bleeding lumbar arteries are suture ligated. *(From Ouriel K, Rutherford RB: Atlas of Vascular Surgery: Operative Procedures. Philadelphia, Saunders, 1998.)*

> Pulsatile back-bleeding through the inferior mesenteric artery orifice suggests robust collateral flow.

both internal iliac arteries is in question, or if one internal iliac has been sacrificed, it should be reimplanted (Fig. 25-4).

Q. Perfusion to the bilateral legs is assessed next, by palpation of the external iliac artery pulses at their egress from the pelvis, by palpation of the femoral pulses in the groins, and if necessary, by visual inspection of the feet. If possible, thrombosis of, or embolism to, a leg should be recognized at this juncture, before reversal of heparinization and closure of the abdomen.

R. Protamine is administered to reverse the effects of heparin, the sigmoid colon is inspected to ensure adequate perfusion, and the sac and peritoneum are sutured over the graft to isolate it from the serosa of the intestines and avoid the entirely preventable late complication of graft-enteric fistula.

II. **Retroperitoneal Approach:** Because the liver and vena cava obstruct access to the aorta from the right retroperitoneum, the left retroperitoneal approach is commonly used in patients who have had previous abdominal surgery, patients with stomas, and those in whom suprarenal or higher proximal aortic clamping is necessary. The right iliac artery is difficult to access or even visualize from the left retroperitoneum, so this approach is less attractive in cases of AAA with associated right iliac artery aneurysm.

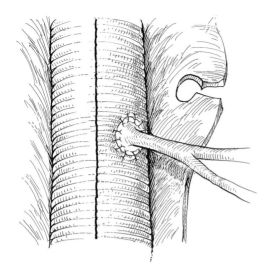

Figure 25-4
Reimplantation of a large inferior mesenteric artery. *(From Ouriel K, Rutherford RB: Atlas of Vascular Surgery: Operative Procedures. Philadelphia, Saunders, 1998.)*

A. The patient is positioned with the table flexed between the iliac crest and the costal margin. Some surgeons attempt to elevate the left shoulder to a 45- degree to 60-degree position, while maintaining the pelvis relatively flat (i.e., parallel to the floor). However, few patients are both thin enough and flexible enough to allow sterile access to the right groin with the thorax positioned vertically enough to allow easy access to the visceral aortic segment. We therefore commonly tilt the entire patient 60 to 90 degrees from the horizontal position and forgo operative access to the right groin. In all cases, a "bean bag" is extremely useful because it allows fixation and support of the patient.

B. The incision is begun at the lateral border of the left rectus muscle and carried cephalad and laterally in a gentle curve to the 10th intercostal space. The external and internal abdominal oblique and transversus abdominis muscles are divided, allowing access to the retroperitoneal space. This potential space is developed bluntly with the surgeon's hand. It is most easily freed posteriorly. The parietal peritoneum is then swept off of the inside of the transversus abdominis muscle. At the cephalad extent of the incision, the dissection is carried into the 10th interspace, at which level access to the supraceliac aorta is easily accomplished. In opening the intercostal muscles at this level, the thoracic cavity is frequently entered. Care is taken to protect the lung parenchyma.

C. Once the incision is entirely opened, dissection is carried posteriorly and deeply in a blunt manner until the lumbar vertebrae are identified. Then it is continued more anteriorly until the pulsatile aorta is identified.

D. The left kidney is generally brought anteriorly with the abdominal viscera; if left posteriorly in the incision, the left renal vein will generally impede access to the aorta. The left ureter is dissected off the aorta and the left iliac bifurcation and is protected behind self-retaining retractors. There is usually a lumbar branch of the left renal vein that overlies the juxtarenal aorta when the left kidney rests anteriorly in the wound; this vein should be ligated and divided before clamping.

E. Access to the visceral segment of the aorta and to the supraceliac aorta is facilitated by division of the left crus of the diaphragm overlying the left side of the aorta. The left renal, celiac, and superior mesenteric arteries are easily identified with this exposure (Fig. 25-5); the ostium of the right renal artery will be evident once the aorta is clamped and opened.

F. Heparinization, clamping, and anastomosis are undertaken in a manner similar to that used for aortic repair through an anterior approach.

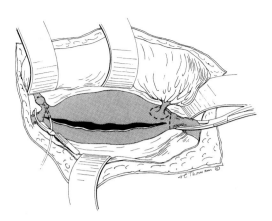

Figure 25-5
Left retroperitoneal approach to the abdominal aorta, with the left kidney retracted anteriorly and balloon control of the right common iliac artery. *(From Rutherford RB [ed]: Vascular Surgery, 6th ed. Philadelphia, Saunders, 2005.)*

POSTOPERATIVE COURSE

Patients undergoing infrarenal aortic aneurysm repair are typically extubated in the operating room and recover in the surgical intensive care unit (SICU). Consideration should be given to keeping patients who undergo suprarenal or supraceliac clamping intubated until adequate resuscitation, warming, resolution of coagulopathy, and urine output are confirmed. It is especially important to remember that supraceliac aortic clamping results in hepatic and intestinal ischemia; as a result, derangements in metabolism and coagulation are common for a period of 24 hours after surgery.

After extubation, pain control is essential to ensure adequate respiratory effort and clearance of secretions. Incentive spirometry is of proven benefit. Use of thoracic epidural analgesia is recommended for 3 to 5 days, until the return of intestinal function allows the patient to take oral narcotics. Nasogastric tube drainage should be maintained until the return of intestinal function. This usually takes 1 to 2 days in the case of retroperitoneal aneurysmorrhaphy and 2 to 5 days in the case of the transperitoneal approach; the longer period of ileus in the latter situation is the result of extensive mobilization of the duodenum. Deep vein thrombosis and gastroduodenal ulcer prophylaxis and intravenous β-blockade should be considered in the postoperative period.

COMPLICATIONS

I. After aortic repair, **bleeding** is suggested by hypotension, oliguria or anuria, an uncorrected metabolic acidosis, or a persistent transfusion requirement, and a return to the operating room is frequently indicated.

II. Strict attention must be paid to the femoral and more distal pulses at the conclusion of the procedure and in the SICU. Both **distal embolization** and **anastomotic thrombosis** can result in limb-threatening ischemia and may require femoral exploration and thromboembolectomy, or operative revision of an iliac anastomosis.

III. Unexplained leukocytosis, fever, left lower quadrant abdominal pain, or bloody diarrhea suggests **colonic ischemia** and justifies an evaluation with flexible sigmoidoscopy. Pale mucosa with patchy sloughing, suggesting reversible ischemia, can most often be treated conservatively with parenteral antibiotic therapy, bowel rest, and observation. Full-thickness necrosis, peritonitis, or shock mandates operative exploration and possible bowel resection.

IV. **Cardiac complications** of AAA repair include myocardial infarction, congestive heart failure, and arrhythmia. The perioperative mortality rate in patients with cardiac complications approaches 25%.

V. **Pulmonary complications,** including pneumonia and respiratory failure, and **renal complications** are unfortunately also very common and are associated with significant morbidity.

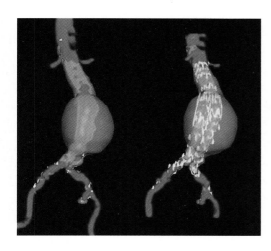

Figure 25-6
Three-dimensional reconstruction of computed tomography angiography of an infrarenal abdominal aortic aneurysm before and after endovascular abdominal aortic aneurysm repair.

AAA STENT GRAFTING

In 1991, Parodi implanted the first aortic endograft for the treatment of an AAA. In subsequent years, EVAR has become a common, and commonly requested, alternative to open repair of AAAs. Currently, four devices have been approved by the Food and Drug Administration for clinical use in the United States; others are being studied and may be approved shortly. Some universal features of the patient evaluation for EVAR, operative planning, and conduct of the operation are worthy of discussion.

Endovascular aneurysm repair is dependent on sealing of the proximal and distal (iliac) attachment sites. The proximal seal zone must be of small enough diameter to accommodate the chosen endograft, must not be excessively calcified or thrombus-lined, and must be approximately 15 mm long. The common iliac attachment sites must not be aneurysmal themselves, unless the surgeon plans to extend the limbs of the graft into one or both external iliac arteries, covering the internal iliac arteries. Finally, the external and common iliac arteries and the aortic bifurcation must be of sufficiently large caliber to permit introduction of the graft and its delivery system. Preoperative planning and device design are aided by CTA, by three-dimensional modeling of radiographic studies (Fig. 25-6), and by software allowing interactive endograft design.

Access is most often accomplished by open exposure of the bilateral femoral arteries. From each groin, stiff wires are placed up through the abdominal aorta and into the descending thoracic aorta to support stent graft deployment. The main body graft is inserted over one wire into the abdominal aorta, and angiography is performed to identify the level of the renal arteries. The main body graft is then deployed so as to land and seal in an infrarenal position. In the usual case when a modular bifurcated endograft is used, the contralateral gate of the device is cannulated from the opposite groin and the contralateral iliac limb deployed inside the main body. The proximal and distal seal zones and the graft overlaps are ballooned. All wires are then removed and the femoral arteries are repaired.

SUGGESTED READINGS

Curci JA, Sicard GA: Open surgical treatment of abdominal aortic aneurysms. In Zelenock GB (ed): Mastery of Vascular and Endovascular Surgery. Philadelphia, Lippincott, 2006.
Schermerhorn ML, Cronenwett JL: Abdominal aortic and iliac aneurysms. In Cronenwett JL (ed): Rutherford Vascular Surgery, 6th ed. Philadelphia, Elsevier, 2005.
Solis MM, Harvey RL, Hodgson KJ: Abdominal aortic aneurysm: Endovascular repair. In Cameron JL (ed): Current Surgical Therapy, 8th ed. Philadelphia, Elsevier, 2004.

Femoropopliteal Bypass

Clayton J. Brinster   and   Edward Y. Woo

Case Study

A 64-year-old mail carrier with a history of smoking and mild hypertension controlled with diet and exercise presents with increasing pain in his left calf muscles during ambulation. The pain has increased in frequency and intensity over the past year, forcing him to limit the distance he walks and compromising his ability to perform his job. Physical examination reveals a palpable left femoral pulse but absent left popliteal, posterior tibial, and dorsalis pedis pulses.

BACKGROUND

Peripheral arterial disease (PAD) is a common but underdiagnosed and undertreated disorder that affects 8 to 10 million Americans and an estimated 20% of the general population older than 55 years of age. The prevalence of PAD increases with age and in the presence of cardiovascular risk factors, such as diabetes, hypertension, smoking history, dyslipidemia, and hyperhomocysteinemia.

Intermittent claudication (IC) is defined as reproducible lower extremity pain on exertion that is caused by inadequate blood flow and is reliably relieved by rest. Classic IC occurs in only 30% of patients with symptomatic PAD, and many older patients with PAD instead complain of lower extremity fatigue, difficulty with ambulation, or other leg discomfort atypical of claudication. A thorough history and physical examination, as well as noninvasive vascular laboratory studies, will usually differentiate IC from other common diagnoses, such as arthritis, nerve root compression, and venous congestion.

> Intermittent claudication is reproducible lower extremity pain on exertion that is caused by inadequate blood flow and is reliably relieved by rest.

> Intermittent claudication most commonly affects the calf muscles and most commonly results from atherosclerotic disease of the superficial femoral artery.

Lower extremity PAD is typically classified as aortoiliac, femoropopliteal, or tibial in distribution. Symptoms frequently correspond to the level of occlusive disease and are localized to muscle groups one joint level below the region of occlusion; calf muscle claudication is most commonly due to superficial femoral artery occlusion, and hip, thigh, or buttock claudication is most commonly due to proximal aortoiliac disease. Multilevel disease can produce symptoms at any level. Importantly, calf claudication is the most common presenting symptom in patients with femoropopliteal disease *and* in those with occlusive aortoiliac disease because of the distal extent of this muscle group.

Patients with PAD often have concomitant comorbidities. Nearly one third of patients with IC die within 5 years of diagnosis of myocardial infarction, cerebrovascular disease, or other cardiovascular events, a rate more than three times that in age-matched control subjects. Based on the presence of risk factors, the global nature of atherosclerotic disease, and the high risk of systemic ischemic events, patients with PAD should be treated with aggressive lifestyle modification, appropriate pharmacotherapy, and when necessary, appropriate intervention.

Interventions for lower extremity PAD range from percutaneous procedures, such as angioplasty, stenting, or atherectomy, to operative bypass. Operative bypass is usually reserved for circumstances in which percutaneous procedures are unsuccessful or cannot be performed because of anatomic factors. **Infrainguinal bypass** refers to any major arterial reconstruction that originates below the inguinal ligament and uses a graft (i.e., autogenous vein, cadaveric vein, or prosthetic conduit such as polytetrafluoroethylene [PTFE]). Proximal inflow sites include the common, superficial, and deep femoral arteries, and target sites include the popliteal (above or below the knee), tibial, peroneal, and pedal arteries. This chapter focuses on femoropopliteal bypass for the treatment of PAD and IC.

INDICATIONS FOR FEMOROPOPLITEAL BYPASS

I. **Disabling or refractory claudication** is the most common indication for surgical revascularization of the lower extremity. Patients with claudication symptoms that significantly limit their lifestyle or compromise their ability to work or perform activities of daily living are candidates for lower extremity bypass. Claudication is deemed refractory when lifestyle modification (e.g., smoking cessation, exercise therapy, cholesterol reduction, blood pressure control, blood sugar control) and pharmacologic therapy (e.g., anticoagulation, antiplatelet therapy, arterial vasodilation) do not reduce symptoms or halt the progression of atherosclerotic disease. The primary reason to intervene in the patient with claudication is to improve lifestyle; the likelihood of a severe decline in cardiovascular status (<20%) or progression to major limb amputation (<5%) over a 5-year period is low, especially with lifestyle modification and appropriate medical therapy.

II. **Limb Salvage in the Presence of Critical Limb Ischemia:** Critical ischemia is defined as ischemic rest pain or tissue loss (e.g., ulceration or gangrene). A significant number of patients with critical ischemia eventually require vascular bypass or major limb amputation during the course of treatment.

III. **Other Indications:** Less common indications for lower extremity bypass include trauma (e.g., popliteal artery injury from posterior knee dislocation), popliteal entrapment syndrome, and femoropopliteal arterial aneurysmal disease.

PREOPERATIVE EVALUATION

The clinical diagnosis of lower extremity ischemia should be confirmed with a thorough physical examination and a noninvasive arterial evaluation. Radiographic imaging of the arterial anatomy should be obtained when an intervention is planned.

I. **Physical examination** of the patient with exercise-induced leg pain should aim to confirm the diagnosis of IC and determine the level of occlusive disease. Palpation of the aortic, bilateral femoral, popliteal, posterior tibial, and dorsalis pedis pulses is essential. Patients with aortoiliac disease will have dampened or absent femoral pulses. Occlusive disease of the superficial femoral artery presents with normal femoral pulses and absent or reduced popliteal and pedal pulses. Palpable femoral and popliteal pulses in the setting of absent pedal pulses suggest infrapopliteal disease.

II. **Noninvasive Diagnostic Evaluation**

A. The **ankle–brachial index** (ABI) is the primary noninvasive study used in the diagnosis of PAD. If occlusive disease is suspected, based on presentation, but the resting ABI is normal, the ratio should be recalculated after a period of exercise. Any decrease in ABI with exercise is considered abnormal. The ABI may be falsely elevated and unreliable in patients with extensive arterial calcification as a result of noncompressibility of lower extremity vessels (Fig. 26-1).

B. **Segmental limb pressures** are obtained with a blood pressure cuff and Doppler probe, comparing brachial artery pressures and pressures at various arterial levels in the bilateral lower extremities. ABI and segmental limb pressure recordings are commonly used in conjunction with **pulse volume recordings (PVR)** of arterial waveforms to further delineate the anatomy of the occlusive disease. A normal PVR resembles an arterial waveform, with a sharp systolic spike and a diastolic downstroke. A change in contour, typically

URGENT SURGICAL EVALUATION IS INDICATED IN PATIENTS WHO HAVE PAIN AT REST, GANGRENE, ISCHEMIC ULCERATION, OR AN ACUTE CHANGE IN PULSE EXAM.

Surgery should be performed only if: (1) the risk–benefit ratio is acceptable, (2) the patient's lower extremity vascular anatomy suggests that a favorable and durable result is plausible, and (3) symptomatic relief or limb salvage is expected.

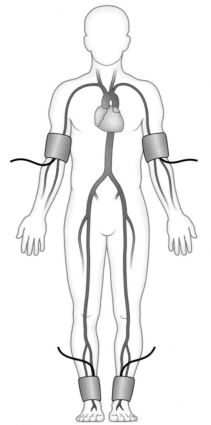

Right ABI	Higher right ankle pressure (mm Hg)
	Higher arm pressure (mm Hg)
Left ABI	Higher left ankle pressure (mm Hg)
	Higher arm pressure (mm Hg)

Interpretation of calculated ABI	
>1.30	Noncompressible
0.91–1.30	Normal
0.71–0.90	Mild obstruction
0.42–0.70	Moderate obstruction
0.00–0.40	Severe obstruction

Figure 26-1
The ankle–brachial index (ABI).

observed as a dampened waveform, indicates proximal occlusive disease. The extent of this change correlates with the severity of disease.

C. **Arterial duplex** ultrasonography can confirm the diagnosis of PAD, identify the level of disease, and differentiate between stenotic and occlusive lesions. Lower extremity examination begins at the common femoral artery and proceeds distally. Arterial stenosis is localized with color Doppler imaging and assessed by measuring Doppler velocities at several arterial levels.

D. **Vein mapping** with duplex ultrasonography is useful preoperatively in the selection of appropriate bypass conduits. In the absence of a suitable greater saphenous vein (GSV), the cephalic, basilic, and lesser saphenous veins can be evaluated for potential use in a spliced vein graft (discussed later).

III. **Radiographic Evaluation**

A. **Computed tomography angiography** (CTA) provides rapid, high-resolution images of the aortoiliac and lower extremity arteries. The utility of CTA, however, is limited by the need for intravenous iodinated contrast, which precludes the evaluation of patients with renal disease.

B. **Magnetic resonance angiography** (MRA) also offers adequate imaging of the arterial anatomy. Intravenous gadolinium, however, is contraindicated in the setting of renal insufficiency because of the high risk of associated nephrogenic systemic fibrosis, a sclerosing disorder of the skin and visceral organs that can result in severe end-organ damage.

C. **Invasive digital subtraction angiography** remains the gold standard in the imaging of PAD. It is, however, an invasive procedure that also requires iodinated contrast.

COMPONENTS OF THE PROCEDURE AND APPLIED ANATOMY

General Operative Principles of Lower Extremity Bypass

There are three basic requirements for successful lower extremity bypass: (1) adequate arterial inflow to the bypass graft; (2) a target vessel that is relatively disease-free and provides adequate run-off, or continuous blood flow, to the foot; and (3) an adequate conduit. The ideal conduit for most bypasses is the GSV. In the absence of an adequate GSV, alternative veins, cadaveric veins, or a prosthetic graft can be used.

In general, the proximal anastomosis is performed at the level of the common femoral artery. If the length of available saphenous vein is limited, the deep femoral or superficial femoral arteries may be used. If the deep femoral or superficial femoral arteries are stenosed, an endarterectomy may allow appropriate inflow. Bypass with **reversed saphenous vein graft (SVG)** is described in the next section. Alternatively, lower extremity bypass can be accomplished with any of the following conduits:

    I. **In situ SVG**, with the saphenous vein left in its native location. Ligation of the tributaries and lysis of the valves are performed without disrupting the GSV vein bed.

    II. **Spliced vein**, consisting of combinations of the cephalic, basilic, or lesser saphenous veins, or portions of the greater saphenous vein.

    III. **Cadaveric vein**

    IV. **Prosthetic grafts;** PTFE is most commonly used in infrainguinal bypasses.

Preoperative Considerations

    I. Lower extremity bypass can be performed under regional **anesthesia** (e.g., spinal or epidural) or general anesthesia, depending on the patient's comorbidities and whether arm veins are harvested.

    II. A **Foley catheter** is inserted.

    III. **Prophylactic antibiotics** are administered intravenously before incision.

    IV. A **radial arterial line** is commonly placed to allow for continuous hemodynamic monitoring.

Patient Positioning and Preparation

    I. The patient is placed in the supine position with the arms extended.

    II. The sterile skin preparation and draping should include the entire groin, leg, and foot. A sterile, clear plastic bag is commonly placed over the foot.

    III. During the procedure, the hip may need to be externally rotated and abducted, with the knee flexed and the thigh supported with a soft bolster or "bump."

Exposure of the Common Femoral Artery

    I. The groin is palpated, and the femoral pulse is located. To expose the common femoral artery, a vertical or oblique incision is made over the pulse. A self-retaining retractor is placed in the wound, and the common femoral artery is located, dissected free of surrounding tissue, and controlled with vessel loops (Fig. 26-2).

    II. The superficial femoral and deep femoral arteries may also need to be exposed and controlled with vessel loops.

    III. To prevent seroma formation and reduce the risk of postoperative infection, care is taken to identify and ligate or cauterize the lymphatic tissue surrounding the femoral arteries and saphenofemoral junction.

    IV. The circumflex femoral vein is a large vessel that crosses the proximal deep femoral artery just distal to the common femoral artery bifurcation. If more distal exposure of the profunda is needed, this vein should be divided to allow adequate exposure of the deep femoral artery.

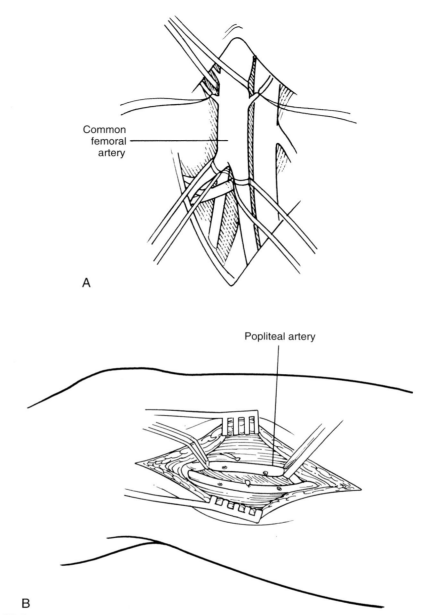

Figure 26-2

A, Exposure and control of the common, superficial, and deep femoral arteries. **B,** Exposure and control of the above the knee popliteal artery with conservation of the greater saphenous vein (inferior). *(From Khatri V, Asensio J: Operative Surgery Manual. Philadelphia, Saunders, 2003.)*

Exposure of the Popliteal Artery

   I. The distal target vessel for lower extremity bypass is determined by preoperative imaging or intraoperative arteriogram. This discussion focuses on the use of the popliteal artery, although the posterior tibial, peroneal, and pedal arteries are used as distal target vessels in appropriate circumstances.

  II. **Above the Knee:**

    A. A longitudinal incision is made along the medial aspect of the distal thigh, below the muscle belly of the vastus medialis.

    B. Care is taken not to injure the GSV during this incision and exposure of the popiteal artery because this vein may be the planned bypass conduit.

    C. The sartorius muscle is reflected posteriorly, and dissection is carried out along the posterior aspect of the femur.

The superficial femoral artery passes through Hunter's canal and the adductor hiatus and then enters the popliteal space; it is then called the *popliteal artery*.

III. **Below the Knee:**
  A. A longitudinal incision is made along the medial aspect of the proximal calf.
  B. The GSV is identified and mobilized.
  C. The medial head of the gastrocnemius muscle is reflected posteriorly, and the popliteal space is entered.
  D. The popliteal artery courses inferiorly in association with the paired popliteal veins, and after adequate dissection and exposure, the artery is controlled with vessel loops.

Saphenous Vein Harvest

  I. The saphenous vein is exposed by connecting the femoral and popliteal incisions or with multiple short "skip" incisions along the medial thigh. The vein is excised, and tributaries are ligated (Fig. 26-3).
  II. After the vein is harvested, it is injected and distended with heparinized saline; leaks are identified and ligated (Fig. 26-4).
  III. The vein is reversed (to permit flow past valves) such that the end originally in the groin can be anastomosed to the popliteal artery and the end originally in the lower thigh or calf can be anastomosed to the femoral artery.
  IV. The vein is marked for orientation to avoid twisting.
  V. The graft is then tunneled with a blunt instrument or a specifically designed tunneling device in a subcutaneous plane shallow enough to allow for postoperative graft surveillance (Fig. 26-5).

> When the bypass is carried out to the popliteal artery below the knee, the graft is sometimes routed via the anatomic popliteal course to avoid angulation or kinking of the graft as it crosses the knee joint.

Construction of the Bypass

  I. The patient is systemically heparinized, and the inflow artery is atraumatically clamped.
  II. An arteriotomy is made on the anterior surface of the artery with a scalpel and extended with angled scissors.
  III. The proximal anastomosis is performed with a running suture. Care is taken to approximate the intimae of the vessels (Fig. 26-6).
  IV. After completion of the proximal anastomosis, blood flow is temporarily restored to confirm unimpeded flow through the conduit.
  V. The distal anastomosis is carried out in similar fashion (Fig. 26-7).
  VI. Before completion, adequate forward blood flow through the graft and back-bleeding from the target artery are confirmed.
  VII. A **completion arteriogram or color flow duplex ultrasound** should be performed to document graft patency before the patient leaves the operating room.
  VIII. After hemostasis is achieved, the wound is thoroughly irrigated to remove any debris. Scarpa's fascia is reapproximated, subdermal sutures are placed, and the skin is stapled or closed with sutures.

POSTOPERATIVE MANAGEMENT

  I. Patients are maintained on **antiplatelet therapy** (aspirin, aspirin and clopidogrel, or systemic anticoagulation), unless contraindicated.
  II. A **pulse examination** should be undertaken at regular intervals. This examination consists of palpation, with or without portable Doppler evaluation. The **graft pulse and distal arterial pulses** should be documented.
  III. If the bypass was performed in the setting of acute severe ischemia, monitoring of lower leg compartment pressures is essential to exclude reperfusion-induced **compartment syndrome.**

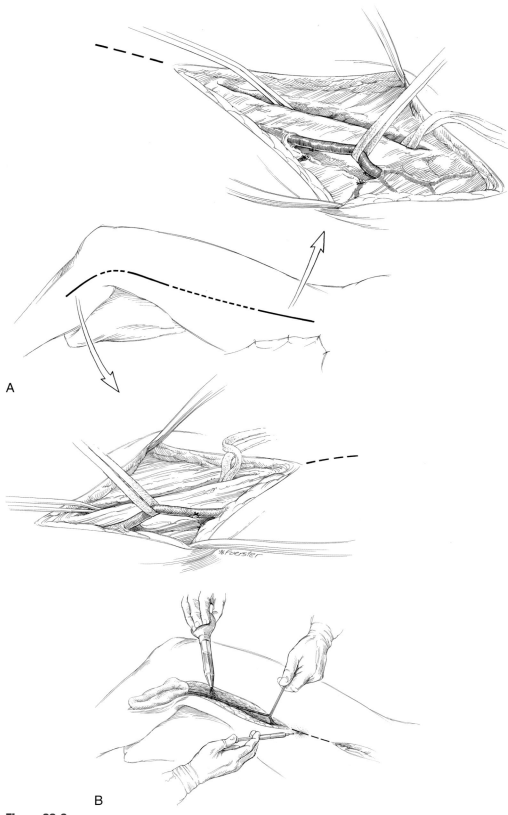

Figure 26-3

Saphenous vein graft harvest. **A**, The greater saphenous vein is harvested from the saphenofemoral junction proximally (top) and to the level of the bypass target distally (bottom). **B**, The surgeon isolates the vein and ligates venous side branches while the assistant irrigates and retracts. *(From Rutherford RB, Ouriel K: Reversed saphenous vein femoropopliteal bypass. In Ouriel K, Rutherford RB: Atlas of Vascular Surgery: Operative Procedures. Philadelphia, Saunders, 1998.)*

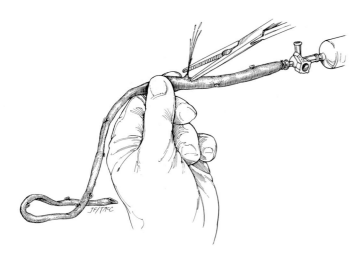

Figure 26-4
Vein graft preparation. *(From Rutherford RB, Ouriel K: Reversed saphenous vein femoropopliteal bypass. In Ouriel K, Rutherford RB: Atlas of Vascular Surgery: Operative Procedures. Philadelphia, Saunders, 1998.)*

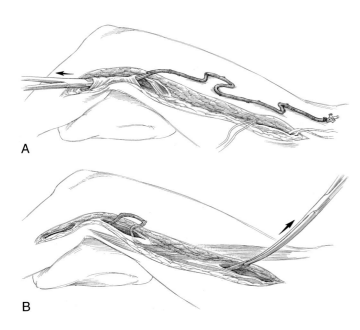

A

B

Figure 26-5
Vein graft tunneling. The vein graft is tunneled to the distal (**A**) and proximal (**B**) target sites. *(From Rutherford RB, Ouriel K: Reversed saphenous vein femoropopliteal bypass. In Ouriel K, Rutherford RB: Atlas of Vascular Surgery: Operative Procedures. Philadelphia, Saunders, 1998.)*

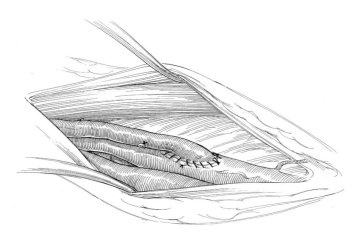

Figure 26-6
Proximal anastomosis. *(From Rutherford RB, Ouriel K: Reversed saphenous vein femoropopliteal bypass. In Ouriel K, Rutherford RB: Atlas of Vascular Surgery: Operative Procedures. Philadelphia, Saunders, 1998.)*

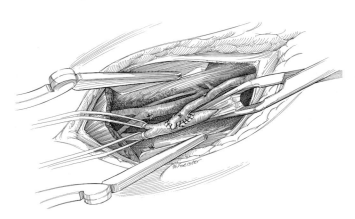

Figure 26-7
Distal anastomosis. *(From Rutherford RB, Ouriel K: Reversed saphenous vein femoropopliteal bypass. In Ouriel K, Rutherford RB: Atlas of Vascular Surgery: Operative Procedures. Philadelphia, Saunders, 1998.)*

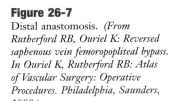

IV. Postoperative vein **graft surveillance** is an essential component of postoperative follow-up. Patient evaluation and duplex ultrasonography of the graft are performed at 1, 6, 9, and 12 months postoperatively, and yearly thereafter. Recurrent symptoms or a change in findings on pulse examination, ABIs, or PVRs may reflect graft stenosis and require evaluation with CTA, MRA, or invasive angiography.

COMPLICATIONS

I. **Cardiac complications** are a major cause of morbidity and mortality in patients with PAD. Preoperative optimization of cardiac status, routine postoperative β-blockade, and judicious perioperative fluid management are critical to minimizing cardiac risk.

II. Patients with diabetes or chronic renal insufficiency are at increased risk for **postoperative renal failure.** Maintaining intravascular euvolemia and minimizing the use of nephrotoxic contrast agents and drugs are important preventive strategies.

III. **Infection, wound dehiscence, and skin flap necrosis** are common because of the length of the incision required and the long case duration. Gentle handling of tissues, avoidance of skin flap creation, use of prophylactic antibiotics, and meticulous wound closure reduce the risk of these events.

IV. **Perioperative graft thrombosis** occurs infrequently and should be treated promptly with surgical thrombectomy and correction of the underlying cause.

V. **Early graft failure** occurs within 1 month of the operation and usually reflects a technical problem. Immediate reoperation is generally indicated. **Late graft failure,** occurring within the first 1 to 2 years, is more likely to be caused by intimal hyperplasia of the graft itself, whereas graft failure after 2 years reflects progression of atherosclerotic disease. Reoperation may be necessary in these cases, but should be preceded by a thorough investigation of the anatomy and cause of the graft failure.

VI. **Pulsatile hematoma or hemorrhage** is usually caused by a dislodged ligature on the vein graft or an anastomotic disruption. This situation can be life-threatening and requires immediate reexploration. Inadequate intraoperative hemostasis may lead to a slowly accumulating hematoma. Large hematomas should be drained expeditiously to prevent superinfection, wound dehiscence, and graft failure secondary to compression.

VII. Disruption of lymphatic tissue in the groin during dissection of the femoral vessels can lead to **seroma formation.** The rate of seroma formation in the groin, leg, or popliteal wounds from lymphatic disruption can be decreased by obliterating dead space during wound closure.

SUGGESTED READINGS

Freischlag JA, Angle N: Reversed vein bypass. In Baker RJ, Fischer JE [eds]: Mastery of Surgery, 4th ed, vol II. Philadelphia, Lippincott Williams & Wilkins, 2001, pp 2160–2166.

Ouriel K, Rutherford RB: Reversed saphenous vein femoropopliteal bypass. In Ouriel K, Rutherford RB: Atlas of Vascular Surgery: Operative Procedures. Philadelphia, Saunders, 1998.

Rosenthal D: Femoropopliteal occlusive disease. In Cameron JL [ed]: Current Surgical Therapy, 8th ed. Philadelphia, Mosby, 2004, pp 777–781.

Page numbers followed by b, f, and t indicate boxes, figures, and tables, respectively.